STO

ACPL ITEM
DISCARDED

HEALTH
AND
THE NATURE
OF MAN

HEALTH AND THE NATURE OF MAN

FRANK S. RATHBONE, JR.
ESTELLE T. RATHBONE
Professors of Health and
Physical Education, Brooklyn College

McGRAW-HILL BOOK COMPANY
New York   St. Louis   San Francisco   Düsseldorf
Johannesburg   Kuala Lumpur   London   Mexico
Montreal   New Delhi   Panama   Rio de Janeiro
Singapore   Sydney   Toronto

JUN 4 '71

This book was set in News Gothic by Monotype Composition Company, Inc., and printed on permanent paper and bound by The Maple Press Company. The designer was J. E. O'Connor. The editors were Nat La Mar, Antonia Stires, and Robert Weber. Peter D. Guilmette supervised production.

HEALTH AND THE NATURE OF MAN

Copyright © 1971 by McGraw-Hill, Inc. All rights reserved. Printed in the United States of America. No part of this publication may be reproduced, stored in a retrieval system, or transmitted, in any form or by any means, electronic, mechanical, photocopying, recording, or otherwise, without the prior written permission of the publisher.
Library of Congress Catalog Card Number 75-148132

07-051206-X
1 2 3 4 5 6 7 8 9 0 MAMM 7 9 8 7 6 5 4 3 2 1

CONTENTS

Preface   vii

PART ONE
TOWARD A CONCEPT OF HEALTH

1. PROBLEMS IN UNDERSTANDING HEALTH   3
2. ON BEING HUMAN   17
3. BASIC QUALITIES OF HUMANNESS   37
4. MAN AND HIS SYMBOLS   57
5. THE NATURE OF EXPERIENCE   69
6. HEALTH AS A QUALITY OF RESPONSE   79
7. SOME CRITERIA FOR EVALUATING RESPONSE   91
8. THE RELATIONSHIP BETWEEN HEALTH AND DISEASE   101

PART TWO
THE DYNAMICS OF HEALTHFUL ADAPTATION

9. CREATIVE ADAPTATION   119
10. IN THE BEGINNING   133
11. VALUE CONDITIONING   147
12. CONFLICT AND THE DEVELOPMENTAL TASK   159
13. THE SKILLS FOR RESOLVING CONFLICTS   171

PART THREE
SOURCES OF CONFLICT FOR COLLEGE STUDENTS

14. ESTABLISHING AN IDENTITY   191
15. TO CONFORM OR NOT TO CONFORM   209
16. COMPETITION AND ACADEMIC PRESSURE   221
17. THE DYNAMICS OF ADDICTION AND DEPENDENCY   233

PART FOUR
SEX AND MARRIAGE

18. SEX AND SEXUALITY   255
19. DATING: EXPLORATION OR EXPLOITATION?   275

20. PILLS, PREVENTION, AND PROMISCUITY   295
21. THE INTIMACY OF MARRIAGE   319
22. THE MIRACLE OF BIRTH   341

CONCLUSION

23. ARE AMERICANS HEALTHY?   365

   Index   383

PREFACE

This book is the result of ideas developed over twenty years of teaching health education to college students. It is based upon the idea that one's true health (not just his freedom from sickness and disease) is a direct outgrowth of his way of life. If that life is rewarding, developmental, and satisfying, he is healthy. It will matter little whether or not he manages to get eight hours of sleep every night. In many cases, clichés about health simply do not apply. What is important is the way in which each individual utilizes the resources available to him in meeting the challenges of life. When people can upgrade the quality of their responses, they are healthier persons. They have developed a resource for living which they did not have before, and the range of possibilities that is open to them for the future is broadened.

College students presumably have been exposed to all the basic information about structure and function of the human organism several times over in the course of their formal education. Whether or not they have remembered it does not matter. We assume they will not benefit from further exposure to this same information. Therefore, virtually none of it has been included in these pages. The exclusion of basic physiology and biology here does not imply that this information is unimportant, but rather that the student is now ready to move on to consider these facts in a broader perspective. An effort has been made to concentrate in this text on aspects of health that are usually not found in a standard volume on health but nonetheless have a direct influence on healthful living.

This book is a philosophic and speculative study of health and human nature. It is not a set of rules for healthy living. Because of the vast areas of ignorance still faced by scientists, a fair amount of philosophic speculation must be undertaken by the student of health. He must speculate about the real nature of a human being, about what he can become and about those things which really influence health. Although we do not presume to have all the answers, we are convinced that, with an adequate exploration of the areas of interest discussed, the student will grow in his understanding of himself, his health, and his fellowman. Presumably, from this growth in understanding he will be better equipped to direct the course of his life and will therefore be equipped to influence his health more favorably.

The areas of interest were selected from two sources. One was a survey of students at Brooklyn College, where an effort was made to ascertain their major sources of concern. The results tended to agree with studies of college students throughout the United States. Students are mainly concerned with the problems inherent in (1) establishing their identity, (2) working out the dependence-independence relationship between themselves and their parents, (3) establishing a set of values about life, (4) working out an acceptable means of dealing with their sexuality, and (5) satisfactorily accommodating to the pressures of academia.

These are areas where most of the real conflicts of college students originate. The conflicts may manifest themselves in the use of drugs, alcohol, and the sometimes bizarre and extreme practices of young adults. To deal with the manifestations of the conflicts may be important, but it is more important in the student's *understanding of himself and his health* to deal with the real issue: the sources of the conflicts themselves. The major portion of this book addresses itself to exploring these sources of concern. Part 2 sets a frame of reference by examining the dynamics of healthful adaptation. Part 3 deals specifically with the sources of conflict for college students. Part 4 examines the problems of sex and marriage.

The second source of information has been our observations about life and our reading in the area of human behavior. Thoughts resulting from a lifelong effort to puzzle out what a human being is and what truly influences his health are organized in the first section of the book. Thus, Part 1 focuses upon what seems basic to understanding man as a functioning organism.

The book is strongly oriented toward what is usually called "mental health" because we feel that one's feelings, attitudes, and values directly influence his physiologic function. There is no escaping this. *Since health is a functional phenomenon, it is impossible to separate those things which are mental from those things which are physical.* Health means wholeness of function and being. All conditions of health have as much to do with the mental as they do with the physical. It is misleading to separate them.

We regard these pages as a transition from the traditional concepts derived from physiology and biology to a broader interdisciplinary view of health and human nature. We seek to provoke discussion and thought, to raise issues which, when discussed, will lead to further insight and help the reader in assessing his own life and health.

The effort of writing this book has made us aware of our great debt to the many people who have helped shape our ideas, challenge our thinking, and puncture our pomposity when necessary. Through the years our students have been the major challengers and puncturers. Without them the ideas expressed here could not have been formulated. The chairmen under whom we have served have been particularly helpful by encouraging the academic freedom necessary to experiment with thoughts, ideas, and methods of teaching. To colleagues who have patiently joined us in long hours of discussion and argumentation we owe thanks. Professor Bernard Pollack of Brooklyn College has been especially helpful in the organization of the book's content and in the formulation of some of the methods suggested in the instructor's manual. Professor Helene Sloan, one of the truly outstanding teachers we have known, has helped to develop the ideas in the instructor's manual. Finally, our thanks to Rikkie Cyrlin for her help in the preparation of the manuscript.

Frank S. Rathbone, Jr.
Estelle T. Rathbone

**HEALTH
AND
THE NATURE
OF MAN**

1. TOWARD A CONCEPT OF HEALTH

1.

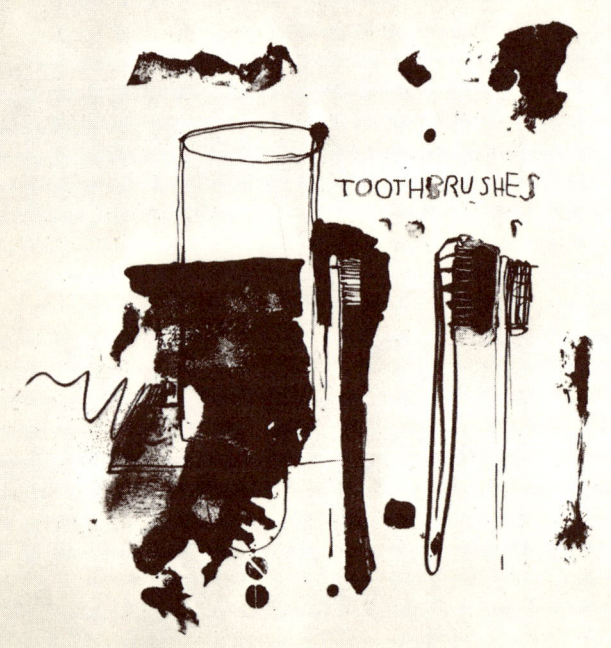

PROBLEMS IN UNDERSTANDING HEALTH

The time has come when we must drastically reorder our thinking about health. We have been reluctant to abandon comfortable ideas; we have been content to live with an intellectual amalgam of old wives' tales, folklore, pseudoscience, and partial truth.

As long as we believed that brushing our teeth twice a day, eating the right kinds of foods, and getting the proper amount of rest resulted in health, we had reduced it to a mechanical formula. But the empirical evidence was that the formula did not work, since many people who followed the suggested practices religiously did not obtain the desired results.

Why weren't people healthy? Formerly, our answer was that when people were exposed to disease organisms, they would become sick. When this reasoning was found to be inadequate, we invoked the term *mental health*, not realizing that in discussing mental health we were most often referring to some aberration from the norm. Most of us were unaware that this was a limited and fractional concept. We were comfortable with the idea of a duality of physical and mental health. Although the concept of health put forth in this book is much more difficult to master, it is concerned with the wholeness that is implicit in the word *health*.

A Dynamic Concept

Most of our thinking about man has been in terms of static ideas; for example, we study history by memorizing important dates. The concept that proper rest, nutrition, and shelter will produce health is a static one. It suggests that disease is solely the result of physical organisms: we are exposed to germs—therefore, we get a disease.

The dynamism of the concept of health discussed in this book is in its emphasis on the quality of one's response to life. It is an existential concept. It implies that man, in his existential set-

Jim Dine, "Toothbrushes #4," 1962. Lithograph. Collection, The Museum of Modern Art, New York. Gift of the Celeste and Armand Bartos Foundations.

ting, attempts to give meaning to his life according to the way in which he sees himself involved in it. If his vision of himself or of the circumstances of his environment is distorted, he cannot respond in a manner appropriate either to his own well-being or to the situation in which he finds himself. As he moves through life with this distortion, he accumulates experience from which he derives distorted meaning. As this meaning is built into his personality in the form of attitudes, he progressively shapes his values in ways which are inaccurate (refer to Chapter 11 to clarify what is meant in this book by the word *value*). Therefore, he finds it difficult, if not impossible, to perceive clearly what the elements of reality are.

To develop this dynamic concept of health, it is necessary to examine some basic aspects of man's nature to see how they influence the quality of one's response to life.

The Reader's Tasks

First, the reader must recognize that the concepts advanced in this volume are not put forth in the interest of academic theorizing. The individual should attempt to apply these concepts to his own life and, through creative introspection, must find his own specific illustrations. The examples given here can only be in the form of generalizations and are never complete.

In order to describe a concept, it is necessary to fragmentize. This, however, takes us a step away from the reality of the situation. Thus, the second challenge for the reader is to be able to recognize that while one aspect of man's nature is being discussed, there are other aspects at work at the same time. Sometimes these aspects operate at odds with one another. For example, by the time a person has reached college age, he has the ability and desire to engage in sexual intercourse. But he has also been strongly indoctrinated by strictures against the free expression of his sexuality. It is important for the reader to know what factors are at work in any given situation.

A third task for the student is to free himself from the limitations of previous conditioning about the nature of health. He is asked to set aside much of what he has learned, to divest himself of certain ideas that have been easy to handle, and to examine the context from which these ideas have developed. If he is able to do this, he will come to understand how these ideas were passed on to him.

One last task: the student must be able to read with discrimination and critical judgment. Much of the research on health, disease, and man's nature is fragmented. When a doctor with a particular orientation toward nutrition conducts research on the heart, his findings must of necessity be limited. It stands to reason that he cannot have carried forth research on all aspects of the human organism relative to eating habits, living habits, and the complex subjective context in which the individual lives. The discriminating scientist knows this and does not jump to conclusions based upon partial truth.

What Is the Good Life?

More than ever before, Americans are now concerned with living a qualitatively satisfying life. Most of us are no longer concerned with the essential task of survival. We want a better standard of living, a better job. Some of us are concerned with status or are seeking new challenges to our talents.

We see this concern for quality of living in many segments of our society. College students are actively, sometimes violently, protesting the values by which most of us are living. Blacks no longer are willing to be treated as second-class citizens. Labor leaders are justifying strikes to obtain better working and living conditions for their constituents. Vast numbers of people are disturbed by governmental policies which influence the quality of living of the American public.

In all these efforts two basic challenges lie before us: The first centers about the question of what determines the good life. What concepts are basic to describing the good life? What frame of reference should people live in to accomplish the quality of living which will be most satisfying to them? These are primarily philosophic questions. They are as old as man himself. The great religions of the world have dealt with them to give meaning to life and to enable man to develop a pattern of living which will make that meaning clear.

The second basic challenge is of more recent origin. Science has made it possible for us to move forward in our understanding of the mysteries which surround us. It is not so much that we solve the mysteries as that we are able to ask questions which are more and more refined. We have learned that behind every important discovery lies another great question.

It is important to understand the value of asking the right question when seeking meaning in life. Too often men are satisfied with easy answers that enable them to avoid the frustration of living with questions. But when men give up questioning, they give up growing. Such a surrender is tragic.

A look at history reveals that whenever societies become content with what they are and cease to question what they are doing, they are in the process of disintegrating. When individuals settle for easy answers, they commit themselves to rigidities which lock them into patterns of response that are limited and limiting. It is as though they are afraid to move forward into the process of personal growth and development.

Questions about the good life are essentially questions about health. It is in the context of struggling to achieve the good life that men build or break themselves. The quality of our response to the circumstances of life as we see it determines our health. In finding what we believe important, we create the context in which we live. If that context is consistent with our nature, we are fortunate. If it is not, damaging stress results.

The concepts presented in this volume grow out of asking basic questions about man's nature. The answers suggested are offered tentatively. They seem to be merited on the basis of scientific knowledge now available. The position now held will probably have to be modified tomorrow. The science of the future will make this necessary.

These constructs should provide a new position for thinking about health. They should lead the reader toward an integration of thought about man and his health which is more comprehensive than that which he previously held. They should even force him to change his way of viewing himself. If this is done, this book will not be read easily. It should evoke feelings which are not comfortable to hold. If the reader asks himself why he feels as he does, he will come to a deeper understanding of himself. He will also develop a more realistic understanding of man and his health. The process of questioning is useful personally as well as academically. If a realistic understanding of man does not develop in both areas, this should also be questioned as to possible resistance to the task posed.

Variables in Life Style

The good life is seen differently by different philosophies, by different societies, by different individuals. Through the ages the concepts about man and his way of life have been reflected in the great classic formulations of philosophers. Each of these is reflected in the life style of individuals today. The hedonist believes that happiness is the chief goal of life and that man achieves his highest meaning in the search for it. For many Americans today there is a strong tendency to find meaning solely in this. Affluence has made us reluctant to engage in protracted efforts to achieve our ends. Immediacy is the order of the day.

The Protestant ethic, strongly set among us by Puritanism in the United States, has taught that frugality and hard work are essential to the realization of the good life. When carried to an extreme, the limitations of this philosophy are humorously apparent. For example, a thrifty housewife scrupulously tries not to waste the apples stored in a barrel. Every day she carefully picks out those that are going bad to serve to her family. Thus by the time the barrel is empty, her family has eaten only apples that were beginning to rot.

The contemporary existentialist philosophy suggests that the meaning of life is to be found in the living of it. As we experience life, so we find its meaning. This thinking strongly dominates contemporary thought. In fact it is so much a part of our way of looking at things that when it is pointed out as a special philosophy, we are surprised to recognize that another way of looking at things could ever have existed. The modern mind would say, "Of course the meaning of life is found in the way we experience it." Freudian psychologists, and most others as well, have discovered that our view of life is so strongly influenced by our experience that it is virtually impossible to ignore the importance of experience.

Existentialism and Health

Health is an existential phenomenon. It is an outgrowth of the way in which we live our lives. The experience we create for ourselves results in the attitudes with which we view ourselves, our fellowman, and the circumstances of life. These attitudes then shape the responses we make to life situations. Through the living of our lives we come to see ourselves as more or less successful at performing the tasks of life. If we see ourselves as generally successful, frustration and stress are minimized. When we see ourselves as failures, we not only increase the stress of life, but we also play out the drama of our lives in a way that will confirm the expected failures. When our sense of self is one of rich, exuberant enjoyment of life, we are healthy people. When it is not, we are unwell.

Whatever philosophic construct we act out in our lives, it is important for us to understand what we are doing. The central questions of this book are directed toward this end. It is assumed that every person seeks to answer the question "Who am I?" His life style is designed to help him find the answer. Many of us, however, have become engaged in endeavors which tend to obscure this insight. We fail in our central task; because of this we begin to expect failure and then tend to work against our own central purposes.

Importance of Attitude

A young college student sums up his attitude toward himself and toward life by saying simply, "Life is frustrating." His life *is* frustrating, but it is frustrating more because of what he feels about himself than by virtue of what he does. He lives his life in such a way that his belief is made a reality; he acts out his belief.

Victor Frankl, speaking out of observations made while a prisoner in a German concentration camp, formulates the "will to meaning" as a primary force in life. He says[1] the will to meaning "is not a secondary rationalization of instinctual drives. This meaning is unique and specific in that it must and can be fulfilled by him alone; only then does it achieve a significance that will satisfy his own will to meaning." He further points out that the meaning man finds in life is so important that it influences his health. In the concentration camp "We were unable to clean our teeth," he writes,[2] "and yet, in spite of that and a severe vitamin deficiency, we had healthier gums than ever before. We had to wear the same shirts for half a year until they had lost all appearance of being shirts. For days we were unable to wash, even partially, because of frozen water pipes, and yet the sores and abrasions on hands which were dirty from work in the soil did not suppurate."

Dr. Lawrence LeShan also concludes that our purposes in life are important factors in preventing disease.[3] His study of the contrast between the incidence of cancer of nations at war and the cancer rates of the same nations at peace is startling. The results show that the cancer morbidity rate is lower when nations are at war than when they are at peace. He theorizes that the reason lies in the unifying purpose felt by the people in their fight for a common cause.

Both these conclusions urge us toward recognizing that attitudes are important in protecting against disease. Chapter 8 treats the relationship between health and disease more fully, but it is important here to note that attitudes are a determining factor not

---

[1] Victor Frankl, *Man's Search for Meaning,* Beacon Press, Boston, 1959, 1962, p. 99. Reprinted by permission of the Beacon Press, copyright © 1959, 1962 by Victor Frankl.
[2] *Ibid.*, pp. 15–16.
[3] Lawrence LeShan, "Loss of Cathexes as a Common Psychodynamic Characteristic of Cancer Patients: An Attempt at Statistical Validation of a Clinical Hypothesis," *Psychological Reports,* vol. 2, pp. 183–193, 1956.

only in mental health but in the physiologic functioning of the body as well. No sharp distinction can be made between the biologic and the attitudinal in its influence upon our functioning.

Again we see that we can no longer remain content with the old ideas about health. If attitudes are important in the phenomenology of health, we must make a place for them in our conceptual thinking. We must be able to reorganize the insights previously held in such a way that a closer proximity to the truth results.

Attitudes are variable and complex. An attitude of self-confidence in one context of life may change to an attitude of inadequacy in another. The young person who feels himself to be a success in the intimacy of his own home may feel himself to be quite inept when relating to people outside his home. In both situations the attitudes relate to the self, but the attitudes are different. An example can be found in another area: An individual may be comfortable with members of his own sex but quite anxious with members of the other sex.

Finding Meaning in Life

From the limitless variability of attitudes according to context, it follows that an individual's responses too will vary in the multiplicity of life's circumstances. Our ways of thinking about our own life experience therefore need to be quite sophisticated to make it possible for us to discover the meaning of life. In an age when there are so many demands upon our energy and time, the tools of critical evaluation of the resulting experience must be sharpened. Too many of us are baffled by the challenges in our lives. Too often we are led to make inappropriate responses to these challenges. Too often the responses are not only inappropriate but downright destructive.

It is interesting to speculate on the contemporary phenomenon called *dropping out*. What are the dropouts dropping out of? A casual examination of the situation seems to indicate that the dropout has surrendered to the frustrations inherent in finding a satisfying meaning to life. The resultant anxiety is frightening, and the guilt at not being able to find meaning when he feels he should is depressing.

Unable to reconcile the difference between the need to find purpose and the inability to do so, the individual drops out. There are many forms of this, ranging all the way from the indifference of some members of hippiedom, through the flunking college student, to the drug addict, the alcoholic, and the suicide. Even a casual look at the statistics in each of these areas indicates a startling rise in incidence. The more astonishing rises are in alcoholism (now among the top four of national public health problems), drug abuse, and suicide (a leading cause of death among college students). Obviously there are serious health problems associated with our lack of ability to find a satisfying meaning for existence.

While it is apparent that this is a problem in the realm of health, it is difficult to pinpoint the specific nature of the problem. In the first place, meaning for existence is vague—even when found. In the second place, its specific relationship to health is not really defined.

Protection versus Promotion

A further problem in defining health lies in the fact that for generations we have concerned ourselves with the *protection* of health. While this has been important, the effort has limited research to those endeavors which are disease-oriented. Traditionally we have concerned ourselves with disease after it has developed. So much energy goes into plugging holes in the dike that no attention is given to building a better dike.

Modern public health began with the great plagues of medieval Europe. They were so destructive and so frightening that the effort to control infection was imperative. From that point on, for several hundred years, strenuous efforts were directed toward curing disease and limiting the spread of infection. The rewards of this effort have been manyfold. The most dramatic, perhaps, has been the increase of life expectancy. Furthermore, the picture of public health problems today is vastly different from what it was even seventy years ago. Contagious disease ranks well down on the list of causes of death. It is no longer the scourge of mankind that it once was. Problems of a different nature have achieved ascendancy, as can be seen from the table on page 11.

In the past fifty years sporadic work has begun on the *promotion* of health. Only in the past twenty years have any comprehensive efforts been made by public health agencies to promote health. Much of the effort in this direction has been to discover those factors in the lives of individuals, families, and communities that precipitate health problems and/or stand in the way of the success of health programs.

Promotion of health is still a frontier of public health work. One of the newer impressions of the nature of disease has come from the analysis of the effect of crisis on an individual. The assumption is that crisis precipitates health problems. Current research indicates that it matters little what the crisis is. It may range from

The ten leading causes of death in the United States in 1900 and in 1967

	1900*		1967	
RANK	CAUSE OF DEATH	RATE PER 100,000	CAUSE OF DEATH	RATE PER 100,000
1	Influenza and pneumonia	202.2	Disease of heart	364.5
2	Tuberculosis (all forms)	194.4	Malignant neoplasms†	157.2
3	Gastritis, etc.	142.7	Vascular lesions of central nervous system	102.2
4	Diseases of the heart	137.4	Accidents	57.2
5	Vascular lesions of central nervous system	106.9	Influenza and pneumonia‡	28.8
6	Chronic nephritis	81.0	Diseases of infancy	24.4
7	All accidents	72.3	Arteriosclerosis	19.0
8	Malignant neoplasms	64.0	Diabetes	17.7
9	Certain diseases of early infancy	62.6	Other diseases of circulatory system	15.1
10	Diphtheria	40.3	Other bronchopulmonic diseases	14.8

* Rates for 1900 apply to death-registration states only.
† Includes neoplasms of lymphatic and hematopoietic tissue.
‡ Except pneumonia of newborn.
Source of 1967 data: U.S. Bureau of the Census, *Statistical Abstracts of the United States*, 90th ed., Washington, 1969, p. 59.

economic problems, through accidents, illness, and emotional disturbances, to marital problems. In any of these, stress is produced. This in turn causes reactions which render a person open to disease and infection. This reaction depends on the individual and his ability to withstand stress.

Some efforts in public health have been directed toward helping people deal with crisis. Crisis is a common experience for everyone. For some, the fact of life itself is a crisis of major proportions. Dealing with crisis demands adaptation, change, and adjustment. Those factors, then, that aid the individual in discovering adaptive behavioral patterns which reduce stress are of great significance.

An effort toward changes of behavior must be multifaceted. A program for supplying information on birth control in a ghetto area, for example, must consider how and where the information will be distributed. Will the people be able to afford to buy the contraceptive? Will they want to use it? Could the citizens of the area be supplied through clinics? What are the existing attitudes toward the neighborhood clinic? Is it looked upon with trust? What have past associations been? These are but a few of the many questions that would need to be answered.

In the promotion of health, the issues too are many. What factors in the social experiences of a person predispose him to disease? What causes the breakdown in the body's natural resistance? What behavioral patterns help growth and development of potential? Which hinder? How does the spirit of man affect his health? Underlying most of these queries lies a basic assumption that there is a better, fuller level of experience. Toward what sort of life are we heading? What kind of existence can we hope for? What can we reasonably expect to find within ourselves? What are our potentials?

The Unknown Potential

The problems in teaching people to move toward their potential are manifold. One major difficulty lies in our ignorance of human potential. The behavioral sciences have begun to place signposts for us to follow. But for most of us the self is a vast unknown realm. We are almost completely unaware of the potential we have for abundant living. We are ignorant of the many resources which are an inherent part of each person's armamentarium for dealing with life.

We do not know the values or the limits of our capacity for rational thought. We do not know if this is a weapon for protecting or promoting our health. Our formal education has usually been irrelevant to the promotion of health. The methods of too much of contemporary education are altogether irrelevant to the development of the kind of critical evaluation of experience which is important in promoting health.

Only coincidentally do we learn how to improve the quality of our interpersonal relationships, often the source of the crises of life. Frequently the coercive efforts of parents have induced guilt as the basis for effective human relationships. For too many of us love is a matter of form rather than of genuine feeling. Anger, jealousy, and hate are powerful motivating forces. Frequently these emotions are dealt with in our homes or in our educational experience by our ignoring or suppressing them. This in itself is enough to precipitate severe crises in the lives of most of us.

Often we fail to develop the sensitivities to our own feelings or to the feelings of others that are vital for communication and evaluation of what we are experiencing. College students, when asked to tell what they *feel* about a particular experience, frequently give all sorts of intellectual answers about what they *think*. They will not even be aware of the fact that this is vastly different from what they *feel*. Hence, the great well of human feeling is totally unused as a source of insight and understanding.

Our attention to the physical aspects of life has dulled our capacity to use the resource of intuitive knowledge available to us. We are too often unwilling to trust the impulses we have to behave in particular ways. We leave to chance the acknowledgment of the inner voice which informs us of solutions to problems, directions to follow, and definitions of purpose.

We have been so firmly conditioned to the idea that man is strictly a physical organism that we ignore altogether those sensitivities which are inherent in human nature in its totality. We rely more upon the findings of science than on the personal discoveries of experience to guide our lives. The Western mind discards what it has learned from experience when a limited bit of research appears to contradict its personal discoveries.

A dramatic example of this tendency to follow the scientist lies in the American worship of pills. We take pills for everything—to speed us up, to slow us down, to supplement our diets, to regulate our bowels, to help us sleep, and to calm our nerves. In the absence of critical thought we are subject to every huckster who offers a panacea for the problems of life. Health is not to be found in following this path. In fact, it may lead us away from the commonsense road to health.

Why do we abandon common sense? To some extent it is because we lack knowledge about ourselves, but to an equal degree it is because we lack faith in our ability to deal with life. Both these problems are rooted in the values of our society. The problem of lack of knowledge has several foci: One is that information from research centers is not adequately mediated to the public. Another is our tendency to reject information which does not fit comfortably with preconceived notions about ourselves. If that information demands change in belief or behavior, as in psychotherapy, resistance sets in. Although we may consciously recognize that change may be necessary, to change is difficult and threatening.

The lack of faith in our ability to deal with life has grown in direct proportion to the rate at which responsibility for living has been taken over by institutions. For example, to some extent schools have taken over the role of the parent. Law and the legislative process have established restrictions on personal behavior and removed responsibility for the consequences of one's behavior. Many people operate within the law but in a manner which is completely unethical. The attitude toward the circumstances of life which prevents a direct confrontation with its essentials is a crippling one. No person grows through avoiding responsibility. A society which encourages us to "cop out" is contributing to our lack of growth and making it difficult for us to understand what we are and what our potential is.

A Qualitative and Unique Response

Health is relative. An individual has a degree of health; he is more or less healthy. He is never healthy or unhealthy in an either-or sense.

In an age when survival was the major factor which distinguished between the quick and the dead, the individual who lived and was likely to continue to do so was healthy. When the individual's survival was threatened, as by a fatal disease, he was said to be unhealthy. His health was restored when he was freed of that which threatened his existence.

As man has learned to protect himself, health has become more difficult to define. Clearly, to be free of disease is not the only criterion. Is there a particular condition of living which must be in effect for one to be healthy? Does an individual exhibit signs that mark him as healthy? If so, what are they?

There is a qualitative value in the life of every individual. If our term is to have some meaning, it must have some value (see Chapter 11). But who is able to set down hard-and-fast rules about these values? Can these rules be established so that they apply to all individuals under all conditions and at all stages of life? If we were not concerned with establishing a term which has universality, we would have less difficulty. Our interest is in finding a term that is realistic and can have universality of meaning, and therefore we must search carefully for a meaning that is valid.

The uniqueness of each individual further complicates the problem of defining health. No two people have the same experience. Each sees himself in life differently. Each has his own set of subjective standards for evaluating his success. What would be a success for one person would not be for another, even though the external manifestations of the achievement were similar. For example, the student with a C average and the A student view a B grade in different lights. For the one it is an accomplishment, but for the other it is a matter of humiliation.

If health has a qualitative value and if it is determined by the qualitative effectiveness of one's responses to life situations, then the standards to be used in judging the quality of our responses must be suited to the uniqueness of the individual. In other words each of us has his own ways of determining the quality of his responses. Therefore, each man's health must be judged individually.

Who, then, is qualified to judge? The problem is obvious. Our knowledge of all the variables in human response is so limited that it becomes extremely difficult to arrive at a judgment. Our knowledge of our own variables also is limited. Therefore, it becomes difficult to assess our own response. The limits of our knowledge about man and about ourselves determine the limit of our ability to assess our own health.

Judging the quality of one's responses, then, is not simple. For example, the student who fails a college course may be making a poor quality of response to that life situation. On the other hand it is possible that he is flunking out of college in order to free himself from the control of his parents. In the long run his freedom may be more important for him than to continue in college. Even if he grants that there are better ways to accomplish his purposes than through failure, the dynamics of the situation are such that this appears to him to be his only out. At the same time the student may be subconsciously using this means of self-punishment to buy off his sense of guilt that has resulted from his animosity toward his father.

As each of these factors becomes operative, some aspect of his personality is being appeased, and the situation changes. It is quite possible that after a year on his own he will be able to return to school to do superior academic work. The dynamic elements of his own inner structure will have shifted, and he will have taken a giant step toward maturity.

Summary

In the foregoing pages we have attempted to skim the surface of the task which lies before anyone who seeks to understand health, a task related to every aspect of man's nature. Health touches every action, thought, feeling, and hope that man has. Each of these influences the quality of man's responses. Because our study is not centered about an interest in mankind but is more concerned with an examination of ourselves, we must move toward developing a keen awareness of ourselves.

We are faced with problems of ignorance. Our lack of knowledge is both general and specific. The generalities have to do with man as a species. The specifics have to do with ourselves as individuals. The problem of ignorance is compounded by the fact that our educational experiences have not led us toward introspection nor have they prepared us adequately for the task of assessing our dynamic natures.

While the task is formidable, it is also exciting. In embarking upon a study of health we set out on a journey which can lead to exciting discoveries about ourselves. Furthermore, it may lead us toward the development of increased efficiency in dealing with the other tasks of our lives. It makes possible the unfolding of the potential in us which lies waiting to be actualized. It brings into being that which we were born to produce.

2.

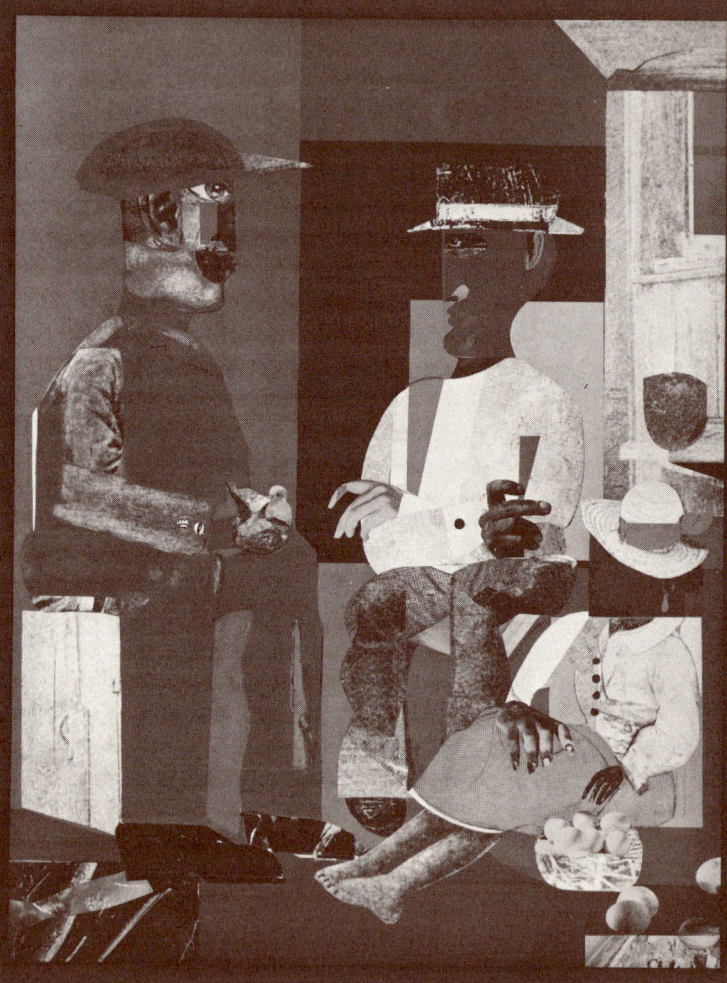

ON BEING HUMAN

Understanding health demands an understanding of the human organism in its totality. The challenge is enormous. The threads of any individual's life are so intricately interwoven that it is impossible to unravel all of them. It is difficult to establish what is the result of nature and what is the result of experience. Living a consciously directed healthy life is equally difficult. It demands that we understand, and differentiate between, two important aspects of experience: what has developed from the past and what is unfolding in the present.

The student of health must continually reexamine his insights and allow for an expanding knowledge and an expanding experience. He must be more than just an observer of mankind. He must become actively engaged in assessing what happens in his life. It is important for him to put his talents and his insights to the test in living situations. If he attempts to develop his knowledge from books alone, his insights will frequently be irrelevant to his life.

The remaining pages of this book will focus on healthful human function, in its live setting. Because of its complexity, the subject cannot be covered completely. Since this is a study of health rather than a set of rules for healthful living, no attempt will be made to direct the reader to follow certain practices as a means of protecting or promoting health. Nevertheless, the reader may be moved to apply some of the insights he develops from reading these pages.

This book, for many, may serve as a mirror. The reader may not like what he sees. If this happens, he may ask questions about what he has seen and thereby develop a new and better self-understanding.

Environmental Control

Each characteristic that belongs uniquely to the human animal has the potential to develop in ways which are either constructive or

Romare Bearden, "Eastern Barn," 1968. Collage of paper on board. Collection, The Whitney Museum of American Art, New York. Geoffrey Clements, photography.

destructive. An example of this is man's control of his environment. Man's ability to control his environment is different from that of other animals more in degree than in kind. However, the degree of difference is so great as to make it almost a difference in kind.

Animals are much more bound by the environment in which they live. While man is not entirely free of this limitation, he does have the ability to collectively establish mutually supportive communities. Through the development of his technology, he has gained manipulative control over many more elements of his environment than the animal. Not only has he developed clothing to protect against the weather, but weather itself is subject to his control. Although this control is not complete, it has been possible to precipitate rain. Presumably it will become possible to influence cloud formation according to need.

Many diseases are controlled or prevented through techniques such as inoculation, drug use, supervisory control of food and living conditions, and destruction of disease-carrying organisms. The cure of disease has been one of the startling developments of modern medicine, eliminating many of the great killers of mankind and increasing life expectancy by nearly half a century. Through this element of environmental control man has made it possible for millions of people to come closer to living a life that is consistent with the potential with which man is born.

The increase in life expectancy is an achievement of which man can be proud. But increased longevity alone is not enough. Unless man succeeds in upgrading the quality of his life, his added years will become little more than a burden for him. The realization of this has moved man toward further study of himself in his environment. Through this study he has begun to recognize what features of his environment threaten and what features enhance the development of his potential. The discipline of psychology, for example, makes it possible for him to control his social environment in many ways. While this science is still in its early years, experimental efforts have led to more effective means of enhancing learning and living. The principles derived from this study are applied in the home, in the school, and in business and industry. Motivational research makes possible the manipulation of entire segments of our population. Packaging of foods in an attractive manner makes them more desirable to the housewife. The development of a political personality through presentation in the mass media controls the votes cast.

Man's study of himself has led to the discovery of many means of influencing himself in his environment. More and more he has demonstrated an ability to control the social context in which he lives.

Self-determination

Some recent literature would indicate that man is strongly controlled by his animal origins and his instinctive drives,[1,2] but it should not be overlooked that these drives and instincts have been translated into refinements which result in self-determination that far exceeds that of animals. While the animal, impelled by the sex drive, can only reproduce, man has translated this drive into art, love, athletic prowess, and cultural achievement. The mechanism of sublimation has enabled man to do similar things with many of his basic drives. The drive toward safety has created civilizations. Our vast technology has developed from the drive to protect ourselves.

As these basic drives have been satisfied, man has discovered other areas for concern. He has found that there is a drive within him which moves him toward the expression of his potential. The creative tendencies in him have become manifest. When he has found that he has potential in several areas, it has been necessary to determine what paths of endeavor he will follow. He is forced into self-determination. His own nature demands this of him.

When we recognize that all man's accomplishments to date are the outcome of the struggle to meet his needs and fulfill his drives, as these become apparent to him, we are impressed with the phenomena involved. We tend to overlook the capacities with which we have been born, to ignore the fact that we have the ability to accomplish astounding things. When we fail to recognize how much potential we have for becoming self-determining, we surrender one of the essential elements of our unique endowment.

Belief in Self

Self-determination depends upon one's belief in his ability to accomplish what he wants. It is necessary to believe that space travel is possible before a project for this can be started. One must believe that the learning process can be fulfilled before schools can be changed or principles of learning can be formulated. Basically, it is necessary to believe that human beings are self-determining

---

[1] Desmond Morris, *The Naked Ape*, McGraw-Hill, New York, 1968.
[2] Robert Ardrey, *Territorial Imperative*, Atheneum, New York, 1966; *African Genesis*, Atheneum, New York, 1961.

before one undertakes the challenges inherent in any task of self-determination.

This belief in self usually does not exist at the conscious level. Rarely can one who does believe deeply in himself articulate his belief. In essence it is built on faith and experience. When one has learned that when he undertakes things, there is a good chance for success, his faith in himself develops. Even when he fails, his experience tells him that no great tragedy has taken place: he knows that he will recover from most failures he experiences.

His faith has freed him to live experimentally. Through his experiments in living he has learned what he can and cannot do. He sees things in perspective, and he has a basis for self-determination.

When man does not have a belief in himself, he acts in ways which are limiting or self-destructive. Every doctor is aware of the importance of the will to live. Patients in critical condition must believe that they can survive if they are to fight for life successfully. Athletes must believe in themselves to succeed. Students who cannot (or will not) believe in their ability to succeed often do not. No area of life is untouched by the principle of belief in oneself. Human relationships, personal achievement, and even physiologic function are influenced by this belief. When persons believe themselves to be unified, effectively related to others, secure in their life setting, and moving toward personal fulfillment, they maintain a physiologic balance that enables them to fight infection, ward off disease, and adapt so that dysfunction does not occur as often.

Seeing Possibilities and Making Choices

The ability to see the various possibilities inherent in a situation distinguishes not only man from animal but the mature, healthy individual from the underdeveloped one. To respond effectively to a life situation it is necessary to see the various possibilities in it. One needs to recognize that in any situation there are always several alternative courses to follow. These can be broadly categorized as retreat, attack, and compromise. A student, for example, faced with a difficult teacher can retreat—drop the course; attack—attempt to gain dominance over the teacher; or compromise—attempt to engage the teacher in some dialogue through which a mutual understanding can be reached.

In order to examine a problem some degree of objectivity must exist. Persons who are able to free themselves from the emotions inherent in a situation have learned the skills of conflict resolvement. All of us have experienced situations in which it seems impossible to separate reason from emotion. A conflict with a parent over one's rights and privileges is so fraught with emotion that it becomes extremely difficult to assess the various alternatives open to us.

Because of the complexity of modern life, it is often difficult to make the choice which is in our own best interest. Obviously there are confusing factors. Too often factors are obscured by our inability to assess the consequences of our actions. Emotions often so color what we see that we cannot choose appropriately.

The person who is not capable of seeing the choices that are available to him follows the emotions which dominate him at the moment. He is not exerting his humanness in its fullest sense.

In this confusion he defines for himself the kind of person he is. Feeling guilty about the actions he may be involved in, he formulates attitudes about himself which are destructive and difficult to deal with as time moves forward. In addition to this there are often physiologic and functional consequences of such circumstances.

An unfortunate reality of a world in which the pace of living is increasingly accelerated is that important decisions often seem irrevocable. For example, a student who would like to choose a particular line of study recognizes that the specialization is so great that he may be well along the path of preparation before he realizes that he has made a mistake. He may therefore be reluctant to make this important choice.

The Watchful Self

The term *watchful self* means that function of personality which observes what we do. Each of us, in every moment of life, has the ability not only to participate in the events of life but to stand aside and observe the performance. In this process of observation we not only see ourselves, but we see ourselves (1) in relation to others in the situation with us, (2) in relation to the image we hope to create in the situation, and (3) in relation to the goals we have in life.

The watchful self usually operates at deeper levels of consciousness rather than functioning at the conscious level. Thus we are not always aware that it is at work. But when we become aware of its existence, the watchful self often gives us clues to our motivations.

Seeing Ourselves in Relation to Others

From childhood we develop ideas about our role with other people. We learn how to behave toward our fathers and mothers. We carve out a niche for ourselves with our brothers and sisters. In each situation we learn what other persons expect of us. We also learn what we expect of ourselves in relation to them. For example, a father may expect obedience, respect, and admiration from his children. While he may never tell them this in so many words, it becomes apparent to the children that these qualities are expected. Rewards are meted out when these qualities are displayed, punishment when they are not. The rewards are not necessarily material; more often they are in the form of friendship, approval, and encouragement.

To obtain this approval children expect themselves to behave with deference toward their father. When they do not function in this way, they feel disappointment in themselves and guilt in having let their parent down.

Children frequently apply the same ideas to other adults in authority that they apply to their parents. They expect of themselves that they will behave in the same way toward a teacher, for example, that they behave toward their parents. The watchful self takes note of what occurs.

Seeing Ourselves in Relation to the Image We Hope to Create

This function of the watchful self is not different from the previous one, merely a continuation. As we learn roles, we create an image of ourselves. In effect, we say to ourselves, "I am a person who should be respectful toward adults." In a discussion with a teacher, for example, we attempt to create the image of respectfulness. When we are successful, we are pleased; when we fail, we experience disappointment. Anxiety and guilt may follow.

A problem enters when we find ourselves in a situation in which one image we wish to create conflicts with another. For example, the college student may wish to create the image of respect toward adults. He may also wish to create the image of mature autonomy. A part of this autonomous image may be that he feels he should speak up when his rights have been challenged. It may be impossible for him to be respectful (as he learned to be with his father) and at the same time autonomous. Confusion of feelings results from the precipitating situation.

Seeing Ourselves in Relation to Goals

The kind of image we wish to create and the way we wish to relate to others is usually determined by the ultimate goals we have set for ourselves. The first two concepts are functions of the third.

Judgmental Function

In addition to observing what happens to us, our watchful self also judges our actions. For many the watchful self is a tyrant that can rarely be satisfied. It creates a context which guarantees frustration, undermining confidence and flooding every situation with so much emotion that objectivity is impossible.

The watchful self develops its values through the experiences of life. When these values are beyond reasonable expectation of achievement, we live in constant fear of failure. Unless we cumulatively build up experiences of success, the tyrannical watchful self begins to set expectations of failure for us. We then adopt the role of being failure-prone. In order to satisfy the expectancy of failure we engage in endeavors which are bound to produce a sense of failure for us. Usually this does not apply to every area of life. For example, a young woman may have developed an expectation of failure in every relationship with a male peer. She then acts vis-à-vis all males so that it is impossible for them to accept her. In effect she fails in this area of life because she has built up an expectancy of failure. Her watchful self judges her in terms of her ability to fail. This leads to the interesting phenomenon that when she fails to fail, she experiences disappointment.

If the watchful self continually applies the rigid standards of the past, growth is difficult. When it functions so that new attitudes cannot be developed, the person is locked into a pattern of viewing himself that makes it impossible to develop the resiliency demanded by life. One of the major tasks of gaining satisfaction in life is to develop a watchful self which functions with flexibility.

Health and Humanness

Whenever a limitation is placed upon the opportunity for man to achieve his unique potential for full and enriched living, then a limitation has been placed upon his health.

Without understanding this concept, one cannot fully know the nature of health. Health has to do with the qualitative adaptation to all life's challenges. That quality is relative to the potential one possesses, among other things. It would be ridiculous to expect a one-legged man to respond to the challenge of a foot race in the same manner as a normal person. Expectation should be in accordance with potential. When one cannot fully, satisfyingly, and effectively utilize his own potential for appropriate response, his chances of achieving full humanness are limited.

Some people are endowed more fully than others. Some have had the development of their potential limited by environment or by experience. It is assumed in this book that each of us has a potential for rich and full living.

Achievement of Full Humanness

For some people the concept of full humanness may be a strange one. It may never have occurred to them that a human being can be anything but fully human, that simply being born of the human race does not in itself make one a whole human being. To develop beyond a level that is only a little higher than that of an intelligent animal, one must have humanizing experiences.

Ira Progoff[3] presents the idea that man has the potential for wholeness. He defines potential for wholeness as "potential on the way to fulfillment," suggesting that wholeness is a process as well as a goal. When an individual is in the process of enhancing his potential, he is in a state of wholeness. Progoff goes on to say that in each man there is an inner sense of what must be manifest in his life. To the degree that one is able to recognize what this is and then make it known in his relationships, he is on the way toward wholeness of being.

As we move toward the fulfillment of our potential, we move closer to full and rich living. But when we become involved in earning a living, in climbing the professional ladder, and in accumulating material things, we are frequently diverted from the central task of discovering our human potential. This does not mean that vocational endeavors are inconsistent with discovery of potential. It does mean that we can become lost in the rat race of high-paced, competitive living.

How do we discover the potential which lies buried within us? Usually through experience. The child with a talent in art will not discover it if he has no opportunity to experiment with this talent. While it may emerge in time, unless a value is placed upon it by his home or his culture, it has no value to him. He has no way of assessing its worth. It does not become a valued part of his personality. It may even become a burden to him, for others may consider him strange because of his interest.

Any capacity we possess must be *utilized* to become an ability. The qualities we value most highly as human qualities lie dormant within us. The quality of love, for example, lies undeveloped unless we have experience with love. This experience must be both in being loved and in loving. Virginia Axline tells of the painful emergence of this human characteristic in her beautifully written

---

[3] Ira Progoff, *Depth Psychology and Modern Man*, Julian Press, New York, 1959.

book *Dibs: In Search of Self*.[4] Dibs, a preschooler of gifted and intelligent parents, had been so deprived of love that he was completely unable to function with other children or with his nursery school teachers. He was fearful, withdrawn, and antisocial. Only after months of psychiatric play therapy with a child psychiatrist, who showed patience, acceptance, and undivided attention to his interests, did Dibs begin to emerge as a person.

Through the weekly sessions with his doctor, Dibs came to value himself. Having his thoughts and the expression of them accepted, he came to realize that he was worth loving. He discovered that his thoughts and feelings could be communicated to, and understood by, another person. Finding himself understood, he grew in the confidence that he could be understood. A self emerged which was valued not only by the doctor but by Dibs himself.

The unfolding of his personality profoundly influenced his par-

[4] Virginia Axline, *Dibs: In Search of Self*, Ballantine Books, New York, 1969.

Sculpture by James Cody owned by the Sovereign Life Insurance Company. Helen Russell, photography.

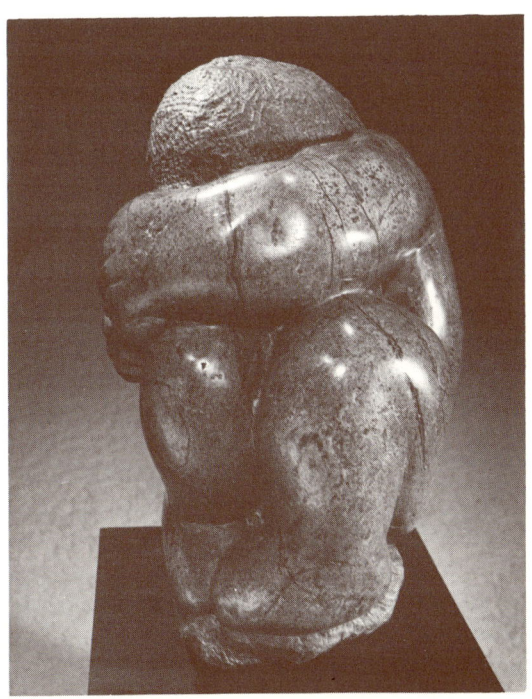

ents. Because he was able to love them, they came to feel that they meant something to him as well. His uniquely human characteristics became a reality. He discovered himself.

Some readers might say that since Dibs was such a remarkable little boy, his potential might have manifested itself in time without the help of the psychiatrist. This is doubtful. Until he was exposed to her he could not function. His own parents, with all their education and intellectual brilliance, had been unable to understand him or to help him on the road to personhood.

As it was with Dibs, so it is with most of us. We need the arena of human interaction for the discovery of self. Extending feelers and examining the feedback is important in the emergence of our self. If what we put forward is accepted and understood, it has meaning for us. If our efforts are rejected, they lack meaning for us, and we ourselves place little value on what we are. We too reject ourselves. The path we follow from this point varies with each of us. Some of us become withdrawn. Some of us give up the attempt to become ourselves and resort to becoming another person. We develop a stereotype which seems to have acceptance and seems to be valued. Then we attempt to identify with that stereotype. A true self does not emerge. An artifact develops, is used, but lacks reality. The self lies hidden. It shows itself only when the controls are lowered. Then it is as much a surprise to the person himself as it is to others who have never seen it.

Another example is Holden Caulfield. The lonely, frustrated boy of Salinger's *Catcher in the Rye*[5] is unable to find himself and proceeds to antagonize all around him. He saw the "phoniness" in himself but projected it to those who represented the world around him. Whatever efforts he made to affirm himself met with failure. He was not a success in school and was a failure with his girlfriend. He even failed in his attempt to have an encounter with a prostitute. The cumulative result was that he could see no value in becoming an adult or in growing past the withdrawn realm of existence in which he found himself. A self that was satisfying did not exist. He did not have the experience or the concomitant confidence in himself to become himself. He was nowhere. He was not a whole person. He was not on the road toward becoming one.

Love and Humanness

By most standards one of the most valued human qualities is love. The person who is able to project himself to others with love that

---

[5] J. D. Salinger, *Catcher in the Rye*, Grosset & Dunlap, New York, 1945.

is ennobling is the individual whom we esteem the most highly. Love, in essence, is a matter of relationships and perspective. The person who can establish appropriate relationships with all that is around him sees himself as a person of value in a setting that is important to him and in which he is important to all else. When he is able to function in this context, he is a constructive and creative force in the universe.

When we examine love in some detail, we find that we can think of it in three broad categories—love of self, love of others, and love of life and all that it consists of. The Judeo-Christian ethic rests upon this foundation. The scriptures tell us that the great law is "Thou shalt love the Lord thy God . . . and thy neighbor as thyself." If we think of love of God as an affirmative attitude toward all that is a part of the universe and if we associate it with giving ourselves fully to turning all things to great value, then we are responding fully to the first part of the commandment. Furthermore, if we are able to give an active affirmation to ourselves and our fellowmen so that each of us moves forward in appreciation of our self and of others, then the second part of the commandment is fulfilled.

Erich Fromm[6] defines human love as "the active concern for the life and growth of the one loved." He goes on to state that love is composed of four components: knowledge, care, respect, and responsibility. If we recognize the influence of these upon persons involved in a love relationship, we see how they become factors in moving them toward the achievement of full humanity.

Knowledge

Knowledge of oneself has long been valued as one of the most important factors in living fully. Socrates held it as his supreme value. To know oneself is to move forward progressively in the ability to utilize what one has for living effectively. It implies that in the process of knowing oneself, one will be able to establish good relationships between himself and others.

Knowledge of another implies more than the accumulation of facts about him. It means a confrontation, an involvement, a mutuality of being, and a progressive exploration of the self of another. It is upon this deeper knowledge that respect and responsibility rest. Without a growing knowledge, respect has little meaning, for it rests upon superficial aspects of one's being.

Carrying the principles of knowledge further and applying them to universal things, an involvement in, and an appreciation of,

[6] Erich Fromm, *The Art of Loving,* Harper, New York, 1956.

these things develop in the individual a sense of the wonder of the universe, in its completeness and interrelatedness. Through this knowledge the self expands, becomes part of, and sees itself in perspective to, the larger forces of the universe.

Care

The care element of love both contributes to and grows out of knowledge. Unless one cares, there will not be the involvement out of which deeper knowledge grows. There are risks in becoming involved with another. Unless care about the other person exists, those risks will not be taken. Consequently there will be a limitation of the relationship and of the individuals within it. The development of those characteristics which we value in human nature do not take place in a vacuum. They only grow out of caring involvement with other people and things.

While one hesitates to base one's thinking upon sloganism, the words which have been popularized in the greeting card industry apply at this point. When "one cares enough to send the very best," he is giving of himself. Giving oneself is a developmental experience. It is rewarding for the giver and for the one who receives the gift.

What does it mean to care about a rock, a tree, or a breeze? Here again there is the implication of an appreciation of these things. In the appreciation, a knowledge develops. One's life is enriched, one is more fully related to the elements of his environment. His life has expanded. He sees himself in relation to the components of the universe. Through the relationship which he experiences, a new dimension is added to his life.

Respect

What can be said about respect as a factor in developing one's humanness? Each of us has had the experience of being respected and knows that it is ego building. But this is only a small part of what is implied in the meaning of respect. It adds to a sense of self-worth and is therefore an important element in the confidence necessary to experience life more fully. It is vital in overcoming the reluctance we have toward running the risks of involvement with others.

Respect cannot be forced. It is not based upon superficialities. It rests upon knowing as fully as possible. A basic assumption is that in all things there is an inherent value which can be known only through a patient and open-minded expectancy toward all that is not self. The willingness to be patient and open-minded in our relationships with others is in itself a manifestation of respect. What more can we ask of another than that he be patient enough and caring enough to be willing to wait for the value in us to show? What more can we ask than that another is willing to encourage the manifestations of value which reside within us? How much has been contributed to our development when this happens!

The reciprocal influence of respect is apparent. The one who shows it gains in his knowledge of the other. He is rewarded in finding elements of being in another which he did not even know existed. But his reward does not stop there. He finds in himself an inner stability which stands him in good stead in the stress of life. In fact, stress itself is diminished, and the subsequent wear and tear of life is kept to a minimum.

In a relationship which rests upon mutual respect, a faith which surpasses all else grows. This faith manifests itself in all the experiences of life. As it has been experienced, it becomes built into one's personality and is carried forward into the next moment of life. Once gained, it can never be lost.

Responsibility

Finally we come to the element of responsibility in love. Fromm speaks of this in far more important terms than those of conscience. If the word were "respons*i*vebility," it would come closer to his meaning. The one who is responsible is able to respond to another's need. Out of his knowledge he sees this need, often even before the other is aware of it. In responding to it he clarifies it and leads the other toward self-knowledge and a returned respect. In the act of responding to the other's need, he develops the other's faith in him and in the other himself. Each is important in furthering the relationship and in furthering the growth of the individuals involved.

Fromm sums up his discussion of these four components of love in these words:[7]

> Care, responsibility, respect and knowledge are mutually interdependent. They are a syndrome of attitudes which are to be found in the mature person; that is, in the person who develops his own powers productively, who only wants to have that which he has worked for, who has given up narcissistic dreams of omniscience and omnipotence, who has acquired humility based on inner strength which only genuine productive activity can give.

[7] *Ibid.*

Self-actualization

Abraham Maslow provides insight into the healthy personality in his book *Toward a Psychology of Being*.[8] He postulates a concept of self-actualization as an important criterion of achieving full humanness. His term implies a dynamic quality of becoming—an unfolding of one's potential in the process of growth. He defines growth "as the various processes which bring the person toward ultimate self-actualization." He further states that "growth is seen then not only as progressive gratification of basic needs to the point where they 'disappear,' but also in the form of specific growth motivations over and above these basic needs, e.g., talents, capacities, creative tendencies, constitutional potentialities."

In Maslow's thinking there are certain clinical manifestations which the self-actualized person demonstrates. He states them as follows:[9]

1. Superior perception of reality.
2. Increased acceptance of self, others and of nature.
3. Increased spontaneity.
4. Increase in problem centering.
5. Increased detachment and desire for privacy.
6. Increased autonomy, and resistance to enculturation.
7. Greater freshness of appreciation, and richness of emotional reaction.
8. Higher frequency of peak experiences.
9. Increased identification with the human species.
10. Changed (the clinician would say, improved) interpersonal relations.
11. More democratic character structure.
12. Greatly increased creativeness.
13. Certain changes in the value system.

Each of these is worthy of thorough consideration, but, in the interest of brevity, we shall examine only seven of them in further detail.

Superior Perception of Reality

In the subjectivity with which we all view life, it is difficult to define reality. It is not enough to define it in terms of what is commonly accepted by the majority in a culture, because often even people in the same group view an event with some degree of distortion. In the early 1950s the American public was neurotically

---

[8] Abraham H. Maslow, *Toward a Psychology of Being*, Van Nostrand, Princeton, N.J., 1962.
[9] *Ibid.*, pp. 23, 24.

fearful of anything which smacked of communism. This was carried to such extremes that anyone who viewed things in a way slightly different from that of the majority was tagged with the label of Communist. However, there were mature members of our society who recognized that difference itself was not a threat to our national interest. There were many who were even able to determine that communism itself was no real threat to our human goals. These individuals often had a greater perception of the realistic nature of the Communist position. They knew that in the structure of American politics, and in the American mind, communism had an extremely limited chance of taking hold.

The person who has a superior perception of reality sees things in perspective. He is able to recognize the relationship of forces to one another. He knows what is a real threat to himself and what only appears to be. He is aware of a larger number of factors and does not apply blinders to his own vision. His frame of reference is large enough to see all the elements in a situation. He is able to see alternative courses of action. After considered evaluation of the consequences of a particular path of action, he chooses carefully what must be done. While he sees himself at the center of all things, he does not lose sight of the influence of his actions on others. He is not stampeded by the anxious cries which come from the frightened people of his world.

It is central to our concept of health that one's perception of reality should be accurate. Unless this is so, one's responses are qualitatively inappropriate. The cumulative result of an inappropriate response is to create experience which becomes more and more confusing.

Increased Spontaneity

This is a marked sign of maturity in individuals. The self-actualized person is able to shift his position readily. It is his good fortune to be able to assess the circumstances of a situation and modify his stance in accordance with them. He is not bound by previously held positions. He is open to new ideas. He is ready to seize upon ideas and actions suited to the moment so that he can move to a new position of understanding. He has a constructive influence on others as well.

When people are bound by their fears, they are unable to move ahead according to the demands of the situation. In the vigorous contemporary struggle for social change great demands are placed upon individuals to see things in a new light. It does not matter that these demands arise from the struggle for civil rights or from the pressures created by the younger generation. The test of the self-actualized person is in his ability to profit from the circumstances as they develop. The demands for change in the civil rights struggle are clearly stated. When the circumstances of our personal lives demand change, the issues are not so obvious. They require a sensitivity to the subtleties of interpersonal relationships. They require the ability to relinquish outmoded attitudes readily. They create the need to reassess one's position progressively and adapt to the newness of each moment.

The person who can react spontaneously to life situations progressively discovers more about himself. He develops the skills of selecting that which is important and that which is irrelevant. He conserves energy. He directs his attention to the central issues of life.

Increase in Problem Centering

Problem centering is a skill. It requires the careful assessment by the individual of the central issues before him. These issues may have to do with the externals of an interpersonal relationship or the task of solving the complexities that develop within oneself in understanding the etiology of feelings.

The five functions that are useful in problem centering are *recognizing, categorizing, analyzing, reorganizing,* and *utilizing.* These are described in detail in Chapter 13, "The Skills for Resolving Conflicts."

Increased Detachment and Desire for Privacy

These characteristics may appear to describe the person who is an isolate, but this is not the intended meaning here. Rather it is to suggest that one does well to value his private moments. He needs them for the meditation so essential to the creative process.

The person who desires privacy is the one who has found a value in himself. He knows that this value cannot come to fruition in the midst of the stimulation of interpersonal situations and that in the distractions of spontaneous action he may overlook an important alternative. He has found that mature judgment requires some moments of solitude to ripen.

Many people find themselves so involved in social processes that they ignore opportunities for solitude and even avoid them. They fear the solitary moment; their lives consist of an endless scurry to be with other people or to be doing something.

Increased Autonomy and Resistance to Enculturation

The same forces which make a person fearful of being alone are at work to undermine his autonomy. The autonomous person is able to operate with a degree of independence. He recognizes that he must make his own decisions about rightness and wrongness. He is aware that many social customs are not for him, that some of them should be challenged. He has somehow developed the courage to leave behind the values of his childhood and act as an individual. He has come to recognize that while these values may have been of worth when he was a child, they are no longer relevant to his life. He values the opportunity to become a pioneer in living for himself. He recognizes that there are certain hazards in the undertaking but at the same time knows that no important task of personal growth is without risks.

Increased Identification with the Human Species

Many of the characteristics of the self-actualized person, if taken individually and exaggerated, would be marks of neurosis. Taken together, they give the balance which is important for the self-actualizing person to have. If, for example, one were to place supreme values upon autonomy and upon that alone, the social order would crumble completely. Individuals would suffer, and only the strong would profit.

For the reason that readers might jump to erroneous conclusions, we rearrange the order of Maslow's list. Along with detachment and autonomy one must also have a strong sense of identification with others. It is necessary for him to empathize with his fellowman in such a way that he can foresee the consequences of his actions upon others as well as upon himself. This counterbalances the risk of his being ruthless in his autonomy.

The person who identifies with other human beings finds himself growing in self-understanding. He also understands others better. There is good evidence that tolerant people are more accurate in their judgments of personality than are intolerant people. In one experiment, a college student who stood high on a scale of measuring authoritarianism was paired with another student of the same age and sex who stood low on that scale. For 20 minutes these students conversed with each other informally about radio, television, or the movies, as they preferred. In this way each formed an impression of the other, as one inevitably does when thrown with a stranger for a short interval of casual conversation. The purpose of the experiment was, of course, unknown to the participants. After the termination of the conversation each student was taken to a separate room and given a questionnaire to fill out *as he thought the other student with whom he had conversed would respond to it.* This method was used with 27 pairs of students. The results were as follows:[10]

> The results showed that high authoritarians "projected" their own attitudes: That is, they thought their interlocutor would answer the test in an authoritarian manner. . . . By contrast, the non-authoritarian students estimated the attitudes of their partners more correctly. They not only perceived them as authoritarians, which they where, but also estimated more correctly their response to certain other questions revealing other sorts of personality trends. In short, the tolerant students seemed in general to "size up" their interlocutors better than did intolerant students.

Greater Freshness of Appreciation and Richness of Emotional Reaction

One of the charming qualities of very young children is that they are able to see things with an enchanting freshness of vision. How often a parent will be stopped dead in his tracks in the midst of a well-meant but turgid explanation of some natural phenomenon by a question from a child which clearly shows a way of thinking that was lost altogether to the adult. Presumably, the reason for this is that the child is more involved in the process of self-actualization than the parent.

One child, for example, upon seeing his first skyrocket split the night with its brilliance and resounding crack, exclaimed, "They broke the sky!" He had seen the event in all its drama. The truth of his observation was from direct experience. He was not encumbered with adult knowledge about explosions and the abstractions of intellectual sophistication.

The self-actualizing person has this freshness of appreciation. He delights in the phenomena of life. From time to time he is awed by miraculous events which are a part of his daily life. He sees a woman, walking with her child, and becomes filled with wonder at the relationship which exists. He knows the child grew within the body of the mother, he marvels at the mystery of it all. From this appreciation there is no limit to the wonder which can open to him when speculating about the people who are all about him. He may even marvel at himself and the astonishing features of his own daily functions.

[10] Gordon Allport, *The Nature of Prejudice*, Addison-Wesley, Reading, Mass., 1954, p. 407. Reprinted by permission of the publisher. All rights reserved.

Accompanying this is a richness of emotional reaction. The individual feels his emotions in their fullness. In joy, his joy is complete; in sorrow, his sorrow is felt to its depths. His love is full, his wonder inspires awe, his happiness is a source of rich pleasure.

Kahlil Gibran puts it well in *The Prophet*.[11] When speaking of love, he says:

> But if in your fear you would seek only
> love's peace and love's pleasure,
> Then it is better for you that you cover
> your nakedness and pass out of love's threshing-floor,
> Into the seasonless world where you
> shall laugh, but not all of your laughter,
> and weep, but not all of your tears.

[11] Kahlil Gibran, *The Prophet*, Alfred A. Knopf, Inc., New York, 1955.

3.

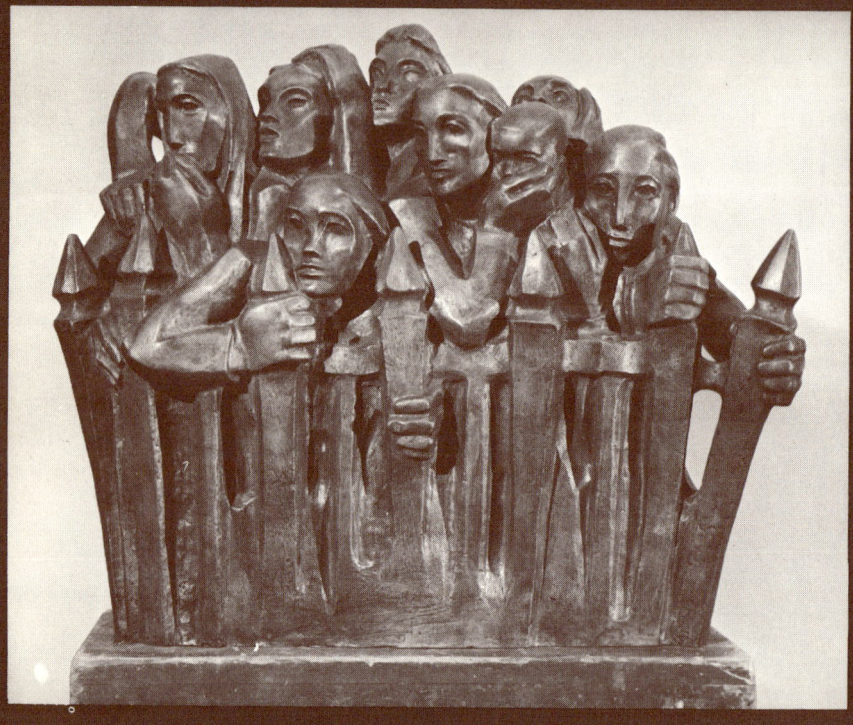

BASIC QUALITIES OF HUMANNESS

If our fundamental concept about health is that it is seen in the quality of one's response to the life situation, then we must examine all that goes into influencing our responses in the qualitative sense.

An example is what happens to a college student when he fails an important examination. A chain of reactions is set off, ranging from disturbed feelings to physiologic changes to behavioral manifestations. These reactions themselves produce further events which demand accommodation. The cumulative effect of the student's past experiential conditioning, as well as the present circumstances, influence his response, and the future too becomes a real influence as the student recognizes the effect of his failure on his future plans.

On the surface this is a relatively simple situation that most students have experienced. But to evaluate the quality of responses to such a situation, it is necessary to develop categories for thinking about what has happened. The succeeding pages attempt to provide categories for critically examining the interaction between a person's environment and his endowment. Only through doing this can he come to a more complete understanding of himself and his health.

Man as a Responding Organism

Certainly one of the central features of man's nature is that he is a responding organism. His capacity to respond is demonstrated in everything he does, feels, thinks, or is. No moment is free of the demand for response. It cannot be avoided. It is as imperative as the need to breathe, itself a response.

The stimuli to which man responds come from both the *external* physical environment and the *internal* physiologic environment. At the same time that he responds to sound, light, odor, and texture,

Berta Margoulies, "Mine Disaster," 1942. Bronze. Collection, The Whitney Museum of American Art, New York. Geoffrey Clements, photography.

he also responds to blood chemistry, stomach contents, and muscle fatigue.

Another set of internal stimuli to which man responds are those which come from the interaction of the various parts of our personality. The id, ego, and superego, to use Freud's terms, constantly interact, causing us to respond in one way or another. The student who feels guilty for not studying must respond to further stimuli which develop from this situation.

Because of the interdependent nature of our stimulus-response mechanism, many systems of the body are brought into play as a result of one set of stimuli. The chain reaction to a frightening situation illustrates this well: Person A, driving a car, approaches an intersection at high speed. He has the right of way and goes through the intersection at the same time that a car from the side street moves through the intersection. Both cars swerve. A avoids being hit, but B, coming from the side street, loses control and slams head on into a stopped car opposite him. A stops and runs to the scene of the crash to find both cars demolished and three people badly injured. He is frightened and revolted by what he sees. On the one hand, he wants to jump into his car and drive away as fast as possible. On the other, he is moved to help the victims trapped in the damaged cars.

Consider the tremendous number of stimuli affecting A. All senses are alert. Hundreds of impulses register on his brain. Feelings are brought into play. Past conditioning activates him. Conscience restrains the impulse to run away. Compassion urges him to help.

Adrenal glands pour forth their hormones. Muscles become tense, eyes dilate, respiration increases along with heart rate. Even his digestive system is activated. In his revulsion at what he sees, his stomach contracts, and he throws up.

These are but a few of the responses which are made to the frightening situation. Each of them is a response to some stimulus which his senses have picked up. Each of these responses is linked to the others. While the responses are sometimes antithetical to one another, the person usually attempts to make some meaningful unity of them, but this is not always possible.

Also to be noted in the stimulus-response cycle is that stimuli are perceived at both the *conscious* and the *unconscious* levels and responses may be made without conscious thought. In the preceding example, A is not fully aware of all he reacts to. Yet he does react. Sweating is a response, though no one consciously tells himself to sweat. Forgetting is a response, and people forget even when they don't want to. They may even utter words and engage in conversations without being fully conscious of what they are doing.

Response and Adaptation

Every stimulus calls for a change within the organism. An increased intensity of light calls for a change in the size of the pupil of the eye. Unless this change—an appropriate response—takes place, varying degrees of blindness may develop. The process of change is an adaptation to the altered conditions of the environment.

Appropriate responses do not happen automatically. For example, each of us at some time has heard a sound that we have located or identified wrongly. Responses we make to life situations may be recognized as having varying degrees of appropriateness. The person who "eats his guts out" is responding to a situation in a manner which is obviously detrimental to him. Many of the functional disturbances to which we are subject are evidence of inappropriate responses.

Since our responses are made with varying degrees of appropriateness, they have a qualitative value to them. *The quality of a response is relative to the effectiveness it has in adapting to the changed conditions which stimulate the reaction.* Our health can readily be measured according to the quality of our adaptive responses.

Learning

Some of our responses are the result of our built-in structure. A muscle can contract or relax. The intensity of the contraction may vary, but the function of the muscle is conditioned by its internal structure and its purpose. Other responses are learned. The combination of muscle contractions and relaxations necessary for throwing an object accurately must be learned. Our reaction to the command of a parent is a learned response.

It is even possible to say that responding effectively is a learned skill. Some children learn that an upset stomach is an effective means of avoiding a difficult situation in school. While such a child may not be able to create an upset stomach at will, the sequence of events which lead up to the crisis is recognized by the child at deeper levels of consciousness. The memory of successfully avoiding crisis by becoming sick may also be triggered by certain events. Therefore, the child in a sense produces the stomach upset in response to critical situations.

Patterning of Response

The sickness-prone child just described has learned a pattern of response. Under specific circumstances it may become automatic for him to become sick. He is locked into a style of response which in this case is detrimental to him even though it works to serve him.

Each of us has certain learned patterns of response. The athlete may have learned to fall in a particular way. The student may have learned to study in an established manner. Prejudice is often a patterned response to a thing, person, or group. Most of our emotions result in learned patterned responses. We often learn to hide our anger or conceal our deepest feelings.

It is interesting to note that, as Allport points out,[1]

> An outstanding result of studies of bigoted personalities seems to be the discovery of a sharp cleavage between conscious and unconscious layers. In a study of anti-Semitic college girls they appeared on the surface to be charming, happy, well-adjusted, and entirely normal girls. They were polite, moral, and seemed devoted to parents and friends. This is what an ordinary observer would see. But probing deeper (with the aid of projective tests, interviews, case histories), these girls were found to be very different. Underneath their conventional exterior there lurked intense anxiety, much buried hatred toward parents, destructive and cruel impulses. For tolerant college students, however, the same cleavage did not exist. Their lives were more of a piece. Repressions were fewer and milder. The *persona* they presented to the world was not a mask but was their true personality.

The well-known endocrinologist Hans Selye has found in his research that people frequently possess learned physiologic patterns to deal with such stress producers as infection.[2] Some people, he says, characteristically underreact to infectious agents, whereas others overreact. They learn these characteristic patterned responses from complex life situations.

Most of us have responses and use them in our daily lives. Problems arise when we rely upon stereotyped responses which have a general application but which are not specifically appropriate to the situation. Under such circumstances our creative potential to be unique is limited. The uniqueness of our responses to situations gives our personality its form and creates our identity. To the extent that we limit ourselves to patterned responses for

---

[1] Gordon Allport, *The Nature of Prejudice*, Addison-Wesley, Reading, Mass., 1954, p. 373. Reprinted by permission of the publisher. All rights reserved.
[2] Hans Selye, *The Stress of Life*, McGraw-Hill, New York, 1956.

similar situations, our lives are narrow, and our appreciation of life is limited.

Man as a Purposeful Creature

There are many words which could be used to describe this aspect of man's nature, but *purpose* is as effective as any. In this section we would call to the reader's attention that the purposes of man range widely: they are consciously and unconsciously held, social and personal, biologic and psychological.

Man's purposes are reflected in the meaning he derives from experience, and they condition the meaning he reads into the events of his life. They are the cumulative result of all past experience and are dependent upon the expectations he has for himself in the future. It is in the realm of purpose that man is unique among all animals.

The grades given in school are interpreted by some students as an evaluation of themselves as people. When grades are used as the sole criterion for self-appraisal, failure in college work means failure as an individual. This is associated with shame and worthlessness. Recognition of other aspects and achievements can offer no compensation for, or mollification of, the sense of failure in a person who holds such standards. Seen this way, passing an examination becomes a test of one's total self. Each test is of paramount importance. Failure is completely unacceptable. It is no wonder that a student may literally get sick at the thought of facing this.

Other students see these situations differently. They think of exams and grades as among the many available self-testing experiences. They see failure in an exam as failure in a particular subject, on a particular day, for particular reasons. Such perspective is freeing rather than limiting. These students see the possibility of changing the grade at some future time and may even be able to joke with friends about the problem. The very same experience in two lives calls forth completely different responses because of the different purpose, or meaning, that each reads into the situation.

Purpose in Biologic Structure

The most basic level of purpose is that which is built into every cell of one's body. Every cell has several purposes inherent in its very structure. Cells can use greater or lesser amounts of energy in performing the tasks for which they are designed. Design establishes purpose, but an accompanying external circumstance initiates the function that is established in the design.

Only when there is a message carried to the cell does it operate according to its built-in purpose. While the element of conscious choice is not available to individual cells, their design is such that a choice must be made according to the stimulus. This choice is related to the purpose that is a part of design.

Walter Cannon, the great American physiologist, postulated the idea that the body and its individual organs and cells function with an inherent wisdom about what is appropriate for their own best interest.[3] It is within this frame of reference that purpose can be recognized as a part of the structure of the body.

When this purpose is thwarted or when conditions exist which prevent the cooperative function of body cells and systems, an element of dysfunction is often established. The organism has an inherent capacity to develop dysfunction, that is, to function in antagonism to itself, as when the body produces conditions which result in ulcers. Obviously this is a condition wherein the health of the organism is destroyed to some degree.

Since it is possible for either effective and coordinate function or discoordinate and destructive function (dysfunction) to develop, it must be assumed that there are reasons for these two phenomena to exist. These reasons are not happenstance. They are the result of some choice-making mechanism within the organism. Hence we can assume that there are purposes built into the very structure of our bodies.

This phenomenon is seen in the way in which different body systems function in interdependence. For a hungry person the sights and smells of food, a sensory function, stimulate salivation and the release of enzymes to be used in the digestion of food. The stomach may even begin its peristaltic contraction in readiness for another part of the digestive process. This is built-in purpose, biologically determined. However, it is not *only* biologically determined, for just the thought of food can produce the same reactions. On the other hand, when we are angry, upset, or emotionally disturbed, we often will *not* produce the necessary functions to aid digestion. Here an emotion inhibits physiologic function.

Sometimes when we have eaten a bit of food and learn later that it was something which is distasteful to us, we automatically regurgitate that food. Again we see the interrelatedness of body systems functioning within a larger purpose for the well-being of the individual. The objective in this is to restore the homeostasis

---

[3] Walter Cannon, *The Wisdom of the Body*, Norton, New York, 1963.

(physiologic equilibrium, or balance) which has been upset by the stimuli to which the organism is subject. Unless these purposes are fulfilled, the organism will die. Hence, purpose functions to preserve life.

Man's Search for Meaning

A more complex aspect of man's purposefulness is seen in the fact that he is a creature who seeks meaning in the experiences of his life and at the same time brings preconceived meaning to the events of which he is a part. Each of us, with a little thought, can recall events which caused us to reflect about what those events meant to us. When a suitor's attentions are rejected, he almost automatically interprets what this may mean to him. He cannot help himself: because he is a meaning-seeking creature, he is compelled to give meaning to the events of his life.

On the other hand, we are often in situations in which events have an impact upon us but happen so fast that we cannot know completely what is happening to us at that moment. However, after the event it becomes apparent to us that the experience did have meaning for us—a meaning we gave to the event. We know this to be so if only from the emotions we experienced.

> In the case of traumatic conditioning, the emotional response is so violent that only a single contiguous connection between the "biologically adequate" stimulus and the "conditioned stimulus" is needed. The following case illustrates the same principle:
> "When I was a young girl, a Filipino houseboy tried to make love to me. I reacted violently and negatively both to the lovemaking and to him. I now actually shudder when I am in the presence of an Oriental."[4]

This is also illustrated in the experience of seeing a disturbing drama. We can be disturbed without understanding why the experience bothers us. We do not even need to recognize that a disturbance in our equilibrium has taken place for it to influence us. The disturbance is itself a response to the situation and implies that meaning has been given to the events we have seen. If there were no meaning, we would not be upset.

Purpose and Satisfaction

Basically, all purpose is related to the drive toward self-preservation. For man, self-fulfillment is an extension of self-preservation. When our responses are self-fulfilling (in terms we ourselves set),

---

[4] Gordon Allport, *The Nature of Prejudice*, Addison-Wesley, Reading, Mass., 1954, p. 298. Reprinted by permission of the publisher. All rights reserved.

the meaning of the event for us is positive and therefore satisfying. If our responses are not self-fulfilling, they represent a threat to us, and further response is initiated to relieve this frustration and threat.

The student, cited earlier, who fails an examination and who gives such meaning to this event that his physiologic and behavioral responses are excessive, responds as though the threat were one against his life. Increased neuromuscular tension is immediately established; alarm bells ring within him; he readies himself for the fight-or-flight response. In actuality, all these responses are inappropriate, but because of the meaning he has given to the failure, he responds with extreme reaction.

When satisfaction is lacking from a specific endeavor or from the general accumulation of life's endeavors, the individual feels the threat of frustration. From that point on a series of responses are established which are designed to remove the threat and relieve the frustration, as for example, in the case of the reporter, unhappy in his job, who blamed all the frustrations of his job on "the goddam Jews who run this paper." The newspaper was not in fact run by Jews; not a single Jew was connected with either the ownership or management of the organization.

These responses are defensive in nature. Even those which are the result of our biologic structure are influenced by the meaning we give to the events of life. Increased amounts of carbon dioxide can be precipitated into the bloodstream simply by our getting excited, and the heart beats more rapidly to assist the lungs in removing the carbon dioxide, because its presence is harmful to the organism. Obviously, excitement may be directly related to the meaning we give to an event; hence, the link between purpose and biologic response.

Purpose and Health

At this point a theory of health is emerging. Since our purposes and the meaning we read into life strongly influence the quality of our response, these become a factor in the maintenance of bodily defenses against any threat to our integrity, or wholeness. Understanding the relationship between purpose and response is important to this theory and to the comprehension of what constitutes the phenomenon of health. To the extent that our responses are qualitatively appropriate, we are healthy. To the extent that these responses are inappropriate, we lack some degree of health. In Chapter 6 we will attempt to identify health in terms of the general and specific responses one makes to life's challenges and experiences.

Man as a Related Creature

All living things exist in a context to which they must relate in order to survive. Unless this is done, death ensues.

Relation to Physical Environment

The most obvious physical law to which man must relate is the law of gravity. It is constant, exerting its forces when we are in any condition and any attitude of body. The importance of this force and our accommodation to it is illustrated in the difficulty men have in getting used to the condition of weightlessness. A new set of relationships have to be established. A new orientation must be made. A new way of behaving must be learned. If we were to live constantly in an environment where the force of gravity was absent, this would be an element of our environment to which we would have to become related and within which we would have to learn to operate.

The phenomenon of becoming effectively related to the physical elements of our environment is so basic and so constant that we take it for granted. And yet, this principle, when understood in its ultimate complexity, has a profound effect upon our health.

First, let us carry forward the importance of relating ourselves to our environment. Every person is aware of what happens when we walk into a strange room. We immediately are on the alert. We sense the atmosphere. We note whether there are people in the room. Without looking at it, we know what the floor is like from the sensations it makes upon our feet. We register temperature, smells, light, size, height of ceiling, placement of objects, and so forth. All this is the process of establishing a relationship with the physical elements around us.

According to the meaning we give to our impressions, we become more or less anxious, more or less comfortable, more or less excited, more or less passive. Interior decorators are fully aware of the impact upon people of color, light, and furniture structure and placement. It would be a rare decorator who would create a bedroom environment, a room where sleep takes place, which was exciting and stimulating. Usually, the tendency is to give it a "bedroomy" look, with quietness, peace, and comfort as the guiding principles in the design and decor.

The effect upon our health begins at the point when we give meaning to the things we find around us. Often, the meaning given is one which comes out of an association with similar things in the past. A graduate student recalled an experience which had produced feelings of deep anxiety for years after. As a young child he was taken to a dentist whose waiting room adjoined a long, dimly lit hall. At the end of this hall was a heavily draped window fronted by a low table upon which rested a bronze bust. From his position in the waiting room this bust took on awesome proportions and assumed expressions of the most hideous sort. It was frightening. Though the student has outgrown the feelings and the associations related to this experience, it took many years, he recalled, to overcome the tendency to look anxiously toward the end of dimly lit hallways in search of the expected monster that lurked there in his imaginative memory.

Many of us can recall more vigorous associations that grew out of our relationships with our environment, associations which had a more lasting effect or which affected us more profoundly. How many of us are made anxious at the thought of eating alone? How many high school athletes can recapitulate within themselves the feelings which precede a competitive event simply by walking into the kind of arena in which the event takes place? How many people have established patterns of response at the thought or taste of certain foods? How many illnesses are precipitated through the associations we have with things and people around us?

Interpersonal Relationships

Although our relationship to the physical elements of our environment is important, our relationship to the people in our lives is of far greater significance. Our initial human relationships are with our parents or those who serve in that capacity. If, in the process of relating to them, we feel that they cannot be trusted, it takes years of experience of another sort to overcome this conditioning. It may well be that because of frustrating relationships with parents we come to feel that life itself is not to be trusted. From this point on we walk through life like the base runner taking his lead from second base. He is wary. He continually expects a surprise attack from an unexpected source. He operates at a level of super-alertness. The cost of this in terms of energy could be exhausting.

Early relationships in life also influence attitudes toward members of a particular sex. It may be that females, if judged by a comfortable relationship with one's mother, are seen to be trustworthy, comforting, and sustaining. At the same time males may appear to be harsh, cruel, and unpredictable. Any combination of feeling is possible. Such relationships are a vital influence in one's life and strongly influence the quality of one's response later.

Relationship and Identity

Our relationship to things and events around us is important in the formation of our identity. We see ourselves in relation to our surroundings and as a result develop certain attitudes about ourselves. The way in which we project our own personalities into life, as with a feeling of being weak and unable to cope with people, is conditioned by the experiences which grow out of our former relationships.

While it is difficult to predict the outcome of these experiences, the generalization can be made that we will use what is effective. For example, two children, unable to cope with life, adopted differing responses to future events: one compensated with aggressive behavior, while the other was inhibited and shy. The aggressive child found that in his relationships with parents, teachers, and friends, his behavior brought attention. Probably some of the attention was the result of negative reactions. But although being naughty may have produced a scolding and being a bully in his peer group was risky business, he did succeed in getting people to notice him. This was his purpose. The attention and recognition that he received more than compensated for the negative results of his behavior.

The shy child found the consequences of aggressiveness to difficult to face. He discovered other ways to get attention without suffering the negative follow-up of aggressive behavior. He found that being shy and withdrawn was a pretty safe position to assume. He wouldn't be hurt; he wouldn't be bothered; there was little element of risk. As for the attention that he sought, he got his kicks from hearing himself described as a "good boy, no trouble at all."

The importance of relationships in personality development cannot be ignored. An infinite number of factors are involved in even a simple human relationship. When two people are together, each is living in his own consciousness with all its past and future concerns. He is also living in the consciousness of the other person and attempting to give meaning to both the conscious and the unconscious projections of the other personality into the situation. Each is concerned about how the other thinks and feels about him. Each is aware either consciously or unconsciously of what he wants from the relationship. Each attempts to respond to the other in a manner that is suitable to his own purposes. Each attempts to realize himself in the situation. To the extent that he is able to do so successfully, he will feel satisfaction and reward. To the extent that he is not, he will experience frustration.

Complicate this situation further by saying that these two people care a great deal for each other. Immediately the complexity of the interaction increases. The intensity of the relationship and therefore the meaning of the relationship for each is increased. With the increase in complexity of the relationship there is a corresponding increase in the possibility of erroneous interpretations.

Relationship and Function

It is not unusual for the purpose in relationship to influence the accurate functioning of the machinery of our bodies. Geriatrists are beginning to recognize that many of the functional disorders of the elderly are not due directly to aging; rather, these are unconscious efforts to block out an environment that is too painful. This phenomenon occurs in any culture where the elderly are shelved as they are in the United States. Functional blindness and deafness are frequent occurrences, and they are associated with purpose as well as relationship.

What does the old person experience? He sees a world in which the relationships he has had up to the present are no longer effective. A man is no longer desired as a functional element in the economy of his world. He is often forcibly retired. As a result of this the entire perspective in which he has seen himself is changed. He must either develop a new way of relating to others, or he must accept that he is useless to those about whom he cares most. This sense of exclusion is one of life's most painful experiences. To protect themselves many old people attempt to close themselves off from the world, and the process of dying is begun.

The drive toward establishing effective, satisfying, and meaningful human relationships is great in all of us. Erich Fromm points out the intensity of human loneliness to which all people are subject.[5] He reminds his readers that this is the source of the insecurity which drives people toward one another. Whenever people cannot effectively relate themselves to others, the sense of threat they experience drives them toward behavior which may be altogether inappropriate to the fulfillment of their needs.

Relatedness and Health

It is important to understand the dynamics of relationships. Otherwise, no accurate understanding of the nature of health can develop, and we are forced to resort to incomplete concepts. Man's relatedness is a fundamental factor of his existence. Since it influences his values, his way of responding, his sense of identity, and his perception of his surroundings—in short, his being—it becomes a vital factor to be considered in any discussion of health.

Man as a Becoming Creature

As each of us looks back upon his life, he recognizes that it has been a continuous process of unfolding. New hopes, new expecta-

---

[5] Erich Fromm, *The Art of Loving,* Harper & Row, New York, 1965.

tions, new talents, new relationships have progressively emerged. New meanings are sought, and in the struggle to grasp them a new self is brought into being.

Each of us has contained within himself the imperative to become more than he is, to reach beyond his grasp, and thus to move forward.

For most of us, however, this is not an unmixed blessing. In the process of fulfilling the drive to become, each person experiences the threat inherent in leaving the old self behind. The college student is fully aware of the problems involved in establishing new values by which to live. He comes to college with a set of values which have been firmly fixed as a result of living in his own home and among the people of his own community.

In the educative processes of college, new horizons are opened, old values are challenged. The limited thoughts which were adequate for the simplicity of living under his parents' supervision are no longer applicable in the new setting of the college life. Most students manage to treat with a certain degree of bravado the problems inherent in throwing off the old values. Nevertheless, the personal counseling services of colleges have files which are loaded with evidence of the struggle to reconcile the old with the new. Apparently the effort is costly.

It is important for people to recognize that there is within themselves the drive to become. The drive cannot be denied even though it is often uncomfortable to live with. The problem for many modern Americans is that so much of life is threatening to them that they are unwilling to allow themselves to become.

The becoming processes of our lives may be classified in three categories: (1) becoming which just happens; (2) becoming as a matter of planning and observation; and (3) becoming as a fulfillment of our inherent potential. These three factors are rarely distinct from one another, but the categories are established arbitrarily as a means of examining the total process of becoming.

Becoming Which Just Happens

Much of our becoming just happens. We have only a limited control over the events of our lives. For example, when a friend who has just quarreled with his fiancé takes his anger out on us and therefore influences the nature of our relationship, we have only limited control of the immediate outcomes. We may be conciliatory, cajoling, humorous, to no avail; he just wants to continue the argument. What happens may be beyond our control, but it will nevertheless influence what we are. If we behave badly in the situation, our estimation of ourselves will be lowered; if we behave well, we value ourselves more. What we become in that situation will have been directed by the circumstances of the moment.

Cultural conditioning has its influence upon the happenstances of our becoming. For many, organic fitness has been sadly neglected as a result of the mechanization of our culture. For others, the results of this mechanization, including pollution of the atmosphere, have had equally unfortunate consequences. What we become, then, is often a happening, the result of things beyond our immediate control.

Becoming with a Plan

Apart from, but operating within, the circumstances of coincidental becoming lies the second category of becoming: what we become often results from both conscious and unconscious observation of ourselves in action. Often as a result of this observation we will plan a campaign of behavior in an upcoming encounter so that we will project a particular image to others. For example, the young woman meeting the parents of her fiancé wishes to ingratiate herself. She acts so that they will come to love her. More than this, she projects herself so that she brings into being, *in her own eyes*, a self that up to now has existed only in her hopes. She seizes upon the test of the encounter to make this hope a reality. She may actually become the person she consciously tries to project.

Becoming Our Potential

The third category of becoming is probably more powerfully motivating than either of the other two. The process of fulfilling our potential is a matter of confusion to many. Some individuals live their entire lives without ever knowing what their potential as human beings really is. This state of being must be learned. We are not human just because we have been born of the human race. Our move toward self-actualization will depend largely upon our ability to identify and manifest the unique potential inherent within our specific nature.

To some extent this necessitates a willingness to experiment in living. Throughout our lives there are demands that we evaluate what we have done and what we are becoming. Our satisfaction derives from the success we have in making ourselves known to ourselves. Often this requires a willingness to wait for ourselves to appear. Too often we lose faith in ourselves, give up waiting, and attempt to be like others. This interferes with the process of fulfilling our potential to be ourselves.

The watchful self is a prime factor in the becoming process. As it observes us in our efforts to unfold what we are, it determines whether or not we have been successful. It sets the stage for frustration if we do not measure up. It creates the opportunity for joy when we do.

When we are not able to find satisfaction in our becoming, we do not learn to value ourselves. We venture less, we hold back from experimental living, and our growth toward full humanity slows down. On the other hand as each challenge to become is successfully met, self-confidence grows. We develop a sense of self-mastery and self-trust. We find delight in ourselves as we become more fully what we have the potential to be. Life, then, becomes exciting, and there is delight in each new challenge.

Man as an Emotional Being

Throughout the preceding pages, many references have been made to the emotional reactions of man. While they have not been named as such, we have called attention to fear, anger, love, and frustration as being integral parts of man's responses. These are basic to human nature and even though repressed or suppressed are present in us in a powerfully motivating way.

While emotions are familiar to all of us, they are also confusing. That element of our emotions with which we are most familiar is the outward manifestation of them. We are all familiar with the behavioral aspects of anger, fear, love, joy, hope, satisfaction. Some of us are familiar with the attitudinal aspects of our emotions. Fewer of us are familiar with the physiologic aspects of emotion. Because we often take ourselves and our emotions for granted, we tend to ignore all but the more dramatic or more troublesome emotions we have.

Our emotions are confusing to us for a number of reasons: First, emotions are both causative agents and resultants of the complex interaction of the phenomena already discussed in this chapter. Second, they are rarely simple and direct. More often they are felt in combination, guilt and anger together, for example. Third, they are capable of being suppressed, repressed, and disguised. Fourth, they flow in a continuum with one emotion following another in an endless sequence, so that it is difficult to pinpoint them. While they are present, we often have no knowledge of them as specific factors, and several series of emotions may be operative at the same time. A fifth factor is the negative-positive classification of emotions, discussed farther on.

Emotions: Both Cause and Result

Our emotions are closely tied with the primitive as well as the evolved aspects of our nature. For example, the emotion of fear brings about the same physiologic changes in the adult as it does in the infant. The degree of change may be different, but the kind of change is the same. Anger produces the same hormonal, nervous, and other bodily changes in animals as in human beings.

Human emotions are closely identified with the values to which we have been conditioned. A child may soon learn that it is "wrong" to show anger toward his parents. Because he is afraid of the consequences of not being able to love (punishment or rejection by his parents), the child may suppress the angry feelings he has.

The word *emotion* comes from the Latin *emovere*, "to move out." In the case above the child has been crossed, senses threat to himself, mobilizes energy through anger, which sets the physiologic adaptive machinery in motion. He then recalls the consequences of becoming angry with his parent and is moved by fear to suppress or hide his feelings of anger. Here we see various characteristics of human nature at work. The child responds to the stimulus of his parent's action with purposes that are related to his integrity (wholeness). He must establish himself as an individual. At the same time it is a situation in which it is important for him to maintain a satisfying relationship. In the process he will use a degree of creativity in handling the elements of the situation, and, to the extent that he is creative, he moves forward on the path of becoming what he must become without doing irreparable damage to the relationship. The entire process is permeated with the symbolizing process (see Chapter 4). The older the child, generally speaking, the more symbolism will be involved. He has already learned that anger-with-parent stands for threat-to-self and may well have learned to hide this anger with symbolic behavior which is retaliative but deceptive.

In this illustration there are other emotions at work. If we add the idea that the child has been so conditioned that he not only feels *fear* at being angry with his parent but also has been made to feel *guilty* about his anger, we see the complexity of the situation. If he feels guilt, the chances are very good that the emotion of anger will not be *suppressed* (consciously hidden) but repressed (unconsciously prevented from rising to the surface). The emotions will be there but at the same time not there. All the physiologic adaptive machinery will have been energized but given no opportunity to show itself. The emotion will have been internalized.

Many of us today are estranged from ourselves because we are not able to follow our true feelings in relation to specific events of our lives. Because we are supposed to love our parents, we may have skillfully learned to hide our anger even from ourselves. We then attempt to respond to a situation as we "ought" to and ignore the natural feelings we have. We expect of ourselves that we should be pleasant when the situation in reality calls for anger. Hence, we judge our response to the situation in terms of the expectation but are puzzled by the uneasiness we experience deep within us. At worst, this internalization of anger is damaging. At best, it is deceptive. It may render us progressively unable to respond appropriately.

The Deceptive Nature of Some Emotions

Whenever emotions have been repressed or the expression of them has been modified, they are difficult to understand. The fear which motivates a college student to study at the expense of fulfilling his need to socialize is usually fairly easy to recognize. But when a generalized anxiety permeates everything he does, the emotions are not easily identified and dealt with. The student who, over a period of years, has found it useful to deny feelings of anger toward himself for not living up to his own grade expectations may make these feelings a part of his identity, carrying them to every aspect of his life and constantly reminding himself that he is worthless, a person to be despised and an object of contempt. In every action, every relationship, every circumstance of his life he may attempt to confirm the negative image he has of himself. Glasser in his book *Reality Therapy* refers to this as "failure identity." In *Schools without Failure* he points out that this phenomenon has played havoc with those who live in ghetto poverty areas.[6]

While the trained psychologist readily recognizes what is at work, the person himself is often completely in the dark about the nature of his problem. Worse than this, he may be incapable of breaking the pattern of his response to the situation. Accident proneness may be a case in point. Some individuals with feelings of guilt learn to use accidents to punish themselves. Such an individual believes that through having an accident he absolves himself of being the miserable creature he believes himself to have been.

Emotions in an Endless Continuum

There is no moment when we are not in some emotional state. Awake or asleep, active or passive, we are living in an emotional context. Recent research on the phenomenon of sleep gives ample

---

[6] William Glasser, *Schools without Failure*, Harper & Row, New York, 1969.

evidence of this. It has been found that individuals create their dreams for themselves in order to alleviate emotional conflicts which cannot be worked out in the waking state.[7] While this is not the only function of the dream, it is an important one. When individuals are wakened as dreams are about to set in and are not allowed to dream, they become progressively more irritable. If the process is continued, varying degrees of neurosis result. The reason is that without dreams we cannot find release for many of the emotional conflicts that remain unexpressed in our waking hours.

Since an emotion is a psychophysiologic response to any situation which either threatens or enhances the self-image and since every stimulus is interpreted by the organism in terms of its threat to or enhancement of the self, even the so-called "passive" state has degrees of emotion in it. Those who do not readily recognize the emotional elements of a passive state might try the following: Imagine yourself to be lying on your favorite couch simply passing the time of day. Try as you will, it is almost impossible to create a total blankness of feeling. Thoughts persist in drifting through your mind. Even if the concentration is to eradicate these, the watchful self makes judgments about your success in the effort. This in itself produces emotional reactions. The degree of reaction may be minute, but it is there, nevertheless.

Negative and Positive Emotions

Emotions themselves are not good or bad—they simply *are*. When they are classified as negative and positive, usually these words suggest a value judgment. Because we are made uncomfortable by fear, for example, it is often classified as a negative emotion, one that is thought of as being bad.

To hold this view is to be deceived. The negative or positive classification should be used according to the degree of movement toward or away from the stimulus causing the emotion. Positive emotions move us toward the stimulus; negative ones move us away from it.

Even this classification is not universally applicable. For example, fear, anger, hate, loneliness, discouragement, shame, guilt, boredom, and feelings of inferiority cause us to draw *away from* an involvement with the causative agents of the emotion. Enjoy-

---

[7] Gay G. Luce and Julius Segal, *Sleep*, Coward-McCann, New York, 1966; *Insomnia: The Guide for Troubled Sleepers*, Doubleday, New York, 1969.

ment of activity, sympathy, love and affection, courage, self-respect, and esthetic appreciation move us *toward* involvement with the causative agents. However, anger, when it mobilizes us to fight and overcome the cause of our anger, may have positive elements, as may fear or any other emotion. An emotion, therefore, is neither all positive nor all negative.

When an emotion has caused us to do that which is indicated by the situation, it has served its purpose. Doubt may cause us to reevaluate. Fear may promote caution. If these responses are appropriate to the situation, they are qualitatively good. It is not the emotion, then, which has the qualitative value, but the response which grows out of the emotion.

It is possible that some emotions are labeled good or bad because they seem appropriate or inappropriate to the circumstances. For example, an individual may become anxious in the presence of strangers. Since most of us meet strangers frequently in our lives, this could be a crippling reaction to normal conditions of life. Again it is not the emotion which is at fault. It is the previous conditioning of the individual and the attitudes he has built into himself in relation to strangers which is the problem. If he perceives strangers to be threatening, it is quite appropriate that he feel fear. The *problem is that he believes strangers to be threatening.*

Purpose of Emotions

It is important to remember that there is purpose behind emotions. Our emotions are designed to facilitate the process of the development of potential. Without them, we would not be moved to accomplish any of the things we are capable of doing. They aid in the accomplishment of long-range goals such as obtaining an education or providing for our loved ones. They also have a protective and preventive function. Without fear, for example, few of us would remain alive for very long.

Many of the great contributions to humanity have been made by people who have been angry, or have felt guilty, or have attempted to compensate for feelings of cowardice. By some standards they have been neurotic individuals; by others they have been great people.

Though our health is related to our emotions, it is not determined by them alone. The degree of creativity with which we express these emotions is a major feature in health. The quality of our *total* response to our *total* life situation is the determinant of our health.

4.

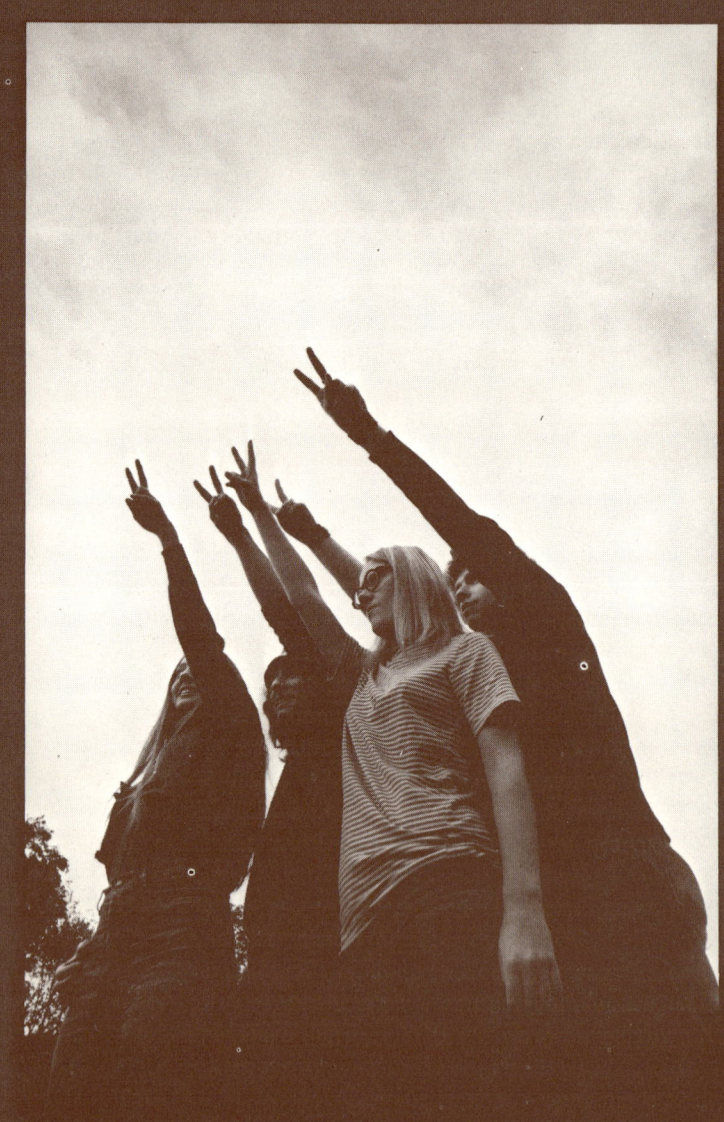

MAN AND HIS SYMBOLS

Through the use of symbolic expression, man projects to others his feelings, thoughts, and attitudes. A symbol stands for, or represents, something else. The most readily understood symbol we use is the word. A word may represent an action like throw, an object such as a stone, a feeling such as love, or something that we cannot fully identify—hope, for example. When we attach a word to an event, it often has meaning far beyond the reality of the event itself. Feelings are then generated which have little to do with reality. A futile cycle is established in which our responses are exaggerated because we have distorted the meaning of the word. Because we use symbols to respond to life, we find ourselves initiating symbolic responses that are unrealistic.

Allport has written:[1]

> An illustration of the craving that people have to attach favorable symbols to themselves is seen in the community where white people banded together to force out a Negro family that had moved in. They called themselves "Neighborly Endeavor" and chose as their motto the Golden Rule. One of the first acts of the symbol-sanctified band was to sue the man who sold property to Negroes. They then flooded the house which another Negro couple planned to occupy. Such were the acts performed under the banner of the Golden Rule.

There are other symbols besides words, such as a smile, a handshake, or a body attitude. Physiologic functioning usually has some symbolic meaning in addition to its basic biologic purpose. A yawn, for example, often stands for more than its purpose of obtaining more oxygen. It frequently exhibits itself as a mark of boredom. Constipation frequently stands for anxiety. A splitting headache is often a sign of repressed anger.

[1] Gordon Allport, *The Nature of Prejudice*, Addison-Wesley, Reading, Mass., 1954, p. 182. Reprinted by permission of the publisher. All rights reserved.

Hugh Rogers, photography, Monkmeyer Press Photo Service.

The Beginnings of Symbolism

Initially there are two parties involved in a symbol-building process. The development of a symbolic structure depends a great deal upon another person. For example, the natural tendency for the infant to cry when he is uncomfortable usually brings forth a more or less appropriate response from the mother. Through the repetition of this experience, the infant rapidly learns that crying can be expected to bring forth some help.

A variety of values develop around this mutually accepted symbol. One is that the infant recognizes that by crying he can influence his environment and those who are a part of it. He finds that *his* cry influences *his* feeding. He recognizes also that his mother usually is the one who responds. Further, he discovers that something in the environment seems to care—in this case, his mother.

On the other hand, let us assume that his cries are often not heeded. A different set of values begins to develop. One has to do with himself. He soon recognizes that he is powerless to influence his circumstances. The environment is hostile and does not respond to his demands. His mother does not always seem to care. He may begin the process of losing interest in his world, feeling that it is not worth the effort to try to fulfill his needs.

Of course, there are many other things which happen to the infant in his early days. From each of these experiences he learns something. Values are accumulated and built into his later understanding of himself in the life situation. Other sets of symbols are developed for communication and expression of himself.

Further experimentation brings about refinement of the symbols he adopts. Most mothers recognize that cries from their children have different meanings. There is an angry cry, a hurt cry, a hungry cry. As the mother responds to these with varying degrees of appropriateness, the infant learns and utilizes these refinements to serve his ends.[2]

Symbols and Growth

Without this progressive refinement of symbolic communication, the growth of an infant is limited. Unless he learns new ways to make his needs felt, his personality remains dormant. He has no basis for learning to cooperate with the forces which act upon

[2] Bruno Bettelheim, *The Empty Fortress*, Free Press, New York, 1967.

him. He feels frustrated in the very task of maintaining his own life.

Sharing is such an important element in the humanizing process that unless a child discovers the means to share what he feels and what he has, he remains at a low level of human development. The experience of sharing is primarily a symbolic one. Basically what we have to share is ourselves. If we find through the early experiences of life that we are nothing because we fail to manage and cooperate with our environment, we have little to share with others. In fact, we have little desire to share ourselves. We do not know the meaning of the experience.

The use of an effective and appropriate symbol is an integrating experience, convincing us that we are able to do the effective thing. It teaches us that we do have worth. It establishes a unity between ourselves and our environment, between ourselves and the other members of our community. When we are unique in our expression of ourselves and at the same time develop a degree of universality, we experience this unifying effect. We move toward the wholeness which is health. Conversely, when we are afraid of violating the conventions in stating ourselves, we stereotype ourselves by using clichéd forms of expression, and we live limited and limiting lives. The frustrations in this are lasting, devitalizing, and debilitating.

Symbols and Communication

Though we have already indicated that symbols are learned in the effort to establish a two-way communication between persons, it is important to underline the communicative function of the symbol. Each of us lives in several contexts. We live in the context of our own inner environment and also in the context of our families. We establish symbols for communication which are mutually understood. Parents become keenly aware of the moods of their children through attending to the symbolic expressions they employ in the context of the home. The child who comes home from school tired and frustrated may slam his books down and retreat to his room without a word. The objective observer would have no difficulty in interpreting the meaning of this behavior. An effective gesture, like a picture, is worth ten thousand words. Problems arise when one does not accurately interpret what is being said through these symbols, which leads to mutual confusion. Feelings are associated with symbolic expressions and may become excessively freighted with supercharged emotion when distortion develops. Each person in the situation becomes progressively confused. Communication breaks down, and emergency measures are brought into action, often with further confusion to both parties.

Each peer group provides a context for living. Each has its own commonly understood symbols for communication. Manner of dress, behavior, style of hair, manner of speaking—all have symbolic significance. They define the degree of in-ness with which members of the group are accepted. The adolescent culture affects many symbols employed by its constituency to express their cohesiveness.

Smoking, drinking, driving, blowing pot, and using dangerous drugs are often entered into for their symbolic value. In certain sections of the country the legal driving age has become a kind of rite of passage. It marks the movement of the individual from childhood into the privileges of adulthood. Similarly, most smokers say that the importance of being one of the crowd was an essential feature in their starting to smoke. Smoking communicates to others in the crowd that they are valued, that the novitiate wants "in."

The kind of symbol employed by the individual to assert himself is of vital significance in his health. When we realize this and know why we are employing the kinds of symbols we do, we stand a better chance of evaluating our actions. Alternative methods then may be undertaken to accomplish the same thing with results more advantageous to ourselves.

Person-to-Person Relationships

Symbols are used in highly individualized contexts. We are one person with our father and another with our mother. None of us employs the same symbols with our intimate friends that we use with our parents. The symbols of communication among men are different from those used among women. Are we the same with a special girlfriend as we are with a male companion? The answer is obvious. Because the contexts are different, because the expectations are different, because the motivations are different, we are different.

Since feelings are important factors in the symbols we choose, preconditioning plays a role in our choice. For example, people are frequently inhibited in their relationship with members of the other sex when they have had a strange relationship with the parent of the other sex in their childhood. Because the roles we learn to play (roles which themselves are highly symbolic) are learned initially in the home through the definitive relationships with our parents, these roles are projected into other life situations in somewhat the same manner until further learning takes place.

In the United States the normal development of heterosexual relationships follows a standard pattern. We move from stages of undifferentiated play with members of either sex to periods of homosexual behavior to a period of increasingly intense interest in the other sex. This pattern and the successes and failures encountered in it structure our symbolic roles. Each of us can recall the strained first encounters in dating when both boy and girl suffered feelings of anxiety about conversation. Frequently, a particular peer group adopts standardized symbols for bridging the gap in understanding the person-to-person relationship. In a group where the mechanical wonders of automobiles is coin of the conversational realm, the girl who cannot discuss compression ratios and carburetors is out of it. It becomes too difficult for young males to make the grade with her. She is a source of too much anxiety. Not infrequently, groups may use physically intimate forms of expression to avoid more direct and more demanding relationships of the deeper personality.

It is tragic when this initial estrangement lasts throughout a human being's life. Because he has never "touched" another person, never allowed another to come close to him spiritually, he lives in perpetual fear of such an encounter. His development is arrested, and he is alienated from mankind. Unless the cycle is broken, he remains doomed to a lonely existence. His symbols for person-to-person relationships remain stereotyped and sterile. Others sense this and hold back from involvement with such a person.

Thought and Feeling

Thought and feeling strongly influence the kinds of symbols we use and the way we interpret the symbolic messages others send to us. The close relationship between feeling and symbolism is seen in the fact that each of us expresses our feelings through unique sets of symbols. Furthermore, there are symbolic behavioral patterns used to express these feelings. Anger is often characterized by strong, violent behavior. Fear, before it turns to anger, is often characterized by uncertain or retreating behavior.

Love too has its own means of being expressed. It is when these feelings become entangled as a result of past experience that we cannot detect the meaning of behavior or expression projected by a person.

For example, the individual who has been thwarted in expressing love in his home environment and has been thus unable to express love without associated feelings of fear shows mixed and confusing symbols in his relationships. Such a person may not be able to understand his own combination of feelings. He may not understand his inability to get really close to the persons he loves. Because getting close represents the possibility of being hurt, he may engage in behavior which actually drives his beloved away from him even though one part of him desires the very opposite. To some extent most of us in our immature years have had these mixed feelings. A young man may be strongly attracted to a particular girl but at the same time may choose every opportunity to ignore her. Confusingly this may occur at times when he feels closest to her. In her turn, the girl may be offended and confused by this behavior and respond in anger which eventually results in breaking off the relationship.

It is only when two people understand what is happening that they are able to bring rational thought into the picture and work through the confusion to more satisfying communication. When this happens, both persons grow in understanding of the other and of themselves. Until it happens, the two are doomed to repetitious and progressive frustration. If the relationship is not terminated, potential lasting damage is done to the relationship and to the persons engaged in it.

Symbols and Physiologic Function

If we are unable to express ourselves in words or behavior, we can do so by body attitudes and body functions. Bodily function or dysfunction as a means of expressing feeling can be learned.

To take an oversimplified situation, anger is usually associated with increased adrenal secretion, a purposeful body reaction. Muscles become ready to act. Reflexes are apt to be sharper if the anger is not excessive and if it is not complicated with other feelings. The total organism is ready for action. Maximum effort is anticipated.

However, when action cannot be taken or anger shouted out,

this readiness remains internalized. As one young woman said to her counselor in college, "I wait in frozen fear all the time for an anti-Jewish remark. I feel a definite physiologic disturbance. I'm helpless, anxious, and in dread." Each of us has known what this feels like. The heart races, the stomach may be "tied in knots," and the muscles ache with tension.

We have phrases which describe these feelings: Unexpressed anger is often associated with "flipping our lid." Every GI of World War II knew the expression "red ass"; because of the authoritarian structure of army life, one's anger often had to be internalized, and the resulting pressure produced piles, or hemorrhoids.

Do we choose, consciously or otherwise, to use these means of expressing ourselves? At the present stage of psychological understanding, it is difficult to give an unequivocal answer. However, circumstances of life clearly indicate that we have learned destructive means of expressing ourselves or of getting what we want or need.[3] Most of us are familiar with these ploys. We have either used them ourselves or have seen others do it.

It does not take many repetitions of the experience of being able to stay home from school because of an upset stomach for a child to be able to induce these feelings when he wants to. He has developed a pattern of response to a critical situation which serves effectively to keep him home and often brings him sympathy and attention at a time when he needs it. No doubt, there is no conscious effort to bring about the upset stomach. But if the child has been unable to get attention in other ways, his unconscious motivation is unquestionable.

Similarly, we do not need to talk very long with a person who has had several operations and who delights in giving us complete and anatomically elaborate descriptions of them to become aware that these operations have been profoundly important to this person. This importance goes far beyond his physiologic need. Every surgeon is familiar with the patient who insists on operations regardless of his counsel. Frequently it is impossible to dissuade such patients from seeking surgery. Sometimes the patient tells the surgeon that if he will not perform the operation, the patient will find someone who will.

For the surgeon these questions arise: To what extent is this operation necessary because of real physiologic conditions, and

---

[3] Arnold A. Hutschnecker, *The Will to Live*, Prentice-Hall, Englewood Cliffs, N.J., 1958.

to what extent has the patient *produced* the symptoms which indicate the need for an operation? Though frequently puzzled by this phenomenon, the tradition-oriented physician finds it difficult to accept that the patient can produce symptoms. Psychiatrists do not doubt it for a moment.

Dr. Faye Lewis tells of a number of patients who have used the symptoms of illness, and often actual physical dysfunction, as a means of solving difficult problems in their lives.[1] An elderly woman was confined to the hospital for about a week with rather vague complaints. "She was weak and tired and not sleeping very well, and sometimes she had chest pain and her heart was irregular." The condition had not varied much for the entire week. One morning Dr. Lewis found her patient "hopping about her room, chipper as a wren. She had her overnight bag open on the bed, and was putting things into it." There was no adequate medical explanation for this dramatic change.

A few minutes later Dr. Lewis met a neighbor of the patient in the hall. The neighbor said, "I believe the thought of all those relatives coming to visit her was just too much for her. There's no reason in the world why some of the rest of her family can't keep them, but they always like to stay at her house. Well, they're all gone now. They left last night."

Here is a case where the reason for the symptoms was unconscious but nevertheless the symptoms served their purpose. The elderly woman had put into operation a set of symbols which succeeded in relieving her of an unwanted burden.

It is interesting to note that illness is a socially accepted means of avoiding responsibilities. In our society special attention is readily given to those who are ill. Flowers and cards are often sent; visits are made—all symbols of concern. For many individuals such symbols are essential to their well-being. If they cannot get them in one way, they will do so in another. These destructive means of meeting needs are all too common.

The literature of psychiatry is replete with case histories of this sort. Symptoms range all the way from those of the common cold to the severely debilitating disorders associated with basic systems of our body.

The major problem in understanding what is involved in the relationship between symbols and physiologic function is that we

---

[1] Faye Lewis, "Patients Who Want to Be Sick," *Today's Health*, vol. 46, pp. 20–23, January, 1968.

have been conditioned to think about these things in other ways; we prefer to use familiar though outmoded concepts. Because of their familiarity, we are comfortable with them. They fit our frames of reference. To change our way of thinking we must relinquish ideas that we have cherished for years. Some of us will have to admit that we have been living in ignorance, a difficult admission for many.

Symbols and Identity

The frustration inherent in not dealing adequately with life is deep and lasting. It is much more profound than the simple frustration of not being able to thread a needle or work out a math problem or pass a driver's test. It is a dissatisfaction with oneself.

A basic characteristic of modern Western man is that when he cannot *be*, he settles for a sort of second-best existence: he finds meaning in *doing*. He measures his worth in terms of what he can do and what he has accomplished. This has become so much the norm that it is accepted as fact—as the *only* fact. Because it is a rare person who examines his life in any terms other than those of doing, many readers may find it difficult to understand the essential issue involved here.

For example, how many students attend college because of their love for learning? American education has become primarily a matter of vocational preparation. Even the liberal arts student is in college simply because he knows that without a college diploma he will get nowhere in the economic world. What is this but a preparation of oneself for the act of doing for the rest of one's life? We know that through the symbolism of the college education we can don the mantle (another symbol) of doctor, lawyer, or social worker. Wearing the mantle, we assume we *are*. And yet, there is a part of us that knows that we are not.

A recent article in *Medical World News* points up the fact that depression is on the rise in the United States today. The age of anxiety of a generation ago is giving way to the age of depression. Dr. Nathan Kline declares that, since the 1940s, diagnoses of neurotic depression have increased tenfold. Dr. Francis Braceland, formerly director and now senior consultant at the Institute for Living in Hartford, Connecticut, estimates that 90,000 depressed patients are annually hospitalized, and the total population for whom family physicians as well as psychiatrists prescribe antidepressant drugs must be in the millions.[5]

What is happening to people today that produces such an increase in depression? One factor is that many people feel that they are living purposeless lives. The very nature of depression is that nothing seems worthwhile. The inability to find a satisfying meaning for life is a dominant factor in producing depression symptoms. The person who cannot *be,* who finds his entire meaning in doing, finds little purpose in existence. He feels that his worth depends entirely upon what he is able to produce in the economic structure. He feels he can be loved only for what he does and not for what he is.

The symbolic structure in which ones lives has much to do with his satisfactions in living. The kinds of symbols he uses to express himself are important not only in terms of satisfaction but in terms of well-being too. Furthermore, he makes himself known through the symbols he uses in life. His very identity depends upon these symbols.

Symbols and Health

Symbolization is closely linked with everything the human organism does. It becomes related to his physiologic processes, it permeates his thought, and it influences his means of expressing himself.

In the complex structure of our personality, the various functions of our bodies assume symbolic significance for us. The way in which we express ourselves through behavior, thought, and body function (the nature of our symbolic structure) influences our health. When we are unable to mediate ourselves in the life situation in a constructive and satisfying way, the quality of our response is distorted. We are able to do neither that which is appropriate to our own well-being nor that which is demanded by the situation. Clearly, then, our health is impaired.

When we have developed a symbolic structure which is utilizable according to the specifics of the existential situation, we have arrived at a state of symbolic organization that is beneficial. We are not bound by past patterns of response. We are not shackled

---

[5] "New Faces of Depression," *Medical World News,* Mar. 22, 1968, pp. 51–54.

by the predominant value structure of our culture. We are free to respond in a manner which will not only fulfill our deficiency needs but will at the same time satisfy our need to grow and to be.

When we are able to be to the fullest extent of which we are capable, we are operating in health and in wholeness. Not only are we moving toward the goal of self-actualization; we are accomplishing this through processes that are efficient and creative. We are healthy people.

5.

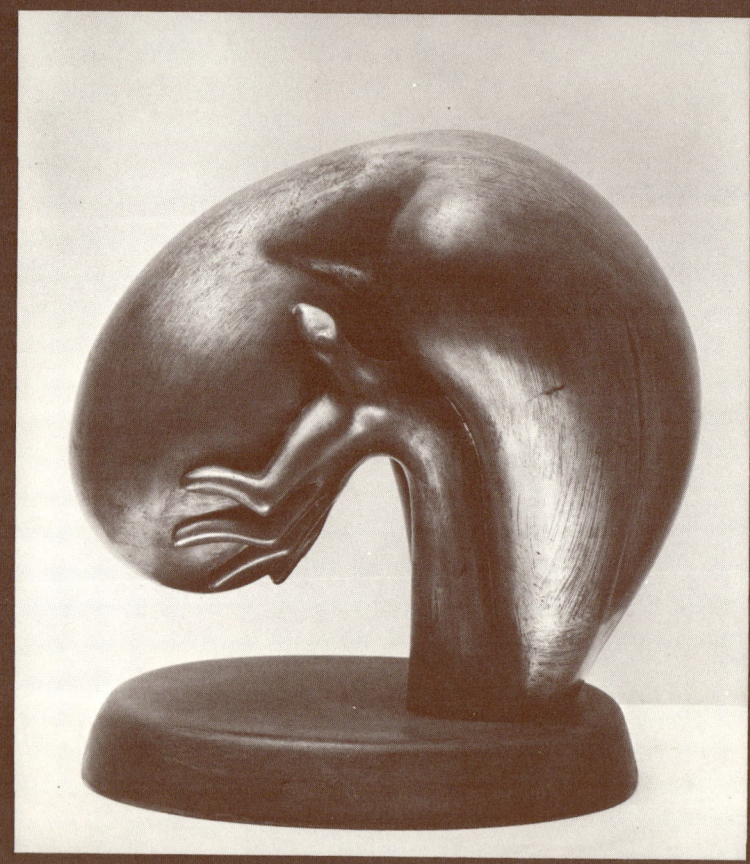

THE NATURE OF EXPERIENCE

The Concept of Experience

The earlier chapters of this book have acquainted the student with the basic elements of human functioning that are most relevant to health. The effort to integrate all these facets of human nature into a single unified concept is, to say the least, difficult.

There is one concept, however, which suggests this unification: The concept of experience implies that there is a unification of all man's drives, interests, talents, hopes, fears, thoughts into one meaningful whole. In the existential moment of experience all our past is applied to the task of bringing meaning to, and deriving meaning from, a complex of interrelated events which comprise that moment.

Our drive toward wholeness is operative in the moment of experience. This drive seeks to satisfy itself in the transactions of life. It does not always succeed. When we actualize ourselves in a block of experience, we feel an enormous sense of satisfaction. When we do not, a sense of frustration inevitably settles out as residue from the experience. From this an attitude is derived and becomes a part of what we carry forward to the next moment of life.

In every experience we test ourselves. The watchful self is the examiner. It determines whether we pass or fail the test. We fail if we cannot make a satisfying unity from the moment. We succeed if we are able to undergo the changes which are demanded of us within that experience.

In the philosophical sense experience implies being affected by what we meet so that to a greater or lesser degree we are changed. Experience is the process in which we perceive all the stimuli to which we are subject. We sort out, evaluate, and give meaning to these stimuli. We scan the value structure that we are. We bring forth that which is relevant, and we react. The result is change.

Hugo Robus, "Despair," 1927. Bronze. Collection, The Whitney Museum of American Art, New York. O. E. Nelson, photography.

The Experience Cycle

If we are willing to settle for arbitrary categories, it is possible to break down the process of experiencing. Though we fragmentize reality by doing this, it is necessary to call attention to what happens in the experiential moment. We may begin by examining the well known stimulus-response (S-R) phenomenon. Every stimulus calls forth a reaction, regardless of whether the stimulus is at the conscious or the unconscious level.

It is useful to postulate two phases of function between the stimulus and the response: Response does not always immediately follow stimulus. There is frequently a meaning-giving phase between stimulus and response. When one walks into an overheated room, he gives meaning to the stimuli he receives. His response may range all the way from "Wow, it's hot in here!" through "What idiot left the windows closed?" to "I'd better open the door." This is attitudinal response.

In addition to the attitudinal aspects of the response there are also behavioral and physiologic adaptive efforts. The behavior may be to open the window, to speak one's thoughts about the heat, to make a gesture indicating that it seems hot, or to ask others in the room if they feel hot, too. The physiologic components of the adaptive response result in reducing the body temperature so that one maintains an acceptable internal condition. Perspiration is secreted, and other mechanisms designed to maintain homeostasis are activated.

Each of these aspects of response are made in qualitative degree. Sometimes the behavior is not appropriate to the circumstances. An individual may verbally attack others in the room for allowing it to become so warm. This only serves to increase internal temperature and further excite oneself. The attitudinal adaptation may be such that because one is fearful of others, he is unwilling to do anything to change the conditions of the room. This in turn requires that a greater physiologic effort be made to adapt.

But before the meaning-giving phase goes into operation, there must be perception by a sensory mechanism. When we enter the hot room, sensors in the skin detect the difference in temperature. They relay the message to other organs of the body. To maintain its internal temperature the organism gives meaning to these messages and responds so that homeostasis is maintained. Associated with this we have the attitudinal meaning giving noted above. We may diagram the entire process as follows:

Stimulus→ Perception→ Interpretation→ Response   { Attitudinal adaptation
Behavioral adaptation
Physiologic adaptation

As a stimulus is perceived by one or more of the five senses, the meaning-giving process (the interpretive phase) is simultaneously at work. This phase is influenced by (1) the context in which the stimulus is encountered, (2) one's past experience with the stimulus, and (3) the way one sees the stimulus and its potential influence.

It is difficult to separate the phases of perception and interpretation. In some instances, the meaning given to a stimulus will influence whether or not the individual will note it at a conscious or subconscious level. In other instances, the stimuli will cause the individual to ignore certain aspects of the situation at the conscious level, the ignored stimuli being noted at deeper, unconscious levels. Those of us who habitually wear a watch have found ourselves looking at our watches without noting the time. Usually this happens because we are attending to other stimuli which are probably of greater significance to us than the time.

Our response to the imbalances that have been created, whether psychic or physiologic or interpersonal, is by attitudinal, behavioral, and physiologic adaptation, which, as already noted, usually results in some form of change in us.

Complexity of Experience

We have been discussing experience in terms of the influence of one stimulus and the corresponding reaction, but, of course, millions of stimuli are inherent in every happening. The student listening to a lecture in class is subject to far more than the sound of the instructor's voice. There are many other stimuli in the room, such as the temperature, the chair he is sitting on, and the other students.

He is also subject to internal stimuli, such as whether he has or has not had a meal, the degree of fatigue present within him, the degree of comfort he feels, his heart rate, and his breathing. Furthermore, his own thoughts provide stimuli to which he must respond. The student who becomes annoyed at the ideas expressed by the teacher may feel moved to respond to his annoyance. His response (annoyance) in itself provides a stimulus in the experiential moment. Thus we see that the phenomenon of experience is extremely complex.

Experience, Learning, and Growth

We are all familiar with the old saw "Experience is the best teacher." It is better said, "Experience is the only teacher," even if it means learning vicariously from another person's experiences. Within the structure of the experience cycle is the concept of *attitudinal adaptation*. Learning is one of the end products of experience. In any experiential situation we learn things about ourselves, the situation, and the stimuli which are a part of the situation. This learning is stored within us in the form of values which are influential in the future. We carry these values forward into succeeding experiences. These values condition our expectations and therefore set the emotional frame of reference through which we view all of what happens to us.

A relatively simple encounter serves to illustrate how learning results from experience. Dave and Mary meet for the first time. They go to a movie together and stop off at the local hamburger joint for something afterward. Later, on the way to Mary's home, they stop to discuss the show and the events of the evening. Soon Dave moves to place his arm around Mary. Being experienced in such situations, Mary avoids the encounter with a witty remark and suggests that she must return home before it is too late. She also suggests another date. The whole exchange has been handled with skill and tact. Dave is also experienced and does not feel unreasonably offended. He respects Mary's wishes and takes her home. What has been learned?

As far as Dave goes, he has learned something about Mary. He draws conclusions about her. He has found her interesting, witty, sympathetic, and understanding. He would like to know her better. He has also learned something about himself. In the context of the occasion, and because of Mary's tact, he has learned that she found him pleasant, normal, interesting, and worthy of consideration. As a result, he feels good about himself. He has not been offended by her refusal to "make out" with him, has hopes that at another time she may be more amenable to his advances. He is able to maintain his respect for both himself and for Mary.

He has learned other things as well. The evening was pleasant. The movie was interesting. The conversation was worthwhile. All this, plus countless other things of lesser significance, has been a part of the evening's experience. Together these factors have created an emotional tone that is favorable for growth and a desire for a further relationship with Mary.

With a few minor changes in the events, the entire emotional context could have changed. The result could have been that he felt himself to be a chump. He could have believed that he had been played for a fool, that Mary was not worthy of any further investment of his time. His confidence could have been undermined, and he might have been unwilling to risk another blind date. Furthermore, things could have worked out so that he would have been unwilling, for some time, to date any girl. His development as a person could have been retarded in the area of his heterosexual relationships.

The evaluation we have made of this situation has been superficial in the extreme. Even so, it is apparent that much has transpired and many things have been learned. Attitudes have been formed which will influence the future turn of events in Dave's life. The whole evening has been a factor in the development of Dave as a person. This experience has been one fragment of the total life experience which has contributed to self-actualization. He has been positively motivated to move toward other dating experiences with Mary and perhaps with other girls as well. The outcome of these future experiences will have been conditioned by these events.

In summary, we see that learning has taken place. More than this, growth has been influenced. Without an experience like the one Dave had, he would have been unable to take the next step ahead in his development. It is important to move forward in the performance of those life tasks which are necessary for full development. In a society which places a premium on heterosexual relationships, the individual who is unable to function in this area of life suffers the consequences of being markedly different from his fellows. The consequences may well be destructive of his general valuation of himself. When one is not able to value himself, he increases the possibility of crisis in his life and the amount of devitalization which he experiences. He runs greater risk of disease and dysfunction. If he cannot stand the stress of this, he is not healthy.

The Existential Moment

This phrase refers to the moment of experience. It is the moment in which we live, the "now" of everyday life. It is another aspect of experience which should be understood.

Usually we think of experience in terms of what is happening in a unit of time, a minute, an hour, a day. With very little difficulty we would be able to see how the physical aspects of one's environment influence his experience. The season of the year, the touch of one's clothes, the aesthetics of the environment all contribute to the content of the experience. Persons who are with us, the relationship we have with them, the feelings we have for them and they for us—all are a part of the experience. It is not difficult to understand this. But there are other factors in any experiential moment.

Both the past and the future are present in the "now." Briefly, our past conditioning and our hopes for the future are represented in the existential moment. Our task is to synthesize a response to the influences of each of these conditions. If we are able to accomplish this synthesis in the interpretive phase of the experience cycle, we can then structure a response which is specifically appropriate to the demands of the occasion.

The Past in Experience

Most of us recognize, in principle, the importance of the past in our reactions. Many of us have weighted this too heavily as a factor of significance in our lives. It should be recognized and clearly understood, but we should not give it more importance than it merits. When we do, we are caught in the grip of conditioning which is totally unrelated to reason. Someone who is prejudiced against Italians says, "Though I know my attitude toward them is unjustified, I still must fight the hold it has upon me. With my Italian friends I lean over backward to compensate, and in doing so I sometimes appear rather foolish."

Both the remote past (our childhood conditioning) and the immediate past play a part in forming our attitudes and influencing our responses. Let us examine the experience of a student attending a class. Entering the class for the first time, he sees an instructor who represents someone he knew in the past. The feelings he has about this may be vague. About all he is able to say is, "That teacher reminds me of someone I know." If the experience of the past has been a frightening one, these feelings of fear are subtly recapitulated in the present. The teacher engenders feelings similar to those he had with the person of whom he is reminded. These, then, become a part of the existential moment.

At the same time, if the instructor is able to tell a joke and put the class at ease, he creates another feeling context which is carried forward into succeeding moments by the student. Without question, what has happened in the immediate past has an influence upon the responses of the student. In this specific situation, however, two sets of feelings are operating within him: On the one hand, he is distrustful; on the other, he is put at ease. Which set of feelings does he believe? How does he reconcile the difference between the two? What he does shows whether or not he is able to make a qualitative response to that moment of experience.

Another significant element about the past in experience is that we have a tendency to want to confirm it in the present. Attitudes formed in the past have become a part of us. Because we do not like to change, we resist doing so. One way of resisting is to confirm what we feel, believe, expect in every moment we live through. If we are unwilling to change, we distort what we perceive and give evidence of not being able to address ourselves to reality in a constructive way. We cannot meet the demands of the existential moment. The quality of our response is poor.

The Future in Experience

Elements of the future are represented in the present. When we meet a friend, we move toward him with certain expectations relative to the immediate or distant future. Usually the circumstances of friendship are related to the immediate future. We look forward to seeing our friend. We know from the past that when we are in his company, we feel comfortable. We expect to be comfortable with him in the moments ahead. We desire to confirm our past experience.

When we move toward an unpleasant task, we anticipate certain difficulties and set ourselve to deal with them. We harden ourselves to be able to withstand the potential frustration in the offing. This, then, influences the feeling context in which we live. It influences the way in which we will interpret what we experience.

Expectations and Experience

More important than the feelings we bring into a moment are the general and specific expectations we have for ourselves at either the conscious or the unconscious level. These expectations are within the very fabric of our makeup. Males, for example, have particular expectations for themselves simply because they are males. A boy expects that he will be treated as such by other people. If this expectation is not fulfilled, he will experience frustration. This frustration may be translated into anger, fear, self-doubt. The strength of the secondary emotions will then influence the way he will experience every other aspect of the situation.

Each of us has a predetermined set of expectations which influence the quality of every experience. These expectations are a large part of what we believe ourselves to be. They are major determining factors in the responses we make in the existential circumstances of life. Since our expectations are so influential, they are major determinants of our health. When our expectations are fulfilled, we are satisfied with the experience. When they are not, we are dissatisfied. At the point of satisfaction or disatisfaction there are other expectations. Some of us have been conditioned to dissatisfaction and frustration in such a way that we can be counted upon to react accordingly in predictable ways. When we are complimented by another person, if we do not expect this reaction, we may not believe that it is sincere, or we may be filled with confusion. For most of us this is only a temporary condition. We may blush, stammer out some unintelligible phrase, and retire behind a silly giggle.

This is a simple illustration of the principle of the centrality of expectations. There are others which have greater and more lasting consequences. These have to do with our ability as students, as men and women, as athletes, as lovers, as persons of worth, as sons or daughters, and so forth. In every experience of life we seek to confirm these expectations. When our expectations are unrealistic, we are doomed to experience frustration, since we cannot achieve them. Most of us have expectations which are more or less unrealistic. Usually what happens is that we learn to modify these expectations. However, upon occasion we are blocked, or block ourselves, from modifying them. The autobiography of Malcolm X[1] sharply points up the blocks which others sometime throw in our way.

> Somehow, I happened to be alone in the classroom with Mr. Ostrowski, my English teacher. . . . I had gotten some of my best marks under him, and he had always made me feel that he liked me.
> He told me, "Malcolm, you ought to be thinking about a career. Have you been giving it thought?"
> ". . . Well yes, sir, I've been thinking I'd like to be a lawyer."
> Mr. Ostrowski looked surprised, I remember, and leaned back in his chair and clasped his hands behind his head. He . . . said, "Malcolm, one of life's first needs is for us to be realistic. Don't misunderstand me now. We all here like you, you know that. But you've got to be realistic about being a nigger. A lawyer, that's no realistic goal for a nigger. You need to think about something you can be. You're good with your hands—making things. . . . Why don't you plan on carpentry?"

[1] *The Autobiography of Malcolm X*, with the assistance of Alex Haley, Grove Press, New York, 1966, pp. 35–37. Reprinted by permission of Grove Press, Inc. Copyright © 1964 by Alex Haley and Malcolm X. Copyright © 1965 by Alex Haley and Betty Shabazz.

What made it really begin to disturb me was . . . [his] advice to others in my class—all of them white. . . . Those who wanted to strike out on their own or try something new he encouraged! . . . They all reported that Mr. Ostrowski had encouraged what they had wanted. Yet nearly none of them had earned marks equal to mine.

It was a surprising thing that I had never thought of it that way before, but I realized that whatever I wasn't I was smarter than nearly all of these white kids. But apparently I was still not intelligent enough, in their eyes to become whatever *I* wanted to be.

It was then I began to change—inside.

When we cannot modify our expectations, we go through life in a state of expectancy that never is fulfilled and therefore with an ever-present sense of failure. Our responses are inappropriate, and we are unable to accomplish the development necessary for self-actualization.

6.

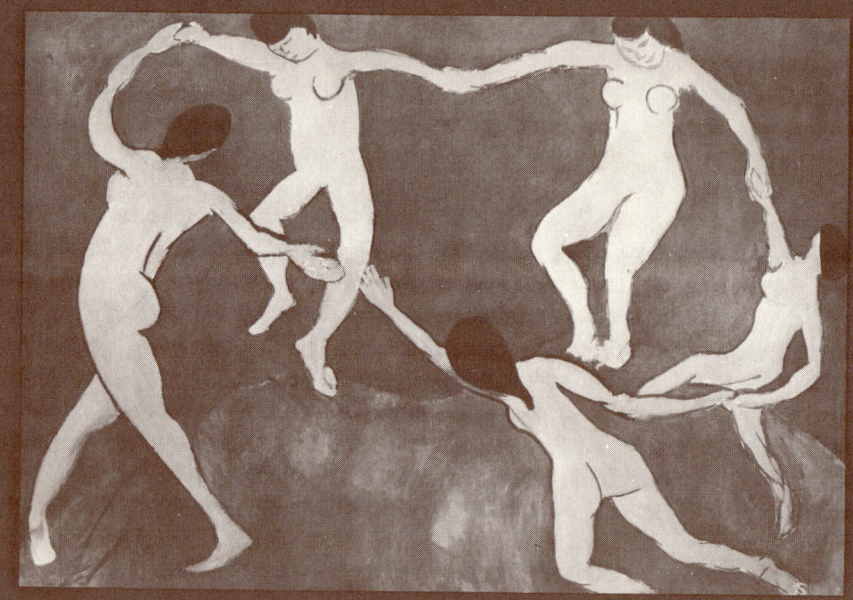

HEALTH AS A QUALITY OF RESPONSE

Traditional Concepts of Health

A variety of concepts of health exist today. Some of them have been around for many years. Among definitions still used probably the oldest is that health is the absence of disease. In an effort to broaden conceptual horizons, the World Health Organization states that health is complete social, emotional, and physical well-being, rather than just the absence of disease.

Jesse Feiring Williams, an outstanding philosopher of health education, developed a concept in the 1920s which gripped the imagination of many in his field. He was aware of the dynamism of health, and he added an important word to our thinking about health by stating that health was the *quality* of living which rendered the individual fit to live most and serve best.[1] In the dynamics of life, Williams recognized that there had to be a balance between the selfish (live most) and the selfless (serve best) tendencies of man. He proposed that if man lived for himself alone and cared not for his fellowman, he created difficult conditions for himself. He also offended, hurt, and alienated his fellowman. Living for oneself alone is evidence of limitation and produces limitation of one's development. It is the way of the child and does not work in the adult world of mutual dependence.

On the other hand the life of selfless devotion sometimes shows a disregard for self which results in destruction. The individual who commits himself solely to the end of serving a goal—business success, academic excellence, motherhood—suffers limitation of self-growth. There is even the possibility of resultant disease and dysfunction. Williams avowed that each goal—self-development and service to others—was worthy, but that there must be a balance between the two in the life of the healthy person.

Many offshoots of this idea developed over the years. One such development is the concept of health as that quality which

---

[1] Jesse F. Williams and A. Kitzinger, *Health for the College Student*, 2d ed., Harper & Row, New York, 1967.

Henri Matisse, "Dance," 1909. Oil on canvas. Collection, The Museum of Modern Art, New York. Gift of Nelson A. Rockefeller in honor of Alfred H. Barr, Jr. Eric Pollitzer, photography.

renders the individual fit to perform happily the personal, social, and familial tasks of life. Again we see the emphasis upon the dynamism. Another thought, implied in Williams's terms but made more definite here, is that health depends on how the tasks of life are performed. To the extent that these tasks can be performed happily and with a minimum of stress, the individual is healthy. It is interesting to speculate upon the kinds of tasks which must be performed for the individual to be considered healthy. Are they tasks which are thrust upon him by society, or are they tasks which he develops for himself? The necessity to earn a living is thrust upon him. To survive he must accept it. On the other hand the tasks of growing are sometimes uniquely those of the individual. The young man who must face up to the crisis created by his own failure has created a task for himself.

The idea that physical fitness is essential for our well-being is clearly not a broad enough concept of health. It fails to recognize that one may be the fittest person alive in a physical sense but have distorted relationships, no friends, and an aggressive manner that alienates others.

Popular Misconceptions

One misconception already discussed is that health is the absence of disease. Each of us has known persons who have been free of the symptoms of disease but who have not been healthy people. The robust weightlifter who cannot get along with other people is far from healthy. The physically attractive coed who brags that she has never been to the doctor a day in her life but who discourages every man she dates is not healthy. On the other hand, if this coed did not discourage men, she might be subject to such stress in her heterosexual relationships that worse things would result. If the weightlifter did not protect himself from others by being obnoxious, he might suffer other, more damaging problems. Each is dealing with life with some degree of value. The quality of the response they are making to the totality of their lives may not be the highest, but it does work to some extent.

Another misconception is that there is a mind-body dichotomy. This dualistic concept once was useful, growing as it did out of research on man. But the easiest things to research are those which are obvious, such as man's body, which can be seen, weighed, touched, and cut up. To some extent the structure of man's body shows its function. Because our bodies have a physical quality, it is easy to postulate man as a primarily physical being.

The more sophisticated research becomes, the more researchers tend to address themselves to the less obvious mysteries. Not all of man's function is explained by his structure. The less tangible elements of man's makeup still pose many mysteries for us. The complexity of emotion is less easily examined than the structure of the body. The intricacies of our value structure pose many research problems. The phenomenon of perception still has us guessing. What means of thinking about these phenomena do we have?

One of the first things we do to bring order to our exploration is to give a name to that which we are trying to understand. Somewhere in the past we created the concept of mind. It was a handy means for categorizing functions we did not understand. The concept of mind was so useful it stuck. We still have it today. We assume that man has a mind and a body and that these are two separate entities. As our thinking has advanced, we realize that mind and body are interrelated, but we nevertheless persist in structuring this dichotomous concept when discussing man's function. We have been unable to recognize that *in terms of function man's mind and body are inseparable.*

"Why must this be a problem?" one may ask. If we recognize that there is an intricate interrelationship between mind and body and if the terms are convenient points of reference, why not use them? The point is well taken, but for purposes of understanding health the mind-body dualism is deceptive.

As long as we remain under the influence of the mind-body concept, we perpetuate another common misconception: that of *mental health* and *physical health* as two distinct entities. Aberrations of the psyche can result in physical dysfunction, for example, ulcers, headaches, asthma. It is also true that bodily dysfunction or deformity can and do effect the elements of psychic development, such as self concepts, confidence, identity formation. To illustrate this interdependency in a most superficial but dramatic way, a director of a play will "psyche up" his actor to set a mood. The actor begins to *act* angry, or happy, or sad and soon begins to feel this emotion within himself. Specific behavior can precipitate a specific emotion. "Whenever I feel afraid, I whistle a happy tune" (*The King and I*) suggests that whistling is a cover-up but at the same time affects the degree of fear that grips the individual. Doctors commonly suggest physical activity to the patient beset by emotional stress and anxiety. Pathways from mind to body and body to mind interweave and should never be treated separately.

Health and Function

To overcome the artificial fragmentation of traditional concepts about health, a number of ideas need to be synthesized. Health is functional. If an individual is termed healthy, he is functioning effectively. In the dynamics of his life, he is able to coordinate many of the features we have already examined in the preceding chapters:

1. Wholeness of function and being
2. Appropriateness of response
3. Movement toward self-actualization
4. Relating effectively
5. Creative use of potential
6. Seeing things in perspective
7. Coordination of attitudinal, physiologic, and behavioral adaptation
8. Use of effective symbols
9. Reasonable freedom from disease
10. Realistic interpretation of experience

When we can unify our responses to life, we eliminate many of the devitalizing strains of life. Energy is conserved, satisfaction is achieved, and self-confidence grows. We see life in appreciative terms, vitality abounds, and we look forward to events with enthusiasm.

All our functional responses to life vary in qualitative value. Few response syndromes are all good or all bad. To the extent that these responses lead us toward developing more and more of our resources for dealing with life in creative and satisfying terms, we become stronger and more sound in the process. To the extent that we are able to unify ourselves with that which is constructive in our environment, we move toward wholeness and the achievement of full humanness.

Degrees of Health

Many times in discussing health we are forced to resort to the use of inadequate terms for want of a better word. To refer to degrees of health is helpful, but the phrase is not as specific as it should be. The word *health* itself implies degree. One is not healthy or unhealthy. He is healthy in degree. As long as we are alive, there is some degree of health in us.

Health is a word like *hot*. It is a relative term. Something is hot in relation to something else. What is a hot day in January may be cool for July. What is a healthy response for one individual may be less so for another. What is a healthy response at one stage in one's life may be less so at another.

Health: A Goal and a Process

Health is both a goal and a process; it also refers to a state of being. It serves as a goal for the person who does not possess it in satisfying terms. When a person becomes ill, he yearns for unity of being and strives to restore the wholeness and effectiveness of function he once had.

There is a deeper meaning of health as a goal. Many do not realize that the drive toward health exists within them. They may often find themselves content with a state of being in which they demand nothing of themselves and in which they simply perform the routine tasks of life. They find themselves so ennervated by this that they are unwilling to venture into the effort required to discover and utilize potential. At the same time the drive persists. The very fact that it persists implies that there is some goal toward which the individual is striving. In this case the goal is to fulfill the need to actualize. Frustration results when this goal is not attained. The individual is then motivated toward behavior which will be little more than tension-relieving. The motivation then is to relieve tension rather than to actualize. There is a blind search for anything which will relieve the depressing sense of guilt about not becoming.

Let us consider the concept of health as a process. We cannot be content with any old process of living our lives. There are some inner demands which must be met. If we meet these demands appropriately, then the process of our life is healthy. If our means of meeting these needs is inappropriate or destructive, then we are not as healthy.

Finally, let us consider health as a state of being. If we could stop a person in a moment of time and examine him, we might be able to determine whether or not his state of being was healthy. But being is not a static condition, so that we have a contradiction of meaning in this concept. In the first place it is unrealistic to assume that we can stop anyone in the process of living. In the previous chapter we discussed life as a continuum of experience. We saw that in experience the individual was synthesizing from stimuli out of the past, present, and future a functional unity for the present. Since these three time factors are represented in the moment of experience, there is no stopping a person in time. His state of being can never be determined except by observing him in the dynamics of his life over a period of time. The word *being* itself implies a dynamism which is lost when static terms are applied to it. In actuality, then, it is inappropriate to refer to health as a state of being unless we place the emphasis upon the being rather than the state. Being is ongoing. It is not associated with the moment of now alone. Being has its eyes on the future. It deals with the past and the present in terms of the future. Being reaches out, not back.

Health has an element of being in it. The healthy person not only assumes that there is a future, he lives toward that future. He savors the present but he looks to the future and moves toward it with hope and affirmation. This does not mean that a reasonable fear of the future is the mark of poor health. But it does imply that when one has a persistent dread of the future, he is in a state of being which does not bode well for him in the long run. He not only has lost hope in a general sense but has lost faith in his ability to manage the future.

Health and Expectation

The quality of looking toward the future with hope and affirmation bears further examination. At other points in this book we have discussed the importance of expectation. In the chapter on experience it was pointed out that the expectations we have for ourselves determine the quality of the experience and influence the quality of our response. Whether we expect that we will succeed in life or that an upcoming encounter will be disastrous for us, the quality of our responses will be markedly affected.

The range of expectations for any situation is varied and complex. We have expectations for ourselves, for others in the situation, for the situation itself. We have expectations for each specific of the situation. As a conversation between two people unfolds, each of them lives through a continuing change in the expectations he has for himself. The following encounter between a counselor and a college student illustrates this.

> The student, Rina, was a young woman, married for six months, who had come to the financial aid office to discuss her needs with one of the counselors. The financial aid program in this large Midwestern university had recently expanded. Some new sources of financial aid had been acquired, and six new persons were employed in the administration of the program. Professor Jones, the counselor in question, had been in charge

of the financial aid program in the years that preceded the expansion. While he was in charge, he felt that things had run smoothly. He was aware of the need for more aid but was unhappy with the transition that was made and the manner in which it had been handled. He was particularly bothered by the confusion which had developed as the new program unfolded. The conference with Rina was toward the end of a particularly hectic day in which it was apparent to many students who had come through the office that things were badly organized. They were inclined to be critical of the program and those who were administering it.

Jones invited Rina in and asked what her problem was. He assumed that he should be sympathetic, understanding, and helpful. He also knew that upon occasion students came in with requests for financial aid which were, in his opinion, ridiculous. Therefore he expected that he should be able to discriminate between a legitimate and a trumped-up story.

Rina had experienced a shattering blow two days prior to the interview. Her husband of six months, who had been in psychotherapy, suddenly announced that he no longer wanted to be married. Rina was in a state of extreme distress. She did not see how she could manage financially. Since she had married against her parents' wishes, they would not take her in. With some fumbling around she told Professor Jones she needed money.

Because she was ashamed, Rina attempted to hide the true reason for her being there. Professor Jones sensed the dishonesty in her story. Within a few minutes he was convinced that the story was a lie, and because his patience was expended from the previous frustrations of the day, he told her that he felt she was lying and he could see no reason for continuing the interview. At that point Rina burst into tears, exclaiming, "Oh, why do I have to cry at a time like this?"

Professor Jones immediately sensed that his judgment had been in error and asked Rina to be seated again. Together they explored the circumstances. Jones recognized that help of several kinds was urgently needed. He used his skill as a counselor to help Rina get things in perspective and the resources of the college to give Rina the financial help she needed.

It is easy to see how the response to the situation developed in each of these two people. Because of his expectation for himself, the counselor started out with one type of response—friendly and sympathetic. When it began to appear (through his interpretive machinery) that he was being taken advantage of, his response changed: he closed the interview and asked Rina to leave.

Rina's responses were also conditioned by her expectations. Her self-image was disoriented. Because of the shame usually felt by a jilted lover, she attempted to cover up the real circumstances, and because of what she had been through in the past few days, she was quite confused. She had resorted to a level of functioning which was basically protective. She wanted help but was not sure that she would be able to get it. She wanted to maintain some degree of dignity but was unsure of her ability to do so. She hoped for sympathy from the counselor. Her expectations for herself were those of one who had some self-pride. This could not be maintained without subterfuge. When the façade was spotted, she lost control and resorted to crying to release the tension which the situation had generated. She became a person reduced to a level of existence which was not satisfying to her.

From the moment Rina cried the expectations of each person changed again, and other responses were manifest. These in turn created another interrelational context, out of which further expectations developed. Each moment was dependent upon the past, and yet each moment had its own uniqueness. The illustration perfectly shows the continuum of experience and the continued effort to adapt to it.

In this situation we see the attitudinal aspects of response. Professor Jones had attitudes toward himself, toward his job, toward the events of the day, toward students and their needs. As he sat listening to Rina, he adapted to the situation by formulating attitudes toward her and her story. These attitudes ranged from sympathetic understanding to suspicion, anger, and rejection. For Rina's part, her attitude toward herself was such that she wished to hide what had happened to her. However, she felt that she had a legitimate need and that it should be met. When it became apparent that her story was viewed with skepticism, her attitude became one of anxiety. Her behavior showed confusion. Her sense of threat increased the amount of neuromuscular tension she felt. Her blood chemistry changed. Her stomach began to cramp. All these were physiologic adaptive efforts. The eventual crying (behavioral adaptation) released some of the tension but increased the shame.

In each case we see the physiologic, behavioral, and attitudinal efforts to adapt. Some of the efforts were successful, others were not. Some were appropriate, others not. The value of each effort to adapt had varying degrees of quality.

Some interesting questions arise at this point. Can we assume that simply because an individual is under stress he is not healthy? The answer must be no, for the presence of stress is not a determinant of health. The indicator of health is how one responds to the stress. If the interpretation of the stress-creating factors is inaccurate, we may raise questions about the person's health. But even then this cannot be the sole criterion. In the professor's case, he had been under pressure for several hours preceding the interview, and therefore it was not to be unexpected that he would be short of patience with Rina.

Another question which arises is, Because the counselor was so disturbed by the events preceding the interview, could questions be raised about his health? Possibly so. If he had made an appropriate attitudinal adaptation to these events, he would have been in a better frame of mind to deal with Rina's problem. Earlier in the day he could have recognized that the expanded program and the large number of inexperienced personnel would necessarily lead to some confusion. He then would have been less upset by it when it developed. He would have been able to keep things in perspective and thereby function more constructively in the situation. He certainly would have expended less energy fuming internally. He would have been able to avoid the anger and frustration which so readily showed in his behavior. His responses would have been qualitatively higher. He would have received more satisfaction from them and would have then projected this in his subsequent behavior.

Health and Unity

Unity of Function

In the above situation we see all adaptive resources of the person being utilized to respond to a normal situation of life. We see how the things which led up to the occasion influenced the response. We see how the self-image each person had became a factor in his and her response. We see the outcome of the continuum of response as it is carried into the future of each individual's life. We see that the responses can be judged qualitatively. In short we see a unity of function within a particular frame of reference.

We see, too, that unity of function alone does not guarantee quality response. The attitudinal, behavioral, and physiologic components of each individual's being come into play. Even when these operated in harmony with one another, still the response was not the best that could be made. Unless the response stems from a reasonable determination by the person of the circumstances, it cannot be qualitatively sound. If one aspect of function is not appropriate, the person is not unified with his environment. Because he distorts the real elements of the situation, some question can be raised about his unity of function. This condition must be assessed within a larger frame of reference than just the individual himself.

Unity of Being

The larger frame of reference is that which comprises the totality of one's life. It not only includes one's motivations and goals but the objectivities of the interpersonal and physical environment. When one is able to relate creatively to all this and is able to make an effective unity of it, he has unity of being; he is healthy.

In part, unity of being comes from effectively assessing the objective reality in which we find ourselves. When we do so, the symbolic structure which we develop in life is reasonably accurate. The devices we use to give meaning to the events of life are appropriate. When we note a statement by another person, we are able to assess accurately what it means. The person who makes the statement and the listener agree on its meaning. We realize its meaning in the context in which it is given. In these circumstances, we have unity of being.

We are unified when our symbols for communication are equal to the task before us. We are able to communicate thoughts, feelings, wishes, and desires to others. We are not at a loss for words or the ability to conceptualize. When confronted with a situation unfamiliar to us, we are able to find the means to explore it and discuss it with others. In doing so we can more efficiently pinpoint the meaning of the new situation to us.

The person who is able to do these things functions with a high degree of unity. Not only does he have himself in reasonable perspective with all that he finds around himself, but he is able to develop more realistic perspective as he moves through life. He does not have to resort to those responses which are damaging or will lead to destruction.

Affirmation of Life

The healthy person sees himself in perspective to the totality of his environment. He attempts to unify himself within and with all that is around him at the same time. He views life with enthusiasm and moves toward it with a hope and expectancy marked by that enthusiasm. He seeks to develop himself in all that he does. He is willing to change when change is demanded. He can shift with the changes that arise.

In short, he affirms life and all that it holds for him. He does not deny the realities of life simply because they are disturbing to him. He seeks deeper meaning in every successive event of life. He is progressively able to capitalize on the meanings he discovers. In doing so he finds himself. His affirmation of life is apparent to all around him. His enthusiasm is contagious. He infects others with his joy in living and with the confident way he handles himself.

This quality of life affirmation is in contrast to the individual who merely exists. So many people today have given up on life. They are willing to settle for minimal rewards. The dominant effort is toward escaping the pain of living rather than finding the challenges in life, performing its tasks, and moving toward the next successive step.

Healthy people are rare. No one is as healthy as he could be, for there is always that which is not developed in the human organism. Furthermore, there are many factors working against the achievement of total health in our society. There is much for which the flower children stand that is patently ill-advised and doomed to failure, but in their affirmation of life they are to be applauded. If they serve to call to the attention of the establishment that its ways are self-defeating, they will have served well in the cause of health.

7.

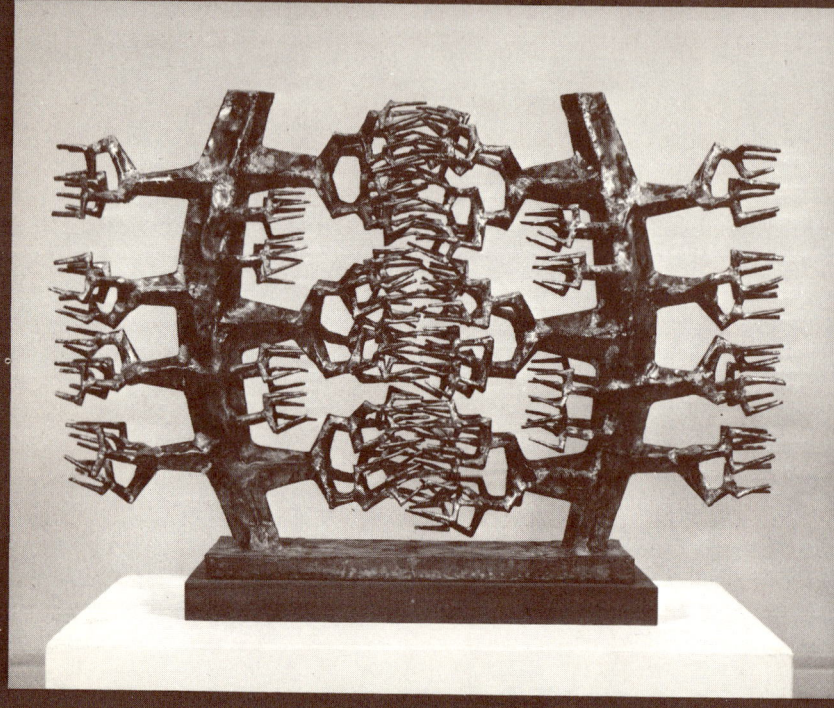

SOME CRITERIA FOR EVALUATING RESPONSE

Since we have problems in defining health, we also have problems in determining what standards should be set to assess health. We can readily set such standards as vitality, exuberance, and recovery rate after fatigue. But the criteria which will enable us to determine the qualitative value of life response are much more complex. No one criterion is adequate.

Since there are so many variables in the phenomenon of health, we cannot be dogmatic about the quality of anyone's response to life. We may, however, ask questions about it. Criteria for health may therefore best be applied in the form of questions.

Even so, we cannot draw specific and unequivocal conclusions from the answers. A particular answer does not tell us that the response is necessarily a healthy or an unhealthy one. It does give us some indication of what further questions should be raised. The criteria, or questions, are mutually dependent. For example, if we ask, "Is this response self-affirming?" the answer "Yes" is not enough. We must also know what has been asserted, whether the assertion is realistic, and whether or not it has been made at the expense of others.

Is the Response Appropriate?

Is the response appropriate to meeting the basic, fundamental psychophysiologic needs of the individual? Is it appropriate to the circumstances? Is it appropriate to the development of the best within the individual? Will the consequences produce in the individual qualities which will be useful to him in the process of self-actualization as he moves forward in his life?

Is the response geared to the development of the best interests of others in the situation? It is important that it develop the best in oneself, but it is of a higher level if its consequences are helpful in the self-actualization process of others in the situation, as well. For example, an individual may do that which satisfies him

Abe Satoru, "Twin Trees," 1961. Bronze, copper, and steel. Collection, The Whitney Museum of American Art, New York. Gift of Mr. and Mrs. George W. Headley, Goeffrey Clements, photography.

but so threatens others that they are moved to isolate themselves from him. However, even this is not necessarily bad; from the situation he may learn to become more aware of the feelings and the integrity of others. As a result he grows.

What Does the Response Proceed From?

What psychological conditions within the individual produce the response? Is the person acting from an emotional impulse or from rational thought? One or the other may be responsible for this action, and there are occasions when both are important.

Most of us have been conditioned to withhold a full display of emotion in particular circumstances. Anger, for example, is an emotion which is not readily accepted in our society. The display of fear by men is frequently not understood. Demonstrations of love and affection are tolerated only in specific circumstances.

The result of bottling up feelings is that they may appear in circumstances where they are highly inappropriate. The person who becomes unreasonably angry over some minor thwarting of his desires is not only acting from his bottled-up emotion but is reading much into the situation that is not there. His response proceeds from sources which he does not understand and over which he has little control.

Another person may respond typically with compulsive coolness. His responses are likewise inappropriate. The person who cannot express love when it is appropriate and necessary is an example of this phenomenon. Another is the person who feels angry but is unable to express his anger. As we have seen, this frequently leads to somatic dysfunction.

When a response results from neurotic needs and further enhances the existence of these needs, then no growth has taken place. Usually patterns of response have been established to protect the neurotic need, and the person locked into such a pattern finds it difficult to free himself. He then proceeds to further the destructive sequence of responses.

Does the Response Indicate Growth?

Growth must be seen in relation to the past performance of the individual, as the following case study shows.

> John had always been a retiring sort of individual. He had been dominated by every member of his family, including his younger brother. When he went away to college, he experienced

an extreme sense of anxiety coupled with an awareness of a freedom which never existed before in his life. He was unable to become involved in the activities of the school he attended. He was hardly known to the students, even among those living in his dormitory.

Though he was not directly involved in school activities, he became interested in some of them. He spent less time studying and more time watching others and observing the things in which they were interested.

When his first semester was nearly over, he received what he thought was an unmerited grade on a paper he had submitted. Acting in complete reversal of anything he had ever done before, he went in to see the professor who had given him the grade and forcefully presented his objections to the grade. He was surprised at his own behavior and found himself secretly delighted that he had acted with what he thought was a new degree of manliness.

For John this response was one which showed a definite amount of growth. It proceeded from a history of diminished self-confidence. It was a healthy response for him.

In another case, with another student, a similar action might not have been a sign of growth. It may have proceeded from a long history of argumentativeness, showing no change. If it was his standard approach, clearly the quality of his response would be considered poor.

Is the Response Consistent with Cultural Mores?

This is another criterion for which there can be no single answer for all situations. To some extent our responses have to be in accordance with the mores of the culture of which we are a part. If they are not, we may suffer unmanageable amounts of stress.

On the other hand the individual who attempts to do nothing more than to conform to the standards of society is doing little of a constructive nature for himself or for society. Frequently, circumstances demand protest and challenge. The protest movement among young people in recent years has many hopeful signs about it. It is a new force which causes the establishment to reexamine its standards. Without a vigorous protest among the black population of our society and without recognition by many whites that changes should be brought about, injustice (an unhealthy condition) will continueto exist.

There is no question that some degree of anxiety will result from bucking society. Protest, in the sense that it stands for a promotion of the best that is within us, is important. Further than that, it is essential for growth.

What Is the Effect of the Response on the Future?

There are consequences to every act we perform, every response we make. However, we can do many things which have no constructive effect on the future, and there are many responses that result in backtracking in development. These responses are qualitatively poor. Too often we become involved in a series of responses which are progressively more destructive. They may meet one or two of the criteria cited but may do little toward a constructive future.

The basic question here is, Will the response have consequences leading to further growth, or will its results be devitalizing and debilitating? A young adult may have effected the necessary separation from his parents and their authority, but if this results in stress which so weakens him that he is rendered ineffective in other areas of his life, it is obvious that he was not ready to do what he did. One may then question the appropriateness of what he did, for it was not truly in his own best interests.

Many young people are not able to make effective choices in this area. They become imbued with the idea that they must assert themselves at all costs. At the same time they fail to make an accurate assessment of the consequences and their own ability to sustain them. The result may be a series of defensive reactions which serve no purpose except to help the person recover from what he has done.

The skill of accurately assessing the circumstances of life and making effective judgments about them is important. But many of us develop this skill only by a trial-and-error method. If the trials and errors are in areas of relative insignificance, then not too much damage is done. If, on the other hand, the experiments are in major aspects of living, then problems arise. The college couple who find themselves impelled toward bringing their relationship to a sexual fulfillment and whose acts result in pregnancy of the girl have done something which will bring about serious consequences for each of them. A moralistic judgment is not being made here. The issues raised are in terms of the cause-and-effect relationship.

If the girl follows the growing practice of obtaining an abortion, the consequences in terms of guilt may be difficult to recover from. If on the other hand they decide to marry and in the course of events the young man must terminate his education in order to provide for his newfound family, his future may be seriously limited. The most difficult limitation may not be the financial one. It may be the more serious one of a lack of challenge in the work he is able to get without a college degree. This, then, becomes reflected in the mariage, with numbing results for both the husband and the wife.

Does the Response Show a Reasonable Perception of Reality?

Meeting this criterion necessitates bringing together all the previous ones. It demands that one become progressively more objective about himself and his acts. It requires that he develop an insight into himself and his motivations. This insight is often beyond the reach of many people throughout their entire lives.

The reality to which we refer is twofold: the physical realities and the interpersonal realities. As far as the physical realities are concerned, the problem is rather simple. Yet, even here each of us has his own personal assessment of what is real and what is not. If the moment of experience we are examining is fraught with emotion, we are apt to distort our view of even the physical realities involved.

Every college professor is aware that many students will hear things differently from the way they were spoken. Dating and courting are replete with examples of distortion of objective events which have taken place between the two people. As each of the individuals reacts to the distortion, there is apt to be further distortion, and then events move toward that which is totally unrealistic for each of them. The effects upon communication are disastrous.

Since subjective distortion of objective events is always possible, the ability one has to assess properly what is happening within himself is important. Furthermore he must be able to evaluate the social context in which he is operating. If at any point he distorts, then his perception of reality is off. From this point on his responses necessarily become inappropriate, because they are based upon faulty perception of the realities involved.

The saving word in this criterion for most of us is the word *reasonable*. Without this word most of us would be in trouble. Few of us are able to be totally and completely realistic in our perceptions. Few of us are able to respond in complete accord with the objective situation. Few of us are able to be accurate in our understanding of our motivations and in assessing the outcomes of our acts. Hence few of us could be judged healthy according to this criterion if it demanded more than a reasonable perception of reality.

Does the Response Lead toward Autonomy?

Some of the earliest signs we show of autonomy appear at about the age of two years. This is so common that some parents refer to these years as the "terrible twos." At this time the child is beginning to use the word no. By his use of it he is testing the strength of his own will against that of his parents. He is attempting to discover how far he can go in making judgments for himself in the direction of his own affairs.

A later manifestation of this testing of one's own will appears in adolescence. When a youngster begins to want to dress in a manner which is more consistent with the values of his peers than it is with the values of his parents, he is exerting some degree of autonomy. He is also testing how far his parents or society will let him go in this endeavor. He may grow a beard and let his hair grow to unusual lengths. He may even begin to appear in what, to the establishment, appears to be bizarre clothing. In these efforts he is exerting a degree of autonomy.

It is granted that this may not be the most effective use of his autonomy, but it is a beginning. Insofar as it does not infringe upon the rights of others, it probably should be encouraged as a means of testing the consequences of being different. In the process the youngster may encounter consequences which make him decide that another mode of behavior or dress is indicated. He may also come to the conclusion that this is not a very mature effort and will reject it himself.

In any event, when a response shows a degree of autonomy or yields promise that the individual is moving toward responsible autonomy, it is probably a sign of health. Naturally the previous criterion of the ability of the person to handle effectively the consequences of his autonomous behavior is a factor to consider.

Does the Response Reflect a Love or a Fear of Others?

Most healthy people view life and others with a reasonable degree of openness. They are willing to move toward other people in an affirmative manner until the others prove that they are not to be trusted.

When individuals demonstrate life responses which show signs of unreasonable fear, we can question the quality of these responses. When an individual is so suspicious of others that he cannot relate to them in a creative manner, he is in a difficult state. He cannot do those things which are necessary to the humanizing task which faces us all.

Many people, for example, have been strongly conditioned to a particular "in" group. They are suspicious of all who are not a part of that group. The dictum "Don't trust anyone over thirty" is an attitude which reflects this kind of suspicion. Prejudice grows from such attitudes. Within the confining influences of prejudice people are unable to appreciate or to understand the values of any person against whom their prejudices are directed. The consequences of this are that they are unable to move toward members of the other group in any way which will dispel these prejudices. They are taking an approach which prohibits growth in particular directions.

Prejudice is bad enough for the group against which others are prejudiced. It is worse for those who have the prejudices. They cannot grow; they are rendered incapable of moving from previously held positions. They respond to life in what could be called a programmed way, as if they were programmed to produce feelings about others regardless of the realities. These feelings then produce responses which are inappropriate to the circumstances or to the well-being of any of the persons involved. Life is seen in distorted ways.

On the other hand the person who operates with a reasonable degree of love for other human beings is more apt to detect the realities in the interpersonal situations of life. Again the key word is *reasonable*. Is the attitude expressed a reasonable one? Will it produce constructive responses? Will it allow enough freedom from past experiences to enable the individual to deal with the conditions according to the objective demands implicit in the situation? The healthy person would give affirmative answers to these questions.

To What Extent Is the Response Creative?

This criterion is based upon an assumption which is not often manifest in our thinking about ourselves or in our thinking about man in general. It assumes that all human beings have an almost unlimited number of resources with which to deal with life. Experience—either the experience of life or the experience the individual creates for himself in *evaluating* his life—produces those forces which will develop this potential.

The creative person is the one who can judge a situation and reach within himself for the resources which are specifically appropriate. Such a person is willing to do that which he has never done before. He is able to utilize capacities which have not been used before in dealing with life. The creative person is discussed fully in Chapter 9.

Hans Selye[1] discusses the importance of developing an "attitude of gratitude" about life. By this he means something akin to the old adage of counting one's blessings. The individual who is able to see in every event of life that which can be capitalized upon develops an attitude of gratitude about the events of his life. He functions in the context of this attitude. He is able to minimize the amount of stress which results from anxiety.

Does the Response Restore Homeostasis?

All response is adaptive in nature, and the maintenance of homeostasis is a fundamental need to which man responds. However, man's needs are complex, and there are times when his responses should not restore homeostasis if he is to fulfill the need to grow. Hence the question may be raised, Should the response restore homeostasis?

In discussing this criterion it is useful to consider two categories of response: The one could be called a defensive response. This is the response which is utilized primarily to defend the individual. It is consistent with fulfilling the need to maintain homeostasis in the psychic as well as the physiologic sense. The other classification may be thought of as an initiating response. This response is designed to push the individual forward into an area which is threatening to him or into an area which is unfamiliar.

In such a case the response ought not to restore homeostasis but rather ought to produce in the individual some reasonable feelings of disturbance. It is probably the initiating point of a series of responses which when brought to conclusion result in growth for the person. Within the series a state of insecurity exists, but at its conclusion there has been marked growth. This series of responses may be somewhat prolonged in nature, lasting a period of days or even months.

When a student goes to college, not out of a desire to learn, but primarily to satisfy the demands of his parents, the pressure of parental coercion is great enough to upset homeostasis. In his desire to appease the parent and to take the heat off of himself, the young person may have acceded to his parents' wishes. Ac-

---

[1] Hans Selye, *The Stress of Life*, McGraw-Hill, New York, 1956.

tually he might be better off in the long run if he had engaged in a series of initiating responses wherein he did not attend college but became engaged in activities which better fulfilled his own needs.

The students who attend college after traveling, attempting to work, raising a family, or serving in the Armed Forces are often able to get much more from their studies in college. The added maturity makes them better equipped to make effective choices of a major program for themselves.

The self-condemnation which follows attending college to meet some demand other than the inner desire of the individual may be damaging for many students. Many students feel they are wasting their time in college. Many blame themselves for not doing something else. At the same time they have not yet found within themselves the courage to do anything different. In such cases the defensive drives are paramount, and the initiating responses are not yet pressing forward.

Is the Response Satisfying?

Again with this criterion there is a qualifying question: satisfying what? This criterion is not too different from the preceding one. It is used because many people feel that the major drive in life should be toward self-satisfaction. This is questionable. Much of what is advocated in this book is toward self-actualization, but this is not to be confused with self-satisfaction.

The self-satisfied state which becomes a basis for life tends to indicate that the individual is not involved in the kinds of things which are steadily leading toward growth. The self-satisfied person shows some signs of refusing to grow. He has found something which is comfortable and therefore is unwilling to run the risks of moving to another position.

On the other hand there is the need to find something in life in which one can take satisfaction. It is important to "do his thing," but in doing it he should not extend himself so much so that he is unable to stand the stress which necessarily ensues, lest he become like the army commander who has pushed so far forward into the enemy lines that he has moved beyond the efficient supply of his troops. He has not only run the risk of the logistics problem but also run the risk of encirclement by the enemy. He has moved so far forward that his entire effort may result in failure.

So it is with each of us. A neat balance between self-affirmation and attention to social standards must be maintained.

8.

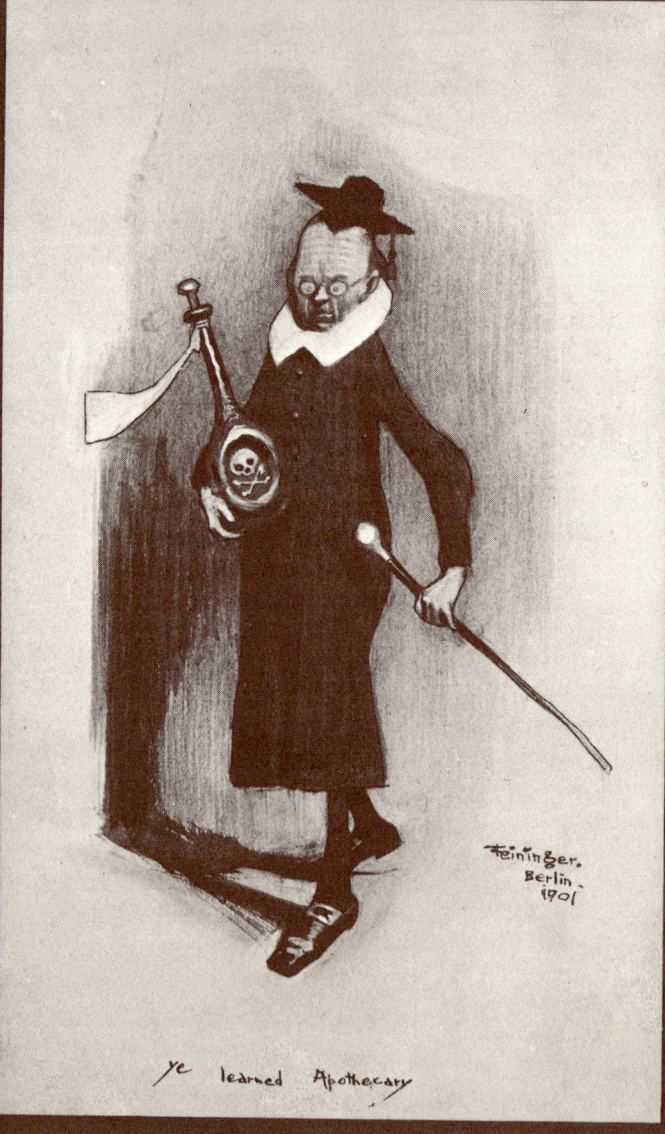

THE RELATIONSHIP BETWEEN HEALTH AND DISEASE

General Adaptation Syndrome

While it is true that certain organisms are factors in disease and that prolonged exposure to cold is devitalizing, Hans Selye[1] points out that there are always "nonspecifics" associated with disease—anxiety, fatigue, and other stress factors which cause the organism to initiate the *general adaptation syndrome* (GAS). The GAS moves through a series of predetermined stages. First, Selye points out, there is the *alarm reaction*, characterized by an immediate mobilization of the body forces to fight off that which threatens its integrity. Hormones are delivered into the bloodstream which in turn initiate other bodily responses designed to ready the organism to fight.

Selye informs us that it makes little difference what the stressor is—it may be the injection of large quantities of disease organisms into the system, a blow which injures some part of the body, a break in the envelope of the skin, or an emotional disturbance. All these stressors bring about the alarm reaction.

Then the organism moves into the *stage of resistance*. In this phase the organism is functioning at maximum efficiency to ward off the influence of the stressor. This stage may last for days or even months, depending upon the vitality of the organism and the amount of rest which it is able to obtain throughout the time of maximum effort. During the period of physiologic adaptation, the organism is not likely to succumb to the influences of the stressor. After the adaptive energy has been expended, the *stage of exhaustion* occurs. In this phase the organism becomes progressively devitalized, and its ability to resist the influence of the stressor diminishes. Every function of which the organism is capable becomes weakened. If this stage lasts long enough, death ensues.

A simple draft, a normal exposure to disease organisms, or the normal anxieties of life are not the only factors that threaten the

---

[1] Hans Selye, *The Stress of Life*, McGraw-Hill, New York, 1956.

Lyonel Feininger, "Ye Learned Apothecary," 1961. Gouache, pencil, pen, and ink. Collection, The Museum of Modern Art, New York. Gift of Mrs. Julia Feininger.

well-being of the organism. If they were, we would all be sick all the time. *Only when there is a combination of factors at work within us do we suffer the defensive breakdowns which are manifest in disease.* When we are emotionally disturbed, for example, and have been so for some time, our defenses against other stressors are weakened. If we then encounter an additional stressor, such as a disease organism or an unusual amount of exposure, our adaptive machinery breaks down. If we cannot summon additional resources for fighting the added stressor, we are apt to succumb to disease. Only when a combination of events persists long enough does the individual move toward debilitation and perhaps even death.

Selye's stress theory is further discussed later in this chapter.

Values and Health

A brief examination of the importance of values in human function will be made here. A more comprehensive treatment of this topic is found in Chapter 11.

A value is a thought, idea, attitude, or belief which results from experience. Since our values result from our cultural experience, they become an established part of our personality.

The superstitions of a culture become a part of the value structure of members of that cultural group, who then function according to these superstitions. Many a person who has been conditioned to the idea that snakes are slimy and repulsive will be unable to stomach snake meat. It is impossible for them to keep the meat down even if they have been able to get it past a gagging throat. This is one example of superstition (value) influencing function.

A. T. W. Simeons structures his entire treatise in *Man's Presumptuous Brain* on the idea that the beliefs man holds about the things and events of his life strongly influence the way he functions.[2] He presents case after case in which he illustrates that these beliefs frequently lead to somatic dysfunction and psychogenic disorders (discussed later in this chapter).

We put into bodily function those things we believe deep within the value structure that we are. These beliefs are subjective and often have little to do with objective reality. In effect, we function according to the subjective realities of our lives. We do this at least as often as we function according to the objective realities of life.

---

[2] A. T. W. Simeons, *Man's Presumptuous Brain*, Dutton, New York, 1961.

Usually we combine the two ways of functioning. The objective realities are colored by the value structure through which we experience them, as in the example just cited of the person who cannot eat snake meat. The objective reality is that snake meat is perfectly edible; it has the nutritional qualities of most other meats. And yet, because of the subjective factors involved, many people cannot eat it. Their stomachs function to reject it.

Since health is the qualitative adaptation to life's challenges and since the subjective phenomena of any individual's life are important determinants of response, it is apparent that these phenomena are important in health. It is therefore necessary to examine the values by which we live to determine the extent to which these values influence our adaptive responses to life. Unless we are able to reorganize these values, we will continue to live according to limited truths. We will have limited control over our health and be limited in our ability to manage our lives.

People in Search of a Disease

Just as there are accident-prone individuals in search of an accident and depression-prone people who seek those things which are depressing, so there are disease-prone persons in search of a disease. Usually these people are successful in their search. The skills we develop in the process of living are directly related to the progressive projection of the inner self. We seize upon those things which will enable us to give outward expression to what we are. The disease-prone person too searches out those conditions which will give affirmation to what he feels about himself.

The person who lives in a cultural milieu which continually impresses him with the fact that he is subject to disease often establishes an identity which is more or less disease-prone. Even specific diseases or physiologic disorders "run" in certain families. This is not so much a matter of a constitutional weakness as it is that the family develops a pattern of response to life which gives particular status and meaning to a specific disease condition. Because of the experiences it has had, this particular subculture (the family) has narrowed down the vast array of choices the members have at their disposal for dealing with life. In other words, only certain ways are acceptable to the members of this family for expressing the feelings they have about life.

It does not matter whether the subculture or the larger society makes this selection and limitation. It becomes a fact in the lives of its members. This is probably the most important reason why we need to examine the relationship between health and disease.

There are also *health-prone* people. If health is the quality of their response to life, they are able, somehow, to transcend the limitations of their culture.

As one increases the variety of resources he has for dealing with the problems of life, he decreases his need to rely upon destructive means of meeting its challenges. It is possible for him to select from among the many arrows in his quiver the one which is specifically designed for the particular task he faces. When his choices are narrowed, he must rely upon the methods of his childhood. He resorts to responses that have worked in the past. Many of these are the methods of weakness. They are not designed for the tests to which the individual is put as an adult.

Our motivations toward disease are not subject to conscious selection. They may be examined at the conscious level if we have sufficient understanding and insight into our motivations. If we are able to recognize the relationship between response and its motivation, we stand a better chance of resisting the inappropriate responses which well up from the deeper levels of consciousness in our personalities. As we grow in this skill, we are better equipped to free ourselves from the conditioning of the past. More control lies in our hands. We are better able to predict what our feelings will be and therefore are able to do those things which will counteract the influence of our feelings at one level so that we may in effect become conscious and active partners with our deeper motivations in the process of self-actualization.

Some Concepts of Disease

The various current concepts of disease that we will discuss here are not mutually exclusive. The intelligent person may synthesize from them a theory which is applicable to the intricacies of human function, and thus begin to approximate the truth about the relationship between health and disease.

The Germ Theory

This concept assumes the presence of disease organisms. When one comes in contact with these organisms, unles he is somehow resistant to them, he will suffer from the disease. The disease organism is specific. It can be seen under microscopic examination. Its life history can be charted. Its influence upon some human beings can be determined under certain conditions.

But disease organisms are not always effective. René Dubos states:[3]

> Many types of microbes can paralyze, starve, or bleed their victims, and are endowed with the power to kill them within a few days or a few years, [yet] it is also true that the same microbes are usually harbored for a whole lifetime by normal, very ordinary citizens, who are not even aware of being infected and who—for all we know—may derive some unrecognized benefit from their infection. The dramatic episodes of conflict between men and microbes are what strikes the mind. What is less readily apprehended is the more common fact that infection can occur without producing disease.

Obviously there are other factors besides the germ in precipitating disease. Does this mean that we must abandon the germ theory of disease? Hardly. There is a relationship between the germ and the disease, but it is not that which many of us have assumed for most of our lives. The protection against diseases of the type associated with disease organisms does not result only from keeping ourselves insulated against contact with the organism. Dubos further states:[4]

> Granted the obvious usefulness of sanitary practices, immunological procedures, and antimicrobial drugs, it does not necessarily follow that destruction of microbes constitutes the only possible approach to the problem of infectious disease, nor necessarily the best.

The Stress Theory

This theory, associated with Hans Selye,[5] was discussed at the beginning of this chapter. Selye's work in the study of the body's adaptational capacities has moved us forward in our thinking about disease. Basic to his thinking is that when the body is subject to a stressor, such as infections, intoxications, trauma, nervous strain, temperature extremes, muscular fatigue, or irritation, it responds in a stereotyped manner to adapt. He states that the response is the same regardless of the nature of the agent provoking the stress.

However, when other nonspecific factors come into the picture, some aspects of the GAS are distorted. Deficiencies or imbalances in the response may then lead to diseases of maladaptation. More

---

[3] René Dubos, *The Mirage of Health,* Doubleday, Garden City, N.Y., 1961, p. 71.
[4] *Ibid.,* p. 70.
[5] Selye, *op. cit.*

simply, it is possible for the body to be mistaken in the specific way it chooses to either combat or surrender to the stressor. Since the stressor may be any agent which threatens the integrity of the organism, it is possible that the germ theory of disease and the stress theory are related. The disease organism becomes the stressor. Either the body in its effort to adapt may maladapt, or it may be under attack for so long that it reaches the stage of exhaustion in the cyclic nature of the GAS.

The Resistance Theory

This theory, held by many, is often linked with the germ theory. It usually states that people have various resistances to disease according to their constitutional strength, their genetic endowment, the amount of fatigue present, and the presence of antibodies developed within their system. To some extent this theory is valid. It can be linked with the stress theory in which Selye poses the stage of resistance as a feature of the GAS.

When the individual is in the stage of resistance, he is capable of resisting the onslaughts of disease organisms which in a later stage of the GAS might do serious damage. Experiments with rats have indicated that minor infections can be eliminated by placing the animal in conditions which call upon him to generate massive resistance to a stressor.

Dubos points out that man has many mechanisms which enable him to resist infection. These mechanisms differ from case to case. They appear to be specific for particular conditions. Some are genetically acquired through heredity.

He points out:[6]

> During a widespread epidemic of tuberculosis, for example, the most susceptible are likely to die young, leaving no progeny. In contrast, many of those who survive are genetically endowed with a high level of natural resistance which they pass on to their descendants. The low tuberculosis mortality prevailing in the Western world at the present time is in part the result of the selective process brought about by the great epidemic of the nineteenth century which weeded out the susceptible stock.

Another of the mechanisms we have for resisting disease is that in which we develop an immunity to the influence of a disease organism by having been exposed to the organism and thereby developing antibodies which effectively protect us against further infection. At one point in our history it was a popular practice to

[6] Dubos, op. cit., p. 72.

expose youngsters to the "children's diseases," so that this natural immunity could develop. However, in recent years our neurotic obsession with cleanliness and our excessive concern for being disease-free has limited this practice. Furthermore children are no longer considered as expendable as they once were. Hence we are reluctant to run the risks involved in this practice.

The Psychosomatic Theory

Lawrence LeShan reports:[7]

> The psychosomatic concept is a very old one, which has gained recognition and lost and gained again throughout its history. In the medieval era, the theory of body humors was a complex and sophisticated theory of mind-body interaction. A letter written in 1402 by a physician, Maestro Lorenzo Sassoli, to a patient has a curiously modern sound . . . "let me speak to you regarding the things of which you must most beware. To get angry and shout at times pleases me, for this will keep up your natural heat; but what displeases me is your being grieved and taking all matters to heart. For it is this as the whole of physic teaches, which destroys our body more than any other cause."

The layman will recognize that there are some diseases which are *not* related to a disease organism but which are influential nevertheless. These diseases he may place in the category of *psychosomatic* disease.

The psychosomatic theory of disease grew primarily out of the work of Freud and his postulates about the emotional motivations which render people susceptible to disease. Emotional disturbance may produce sufficient stress to weaken a person, causing him to be susceptible to infection. Furthermore, the emotional factors may cause certain systems of the body to function at an excessive rate to the detriment of other systems. When there is no ready outlet for these emotions, the subsequent internalization leads to organic dysfunction which may be damaging. For example, when anxiety produces an excess secretion of acids into the stomach and when this condition prevails for protracted periods of time, the stomach lining erodes and hemorrhaging often results. Hence, the bleeding ulcer. It may be healed through a variety of means but can become reactivated during subsequent emotional bouts. When the emotion subsides or an adequate means of externalizing it is found, minor ulcers may heal themselves.

[7] Lawrence LeShan, "Psychological States as Factors in the Development of Malignant Disease," *Journal of the National Cancer Institute*, vol. 22, no. 1, pp. 1–18, January, 1959.

The popular interpretation of the psychosomatic disease is frequently distorted. Often it is thought that this is not a real disease but rather something which is "just in the mind" of the sufferer. It is important to recognize that this is not so, that so-called psychosomatic disease is as real as any other. It is strongly related to stress and results in organic dysfunction and often in organic breakdown. It may even result in death.

The misconception that psychosomatic disease is "all mental" comes partly from a misinterpretation of the word *psychosomatic*. Because the syllable *psycho-* comes first, it is taken to refer to disease that originates in the psyche. In that sense a more appropriate term is *psychogenic*, as noted below. Psychosomatic, from the Greek *psyche* (spirit) and *soma* (body), implies simply that both aspects are involved and that there is a relationship between the two. All diseases are psychosomatic in that they have an influence upon the total organism, both the psyche and the soma being affected. Selye points out that all sick people have in common a sense of "downness," or depression, which seems to be a part of the disease.[8] This feeling of depression can be a forerunner of many different kinds of diseases. From the point of view that health is a functional quality, there is no separation between the psychic and the somatic.

The Psychogenic Theory

This theory postulates that some diseases have their origin strictly in the psyche. An example of this kind of disorder is the stomach ulcer which originates in the feelings of anxiety that are a part of a person's life. The stomach ulcer illustrates, too, that a disease may well be psychogenic and at the same time have psychosomatic aspects.

Like the psychosomatic disease, the psychogenic disease is a real disease. It usually has somatic manifestations. It results in real pain. It may even lead to tissue breakdown and to organic dysfunction. There is no such thing as an "imaginary" disease. What people mean when they use this expression is that the person is suffering from some sort of hypochondria. He may be afraid of being ill, or he may give special significance to rather normal aches and pains, which become exaggerated in his mind.

The psychogenic disorder is difficult to examine in the clinical sense. This is so in part because of the traditional orientation we have toward disease and its physiologic etiology. Dr. Allan Walters

---

[8] Selye, *op. cit.*

of Toronto General Hospital has formulated a concept of *psychogenic regional pain* (PRP).[9] This term

> denotes pain for which clinicians cannot find physical lesions or peripheral cause and does not mean "mental pain" or "pain in the mind." . . . Psychogenic regional pain is a pain signal remotely localized in a field of sensory perception when the trouble is going on in the field of mental perception—in the mind's eye, where we find thoughts and feelings. . . . It is a case of remote localization to one field of perception from another. The site of the remote localization is usually psychologically related to the noxious situation. . . . [A] face pain may occur with every fresh reminder, at the site where the patient was originally slapped or hurt.

Walters further points out that psychogenic regional pain accounts for many of the intractable pains that are "drifting in medical and surgical streams." This is an important finding, for it accounts for much of what may be thought to be imaginary pain. It can be assumed that diseases, such as many colds, which are largely symptomatic may also fall into this category. In such cases the person is able to recreate in himself pain and dysfunction which are associated with some former emotional trauma.

The Symbolic Theory

We often use disease in symbolic ways that express for us what we feel. Walters suggests that the psychogenic regional pain syndrome is a form of symbolization.[10] He points out that "in order to have PRP the patient has to be in a frame of mind wherein emotional life can be expressed in physical and hallucinatory terms." He further states that these conditions apply only at certain times in a person's life and under certain conditions:[11] "Most patients with these pains have declined from a more effective and steadier level of behavior. As we decline we move through frames of mind which are less logical, more emotional, more pictorial and with more remote localization."

The healthy individual is able to select for himself a set of symbols which are appropriate to the conditions of reality in which he exists. He is able to develop those means of symbolic expression which are effective in communicating to others what he feels

---

[9] Allan Walters, "The Psychogenic Regional Pain Syndrome," Paper presented at Henry Ford Hospital International Symposium on Pain, Oct. 21–23, 1964, Detroit; as reported in *Medical Tribune*, December, 1964.
[10] *Ibid.*
[11] *Ibid.*

and, often, why he feels it. The person who functions at diminished levels of health often has a central problem of not having been able to develop symbols which are appropriate to his particular life. Certainly anyone who must resort to pain and dysfunction is operating in a way that is not only ineffective and inappropriate but destructive as well.

The person who finds much in his life that he "cannot stand" may produce symbolic disorders of the legs and feet. The person who cannot "stomach" something may well produce a stomach disorder. When some people have problems which seem to them unbearable, they develop the symptoms of a disorder of the back. "Oh, my aching back!" and "What a pain in the neck!" are verbal statements of what could be physical conditions and may be only a step away from becoming bodily dysfunctions—a back that actually aches or a literal pain in the neck.

Causative Factors of Disease

As we have already mentioned, viruses and other disease organisms are real. Their effects cannot be denied. But they are not the only factors that precipitate disease.

Emotions and Disease

A growing body of research tends to lead us in the direction of recognizing emotional factors as forerunners of disease. For instance, research at the Downstate Medical Center in Brooklyn, New York, has definitely linked asthma to emotions.[12] The conclusions reached have been drawn from experiments in which asthmatic reactions were induced in persons suffering from this respiratory disease by deliberately tricking them into believing that they had been breathing such allergenic agents as dust, pollen, and animal dander.

These persons actually had breathed air containing nonirritating saltwater mist, yet they reacted as if the allergens had been present. A number of the subjects actually developed full-blown asthma attacks. The breathing ability of others tested was constricted to a lesser degree.

The persons who had developed the more serious reactions were then misled into believing that they were to be given a remedy for asthma. Actually they were subjected to breathing the same saltwater mist. The respiratory conditions in all those who

[12] Richard D. Lyons, "Report Links Asthma to Emotions," *The New York Times*, Apr. 6, 1968.

had produced the major asthmatic attacks improved. The conclusion was drawn that beneficial treatment might be as much a state of mind as the disease itself.

Control groups of individuals who were not chronic asthma sufferers did not produce the symptoms of asthma.

Research in other disease areas tends to yield similar findings. An increasing amount of evidence points to the emotion of despair as a predisposing factor in disease. Much investigation of these phenomena is being carried forward at the University of Rochester School of Medicine. Dr. George Engel of that institution reports that periods of gloom, despair, grief, loneliness, and misfortune might predispose people to disease and aggravate their illnesses even to the point of death.[13] At the same time feelings of confidence, tranquillity, and peace of mind might contribute to good health.

At the University of Rochester the phenomenon of the relationship between despair and disease has been termed the *giving-up complex*. At the annual meeting of the American College of Physicians in 1966, Engel reported[14] that accumulated clinical observation has heightened the impression that illness is commonly preceded by some change in the patient's life, a change with which, for longer or shorter periods, he is unable to cope and to which he responds with feelings of helplessness and hopelessness.

"As far as we can tell, the giving-up complex precedes the onset of illness," he said. The giving-up complex appears to entail first an unpleasant, distressing reaction expressed in such terms as "It's too much." "It's no use," and "I can't take it anymore." The patient perceives himself as less intact, less in control, and less capable of functioning in the accustomed manner, although he may continue to attempt to do so.

Relationships with others are felt to be less secure or gratifying, either because the patient has actually suffered the loss or disruption of a relationship or because he feels rejected by others. It may even be that he gives up on himself.

This giving-up complex was referred to by U.S. Army Major William Meir, in a speech[15] delivered in March, 1957. Major Meir was one of a team of psychiatrists who interviewed several hundred American soldiers who had been prisoners of war in the Korean conflict. This investigation was undertaken to determine the reason

---

[13] George Engel, paper presented at annual meeting of American College of Physicians, June, 1966.
[14] *Ibid.*
[15] William Meir, speech delivered at Executive Club of Detroit, Mich., March, 1957.

for the astonishing death rate among Americans who had been prisoners of the North Koreans. In no other conflict had American prisoners of war died at the rate of seven out of ten. These soldiers had suffered from what Meir termed "give-up-itis." In some cases soldiers were known to have crawled off into a corner, covered their heads with blankets, and died.

It was found that these men had been completely isolated from their compatriots (the isolation was emotional rather than physical) and that they had been taught to totally mistrust their fellow soldiers. Through the devices of the North Korean captors these soldiers lost faith in the United States, in their buddies, in themselves, and in whatever cause they may have felt involved in, relative to the war. Not only did these techniques of the captors cause men to die, but they totally eliminated the desire to escape. No Americans were known to escape from Korean prisoner-of-war camps even though these camps were guarded with a minimum of troops. On the other hand, whole divisions were necessary to prevent the escape of North Koreans who had been taken prisoner by the Allied troops.

Another piece of research, under the direction of Dr. Merl M. Jackel at the Downstate Medical Center, reveals that colds are linked to the mental state of the sufferer.[16] "In my opinion, the common cold is the result of psychophysiological changes which accompany depressions in certain individuals," he states. He studied the incidence of colds in ten patients over a three-year period. He found that twenty-five of twenty-six colds were preceded by states of depression. He further found that the colds these patients had never appeared in the absence of depression.

A common finding that runs throughout many of these research projects is that when people have a poor emotional outlet, they suffer from disease and disorder. They find it difficult to put their feelings into behavior, and the only other avenues of adaptive response open to them are those of attitudinal and physiologic adaptation. Unless they can rearrange their attitudes, they are left with the alternative of absorbing all the stress in their physiologic structure. Frequently the task is too great. There is a breakdown, either a symptomatic and symbolic expression of what is felt or a functional or organic breakdown of particular organs or systems.

Michigan State University has looked into the phenomenon of repression as a factor in health and disease. This research would seem to confirm the concepts of emotional causes of disease de-

---

[16] John Leo, "Colds Are Linked to Mental State," reported at American Psychoanalytical Association meeting, The New York Times, Dec. 17, 1967.

scribed above. It was found that persons who had developed the skills of repressing feelings tended to produce headaches, upset stomachs, or skin eruptions. On the other hand, those who were unable to repress feelings tended to put these feelings into words or behavior.

Repression is an attitudinal effort to adapt. It is the process wherein we exclude an emotion from our consciousness. For example, when we are made angry in a situation which we have learned should not call for anger, as when our anger may bring forth the displeasure or disapproval of a loved one, we tend to adjust the attitudes within ourselves in such a way that we do not even recognize that the anger is there. Therefore the avenue of behavioral adaptation is not open to us, and whatever residue of emotional energy is accumulated must be expressed in physiologic changes.

Here, then, we have findings from a wide range of experimental and clinical conditions which all lead toward similar conclusions. There is a close relationship between one's emotions, what he does with them, and the quality of his response to life. When he is unable to handle these emotions and adapt to them in constructive and developmental ways, he then functions in ways which produce one or more of several circumstances: Symbolic symptoms of disease may be produced. Functional disorders may be manifested. Sometimes there is even organic damage which results from prolonged conditions of the type cited above. Usually physiologic stress develops which in itself may be so devitalizing that the individual is open to further attack by disease organisms.

There are times when an individual uses disease to deal with life. Dr. Edith Schulhofer carefully examined a number of college and high school students who had contracted mononucleosis.[17]

> It would appear that mononucleosis is frequently being used by students as a last resort to legitimatize a momentary breakdown of the ego. It is a trigger for dropouts, an excuse for failing to repeat a year, a last straw for requesting medical excuses for postponement of examinations, dropping classes, or changing curricula in the middle of the academic year.

It is interesting to note that all these students were found to be momentarily depressed at the time when they became ill. Several of the students examined even admitted to being depression-prone.

[17] Edith Schulhofer, "Mononucleosis during School Years Called Psychophysiologic Syndrome," *Medical Tribune*, vol. 7, no. 105, Aug. 31, 1966.

Control subjects examined at the same time were found to be less in a state of conflict, less depression-prone, and more optimistic regarding success in school. It would appear, therefore, that when individuals have some degree of faith in themselves and recognize that they are able to cope with the circumstances of their environment, they are able to use more constructive means of responding to the challenges of life. When they cannot do this, they may resort to the use of disease to remove themselves from the difficult situation.

The relationship between health and disease, then, has to do with the way in which an individual chooses, either consciously or unconsciously, to deal with the circumstances of his life. As he is forced to choose alternatives for dealing with life, he may resort to progressively less appropriate means of solving life's problems. He may even turn the hostility generated by his failure to cope toward himself and produce destructive symptoms in his own physiology.

Health and disease are not opposites but rather are points on a scale of quality. In circumstances, for example, where realistic environmental factors exist about which the individual can do nothing but with which he must deal, often the best thing he can do is to develop a minor illness which serves to remove him from these trying events. He then has an excuse for going to bed. He rests. He is catered to. His self-esteem returns. Time has enabled him to see things in better perspective, and he is able once again to reenter the mainstream of life. If he has chosen a minor illness to accomplish this, he can be credited with making a more effective choice than if he resorted to a more crippling disorder like hypertension, cancer, or some other disastrous condition. It goes without saying that the choices to which we refer are made at the subconscious level of being.

SUGGESTED READINGS FOR PART 1

Allport, Gordon: *Becoming,* Yale, New Haven, Conn., 1955.
Barzun, Jacques: *Science: The Glorious Entertainment,* Harper & Row, New York, 1964.
Berg, Jan: *The Changing Nature of Man,* Scribner, New York, 1961.
Bettelheim, Bruno: *Truants from Life,* Free Press, New York, 1955.
———: *The Empty Fortress,* Free Press, New York, 1967.
Bonner, Hubert: *On Being Mindful of Man,* Houghton Mifflin, Boston, 1965.

Boulding, Kenneth E.: *The Image: Knowledge in Life and Society*, University of Michigan Press, Ann Arbor, 1961.
Cantril, Hadley: *The Why of Man's Experience*, Macmillan, New York, 1950.
Combs, Arthur W. (Chairman A.S.C.D. Year Book Committee): *Perceiving, Behaving, Becoming*, National Education Association, Washington, D.C., 1962.
Coudert, Jo: *Advice from a Failure*, Dell, New York, 1965.
Coulson, William R., and Carl R. Rogers (eds.): *Man and the Science of Man*, Merrill, Columbus, Ohio, 1965.
Dubos, René: *The Mirage of Health*, Harper, New York, 1959.
―――: *The Torch of Life*, Simon & Schuster, New York, 1962.
―――: *So Human an Animal*, Scribner, New York, 1970.
Frankl, Victor E.: *Man's Search for Meaning*, Washington Square Press, New York, 1963.
Friedenberg, Edgar: *The Vanishing Adolescent*, Dell, New York, 1962.
Fromm, Erich: *The Art of Loving*, Harper & Row, New York, 1965.
Goffman, Erving: *The Presentation of Self in Everyday Life*, Doubleday, New York, 1959.
Hutschnecker, Arnold A.: *The Will to Live*, Prentice-Hall, Englewood Cliffs, N.J., 1958.
Johns, Edward B., Wilfred C. Sutton, and Lloyd E. Webster: *Health for Effective Living*, 4th ed., McGraw-Hill, New York, 1966.
Johnson, Wendell: *People in Quandaries*, Harper, New York, 1946.
Jones, Herbert, et al.: *Science and the Theory of Health*, Wm. C. Brown, New York, 1967.
Jourard, Sidney: *The Transparent Self*, Van Nostrand, Princeton, N.J., 1962.
Kaplan, Abraham: *Conduct of Inquiry*, Chandler, San Francisco, 1964.
Knutson, Andie L.: *The Individual, Society, and Health Behavior*, Russell Sage, New York, 1965.
Laing, R. D.: *The Politics of Experience*, Penguin, Baltimore, 1967.
Maslow, Abraham H.: *Toward a Psychology of Being*, Van Nostrand, Princeton, N.J., 1962.
Matson, Floyd W. (ed.): *Being, Becoming, and Behavior*, Braziller, New York, 1967.
Medawar, Peter Brian: *The Future of Man*, Basic Books, New York, 1959.
Montagu, Ashley: *The Biological Nature of Man*, Grove Press, New York, 1956.
―――: *Culture and the Evolution of Man*, Oxford, New York, 1962.
Northrop, F. S. C.: *Man, Nature and God*, Simon & Schuster, New York, 1962.
Progoff, Ira: *Depth Psychology and Modern Man*, Julian Press, New York, 1959.
Rogers, Carl: *On Becoming a Person*, Houghton Mifflin, Boston, 1961.
Saul, Edward T.: *The Silent Language*, Fawcett, Greenwich, Conn., 1954.

Sartre, Jean-Paul: *Being and Nothingness*, Citadel, New York, 1965.
Selye, Hans: *The Stress of Life*, McGraw-Hill, New York, 1956.
Sherrington, Sir Charles: *Man and His Nature*, Mentor, New York, 1964.
Simeons, A. T. W.: *Man's Presumptuous Brain*, Dutton, New York, 1961.
Sinacore, John: *Health: A Quality of Life*, Macmillan, New York, 1968.
Sinnott, Edmond: *Matter, Mind and Man: Biology of Human Nature*, Atheneum, New York, 1962.
——: *The Biology of the Spirit*, Viking, New York, 1955.
Whitman, Ardis: *A New Image of Man*, Appleton-Century-Crofts, New York, 1955.
White, Lynn R. (ed.): *Frontiers of Knowledge in the Study of Man*, Harper, New York, 1956.
Williams, Jesse F., and A. Kitzinger: *Health for the College Student*, 2d ed., Harper & Row, New York, 1967.
Wolff, Harold G.: "What Hope Can Do for Man," *The Saturday Review*, Jan. 5, 1957, pp. 42–45.
Young, Paul T.: *Motivation and Emotion*, Wiley, New York, 1961.

2.
THE DYNAMICS OF HEALTHFUL ADAPTATION

9.

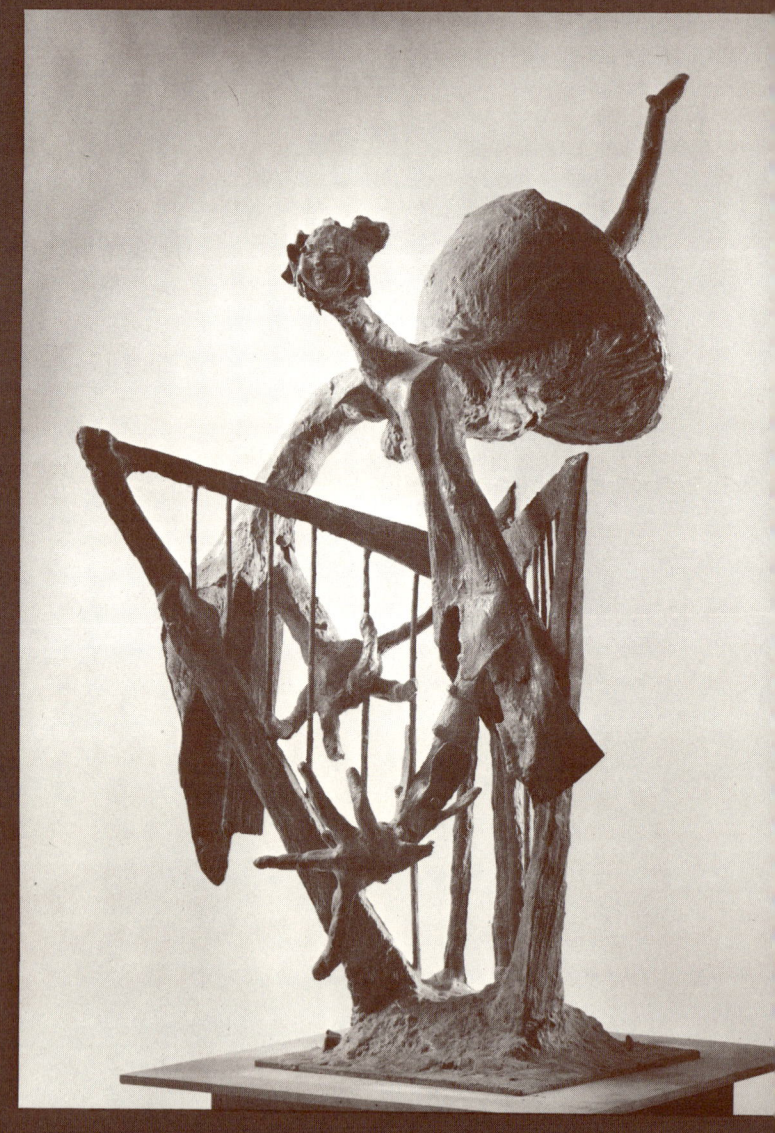

CREATIVE ADAPTATION

The Meaning of *Creative*

When we hear the word *creative*, our immediate association is with the arts. But the human potential for creativity goes far beyond this.

To be creative is to utilize all the ingredients of an experiential situation so that the response one makes is unique and developmental. Briefly, the components of any experiential situation are the circumstances of the moment, the constitutional makeup of the individual, the extent to which his potential has been developed by past experience, the hopes and expectations he has for himself in the situation, and his capacity to capitalize on each of the foregoing.

All people have the capacity to be creative. When our creative skills are developed, we are able to see alternatives in dealing with demanding situations. The more we see, the more likely we will be able to find an effective response. To take an extreme example of someone who can see only one solution to his problems, a person considering suicide is bound to that decision so long as he can see no other. Only when he recognizes that other choices are available is he able to move in another direction. The skills of creative thinking are perhaps the most useful we can find in achieving the fullness of our potential. They are vital in improving the quality of our response to life, and therefore they are vital to health.

There are strong forces at work in our culture which tend to make us fearful of being different, including forces which tend to breed dishonesty in viewing ourselves. A group of young men in a college health class were asked to arrange themselves in order according to the degree of manliness they saw in themselves. Those who saw themselves as quite manly were to place themselves at the head of the column. Those who saw themselves as less manly were to seek the lower end of the line.

Most readers can guess what happened. There was a mass movement toward the center of the line. Rather, there was no

Bernard Reder, "Harp Player, II," 1960. Bronze. Collection, The Whitney Museum of American Art, New York. Charles Uht, photography.

line at all but a huddle of self-conscious and embarrassed young men. After discussing the reactions to the request, it became apparent that feelings of modesty, anxiety, and fear of being disliked prevented them from placing themselves where they thought they should belong. It was further apparent that many of them either had never thought about themselves in this way or had deceived themselves to the extent that they could not recognize what existed in reality.

These men had been subject to the usual experiences and value judgments of our culture. Many of them would go through life without any realistic idea of what they were simply because they had been so strongly imbued with the idea that homogeneity was to be valued and difference was to be shunned.

Whites in recent years have learned about the tragic influence their stereotyped values about blacks have had upon black persons. Ossie Davis[1] writes of the impact Malcolm X had upon blacks and the courage he engendered in them to resist the conditioning of the majority culture of which they were a part in the United States.

> He also knew that every Negro who did not challenge on the spot every instance of racism, overt or covert, committed against him and his people, who chose instead to swallow his spit and go on smiling, was an Uncle Tom and a traitor, without balls or guts, or any other commonly accepted aspects of manhood. . . .
> He would make you angry as hell, but he would also make you proud. It was impossible to remain defensive and apologetic about being a Negro in his presence. He wouldn't let you. And you always left his presence with the sneaky suspicion that maybe, after all, you *were* a man.

Much of the psychology of the past has been directed toward making it possible for people to adjust. Too often, adjustment has meant that one was to avoid the pain of being an individual. To do so, he had to avoid the development of the very characteristics which could bring satisfaction in the achievement of full and unique humanness.

Fitting in, or adjusting, cannot be accepted as an answer to the problems of life without asking first, "Fitting into *what*?" "At what expense?" Should the black members of our society fit themselves in with the prejudiced standards that still exist? Should a child accept the overprotective mother or the dominant, tyrannical father? In some circumstances isn't it better to fight *against* adjustment?

It seems, then, that a bridge must be built between finding one's unique potential and making the adjustments necessary to

---

[1] Ossie Davis, "On Malcolm X," in *The Autobiography of Malcolm X*, Grove Press, New York, 1966, p. 458.

live a satisfying life. These two seemingly opposing forces must be brought into harmonious cooperation by applying the talents of creativity and ingenuity. Adjustment cannot be made at the expense of uniqueness. When man does not address himself to the task of discovering his potential, he not only denies himself the rewards of the rich life but even does things which will eventually lead to disease and dysfunction. At the same time, man must integrate himself into his environment with some degree of adaptation and flexibility. Both our need to fit in and our need to be ourselves must be recognized; the fulfillment of both needs contributes to self-actualization and health. It is man's ability to use his *creative* capacity that will chiefly determine the success or failure of this effort.

Creative adaptation enables us to know what is demanded of us. It creates conditions within us which render us fit to respond in the most appropriate manner to the circumstances of our lives. It is more specifically concerned with the development of the human potentials for living abundantly, loving fully, appreciating deeply, and creating the conditions in which both self and others move toward self-actualization.

Living versus Existing

To adapt creatively is the primary challenge of human life. When people are able to meet it, they discover the difference between existing and living. To exist is merely to maintain homeostasis and to take care of the fundamental biologic processes. To live is to explore the heights and depths of our humanness.

When we view the contemporary scene, we see much evidence that millions of our countrymen are in the category of existing. The effort to blot out the pain of existence is all around us. Drugs, soporifics, alcohol, pills, and nostrums are commonplaces in our materialistic culture. That these things do not work is evidenced in the high incidence of hypertensive heart disease, accidents, suicide, homicide, mental illness, alcoholism, drug addiction, and the vast quantity of functional disorders suffered by the American populace.

Creative adaptation is a concept foreign to the great majority of our people. While many have found the knack of doing it, few recognize that there are skills involved or that we have control over our ability to adapt creatively.

Education has been derelict in this respect. In health education we have allowed ourselves to become disease-oriented. The emphasis upon memorizing has forced us to spend less time thinking in evaluative terms about any of the basic things we must do to live abundantly.

To change this is difficult. Schools are not geared for the kind of work that is necessary. Teachers have not been prepared in their professional orientation to identify the essential areas of life that should be explored with pupils in order to develop the skills of creative adaptation.

As we have seen, stress is a precipitating factor in every adaptive effort. No demand would be made upon the organism without it, no push given toward finding a different way of living. Problems arise when we are unwilling to search out different ways of adapting. When we rely upon old patterns of adaptive response, nothing new develops. When we use only those elements of our being which are physiologic in nature, we often place too much wear and tear upon this adaptive machinery. Other means of adapting must be found.

The Creative Person

A sign of creative adaptation is a general feeling of well-being. However, this can be deceptive. Presumably the mentally ill person who has structured a world of unreality for himself may feel quite at home in it. We must look for more specific phenomena of creative adaptation.

In the first place, the person who adapts creatively feels integrated. He is able to restore homeostasis with a minimum of energy expenditure. He does not condemn himself for having to do what is necessary to accomplish the tasks of his life. His physiology functions in harmony with his attitudes. If he is angry, there is good reason for his anger, and his body systems act consistently with his anger. If he is at peace with himself, his body reactions reflect this sense of peace.

In the second place, the creatively adapting person relates to other persons effectively. He gets and receives satisfaction from these relationships. He is able to communicate what he is feeling to others and to sense what they expect of him. He can ascertain whether these expectations are realistic and whether or not he can meet them. If he cannot, it does not throw him.

His relationship to the physical environment is good. Long stretches of bad weather are not disturbing. Sleep comes easily. Heat does not bother him excessively.

The creatively adapting person is in a continuous act of discovery. He daily discovers things about himself and the world he lives in. His discoveries are integrated into what he already knows. He is able to adjust readily to any new insights which develop.

From this sense of discovery the creatively adapting person finds a sense of direction. As time goes on, he learns where he is going. When he is faced with a situation with which he is unfamiliar, he is able to seize upon those elements in the situation which will help him learn what he must do. In the process he integrates this insight into the general direction of his life. Or, when necesary, he can modify his life direction according to what he learns each day.

The creatively adapting person is himself. He knows what he is and who he is. He is not fearful of projecting that self. He does not attempt to change what he is to others, but is consistent in the projection of himself. At peaks of creative adaptation he is most himself. He allows the inner self to show and utilizes the resources which reside within this inner self.

Because he uses himself effectively, he has a sense of accomplishment in life. He feels strong, and others see his strength. He is strong enough to admit when he does not know the answers to the problems of his life. His strength allows him to seek help from others when necessary, for he is not bound by the need to be all-powerful. He sees himself in perspective.

The Peak Experience

Creative adaptation is not a condition of consistent peak levels of performance. We have seen in earlier chapters that there are varying degrees of effectiveness in adaptation. At the lower levels of creative adaptation the person is able to do the "right" (appropriate, constructive) thing at the right time. From this level of performance the creative person functions upward on the scale of effectiveness until at times he reaches heights which are not easily described. Only when he has had a "peak experience,"[2] an experience in which he is at the peak of his powers, can he understand what this is like.

At peak levels of performance one's experience has a mystical quality—it is not that he *does* the right thing: he *is* the right thing. He discovers that he is related to all there is and feels himself to be closely in touch with mysteries he has heretofore understood only in the abstract. Our biblical literature is filled with references to such experiences. When Moses had the experience of the burning bush, he saw his life in different terms. After years of wondering about the meaning of his life, in that one instant he knew the specific work he must do.

We are all subject to the peak experience, but many of us, because of our materialistic orientation, have little awareness of our real selves and are unable to attend to the inner voice, even when it speaks to us clearly. We believe it to be a figment of our imagination. Because we do not follow the directions set in the

[2] Abraham H. Maslow, *Toward a Psychology of Being,* Van Nostrand, Princeton, N.J., 1962.

peak experience, we rarely reap the rewards of our inherent potential.

When we are able to function at peak levels, we are at the highest points of health of which we are capable. But we must not make the mistake of assuming that functioning at peak levels means to be at the peak of our productivity. Creativity and the peak experience are not necessarily associated with productivity in the materialistic sense. It is not only the *producing* artist who is creative. When health and creativity are related, we are in a condition in which we utilize resources for living that we have not known before. We are fully related to our environment. If that environment is comprised mainly of people, then we are in complete rapport with them. If our environment is one of a natural setting, we are a part of that setting, and we *know it* as we have never before. This is creative adaptation. This is the state of being in which we can say we *are* the right thing.

Is a Psychedelic Trip a Peak Experience?

Adequate research information is still lacking on the significance of one's state of being when under the influence of psychedelic drugs. Dr. Sidney Cohen, chief of psychosomatic medicine at Wadsworth Hospital in Los Angeles, has this to say about LSD:[3]

> Since the psychedelics are taken by some to provide insightful, mystical states, we must ask: (1) whether the insights are valid, and (2) whether the chemical mystical state is the same as the mystical state that comes naturally or is induced by arduous training. The validity of what is seen under a drug like LSD varies greatly. Some flashes of inspired awareness are obviously delusional, and acting upon them can be devastating. Information that comes to the LSD user seems more real than ordinary reality. This does not mean that it is. It may simply mean that he is unable to discriminate and to sort out the exceedingly convincing notions that come to him. He is in a completely credulous, vulnerable state, without the ability to critically examine his thoughts. Some of the ideas may have merit; they should be carefully scrutinized in the days that follow an LSD experience. The world of psychedelia exists in our fantasy; its truthfulness has approximately the same validity as our dreams. Much of it is chaff, but the wheat kernels should be examined closely, for it emanates from our own unconscious and may have revealing things to tell us.

Some mature users of LSD have found that the drug has been helpful in producing insights that enabled them to clear up conflicts or confusion. However, it was not the drug alone which pro-

---

[3] Sidney Cohen, *The Drug Dilemma*, McGraw-Hill, New York, 1969, p. 23.

duced the liberation from their hang-ups but the careful evaluation of what they experienced while on the trip.

Other persons who have used the drug believe that little valuable insight is gained in the long run with the use of LSD and that the same growth can take place in the absence of the drug. They go on to point out that the risks of drug use are not worth the few moments of insight that come from the experience. Apparently for some it works; for others, there is little value to be found.

In the peak experience a clarification of reality markedly influences an individual's future. He knows he has had an unusual experience, and he knows that it was not by a foreign stimulus. One long-range result is that his confidence in himself, his respect for himself and his powers, are increased. In the psychedelic experience one knows that the experience has been artificially induced, and he is likely to assume he is not capable of the experience without some outside agent.

Research still has much to tell us about the influence of psychedelic drugs. It may be that in time drugs may be developed which can duplicate both the immediate and the long-range influences of the peak experience. It is not beyond the realm of possibility that drugs will someday be used to facilitate the developmental processes of life.

Predisposing Factors

There are some preconditions for creative adaptation. One is *naïve expectancy*. This stems partly from the faith that grows out of past experience and partly from the belief that all things are possible in the realm of human experience. One assumes that the unusual is likely to happen. He views life with a childlike wonder.

A second precondition is *readiness*. One does not view life with fear and suspicion. As an apparently difficult situation approaches, he moves toward it, knowing that somehow he will be able to come through it without undue damage. While he may have a plan, his readiness enables him to abandon that plan for what may appear to be a better way on the spur of the moment.

Spontaneity is always with the creatively adapting person. Whereas his life appears to be unstructured, it is quite evident that his personality is thoroughly integrated.

These three qualities, expectancy, readiness, and spontaneity, enable us to learn to *let life live us*. What does this mean? It is useful to make a distinction between fighting the circumstances of life and cooperating with these forces. When we fight life, we attempt to bend people and things to our will. Some of us learn to be successful in this endeavor, but the cost in terms of well-being is exhorbitant. At the same time, the expression *let life live us* does not mean that we blindly stand in the path of oncoming problems that can be avoided or sidestepped. Certain difficulties are avoidable, but when they are not, they are faced squarely and handled creatively.

When we let life live us, we are resilient. We do not expend energy in forcing things which *cannot be forced*. The person who determines that his role in life is to be continually in control believes that if he tries hard enough, he can accomplish anything. He may appear to have an admirable philosophy, but it is one that creates a driving personality which must be strong enough to endure great quantities of stress. Most of us are not this strong.

One example is the typical hypertensive heart patient, a hard-driving determined person who yields to nothing. He is apt to be reasonably successful in his work, but he is not successful in his own eyes, because he feels that he must always work harder to achieve success. He has not learned to let life live him. He has to pass up many of the experiences of life which lead to fulfillment. He has not learned to adapt creatively to the events of his life.

Such persons have superimposed upon themselves a role, or life style, which is narrowly defined. In every situation of life they attempt to live out the specifics of that life style. They are driven to play their role to its bitter end regardless of the consequences.

The following two case studies illustrate opposite extremes of life style. The first shows the role-bound person whose adaptation is limited. In the second we see an individual who adapts creatively to the events of her life.

> Wanda had come to a small Midwestern teacher's college from a farm town in the same state. She had been valedictorian of her high school graduating class and had planned a teaching career from the time she was in junior high school. Her high school guidance counselor recognized that Wanda possessed other talents, and had advised Wanda and her parents of this fact. But her parents had their hearts set on a teaching career for their daughter and, since Wanda seemed to agree, could see no reason to consider anything else.
>
> Wanda had been a "model child." Her life had been hemmed in and shored up by the maxims of her thrifty, hardworking parents. They had achieved success in dairy farming and firmly believed that hard work, honesty, and cleanliness were the cornerstones of the good life, and church and family togetherness were of equal importance. Wanda had incorporated many of these values and diligently practiced them in her own life.
>
> The result was that whereas she achieved academic excel-

lence in high school, she had few other interests besides helping her mother at home. She cooked, sewed, and kept house with the skill of a mature housewife. She had had some dates, but most of her social activities centered around her church youth group and the 4-H club to which she belonged. Her parents believed that there was plenty of time for boys "when she grew up." Just when this would be was questionable; for Wanda it remained in the vague future. She thought she knew what she was looking for in a man and was content to wait until he came along.

Wanda had rigid expectations for herself and spent great quantities of energy in living up to them. She also had high expectations for her friends. Her expectations for the boys she dated were so high that few could meet them. When she found herself suddenly transplanted to college, the standard patterns of behavior did not work. In the new context of her life she began to wonder about what she was, where she was going, why she was different from others, and why they didn't seem to like her very well. She could not fit into social groups as she had at home. Her dates were usually one-time affairs; she was rarely asked out a second time. At the end of her freshman year she transferred to another college.

At the first college, Wanda had neither the expectancy nor the readiness to adapt creatively to her new environment. She had rigid expectations for herself and for others, could not understand why these expectations were not fulfilled, and the stress became increasingly heavy for her. At the college to which she transferred, it was hoped that she would find herself less bound by the role expectations she superimposed on herself and other people.

Nancy had come to the university from a suburban home. She had a wide-eyed naïveté that was at the same time charming and disarming. One was disarmed because it didn't seem possible that intelligence of a profound and practical nature could exist in a creature so free and light as Nancy. Her grades were adequate but not outstanding. Her focus in life seemed to be on the people who flocked around her, and they vied for her affection and friendship.

Within one semester she had become one of the most popular young people on the campus. She was elected as a class representive to the student government, she belonged to the art club and the drama club, and she was a member of the women's intercollegiate archery team.

In the spring of her freshman year she began dating Jack,

an upperclassman of some sophistication. He was something of a wheel at the college. He found himself continually amazed at Nancy's ability to accept everything about him without criticism and without disappointment. He found it difficult to understand how it was possible for her to accept whatever came along, since he himself was not like that. Even on the rare occasions when she was emotionally low, she was able to bounce right back without losing stride.

Jack's idea of success was to drive hard for what he wanted and to let nothing stand in his way. While he had a reasonable regard for ethical considerations of life, he pulled no punches when he was involved in a dispute. He worked hard and expected others who associated with him to do the same. After several months of trying to change Nancy, he realized that hers was the better way in the long run. She seemed to get much more satisfaction from life. As time went on, she was able to impart some of her philosophy to him. While he could never become like her, Jack felt that he was a better man for having known Nancy.

Jack admired her ability to take pleasure out of whatever situation life offered. One day, when his car broke down on the way to an important engagement, Nancy was able to get him over his anger at the situation and turn it into a kind of picnic. They spent a wonderful afternoon enjoying the countryside while the car was being repaired.

Nancy's quality was that of being able to adapt creatively to whatever came up. Nothing seemed to throw her. She was resilient, boundless in energy, and filled with a readiness to adjust to any situation that came along.

The difference between Nancy and Wanda is dramatic. Wanda was bound to a role expectation which limited her function. Nancy anticipated anything and was ready to capitalize on whatever transpired. Her plans could be shifted spontaneously. Her energy was not wasted in frustration but could be expended upon enjoyment. Stress was kept at a minimum, and exuberance was high. Nancy lived fully and joyously. Wanda existed.

Goals and Adaptation

Our goals have a great deal to do with our ability to adapt. Many of us have set goals which are totally unrealistic. When we have expectations which are not apt to be realized, we create stress conditions which have much to do with the responses we make to the various situations of life. One aspect of wisdom is gradually to sort out those goals we have set for ourselves and critically examine them. When we see that they are not realistic, it behooves us to question why we have set them. If we ask ourselves what motivations have driven us to set these goals, we can sometimes see what modification is necessary. The process is one of searching and questioning more than of overt change. When we find the answers, the changes will come about of themselves. We then become more acceptable to ourselves. We are less bound by role expectations and more ready to move through life in a spontaneous manner. We are ready to operate with freedom and to initiate new responses and develop new resources within ourselves.

We then broaden the range of responses we make, increase the possibilities for being ourselves, and activate talents which would otherwise lie dormant within us. We lessen the internal stress that comes from adapting in stereotyped ways and from inhibiting what we are. We allow the inner us to come forth, and we move toward the satisfaction of self-actualization. We become the persons we want to become and cast off the inadequate selves that we have been in the past. The quality of our response is upgraded. Our health improves, and the prognosis for the future becomes progressively better.

The foregoing may create the impression that the answer to all of life's problems is to readjust one's goals, to take a regular assessment and then, as in a new year's resolution, vow to become a better person. On the contrary, what we must learn to live with is our own freedom. We must create this freedom for ourselves. It cannot be given to us by another. Parents cannot bestow it on children. Other authorities in one's life cannot bestow it on us. We must fashion our own freedom by relinquishing those goals which limit the unfolding of our inner nature.

Self-criticism and Change

Creative adaptation is less likely to take place when persons are not self-accepting. In proper proportion the tendency to be self-critical has value. When self-criticism becomes so intense that it renders the individual incapable of action, it hinders the use of creative capabilities.

For those who have been so conditioned to expect perfection in themselves that it is impossible for them ever to live up to their expectations, self-criticism and self-condemnation become a way of life. There is little experience which leads such a person toward valuing himself, for he can never do that which is pleasing to him. Since success is never possible in his own eyes, he develops little confidence in himself. He either gives up about himself or drives himself to compensate for the failures he experiences. The resilience of youth may enable a young person to withstand the strains of his drive, but when the resilience fades, the stress of the drive to succeed takes its toll in the breakdown of one or another system of the body. Unless the person becomes able to see his life in perspective, he continues to hold unsatisfying views about himself and to find it necessary to compensate for his sense of failure.

An essential element of creative adaptation is critical self-acceptance. In a culture which idolizes work, productivity, and material success, self-acceptance is sometimes thought of as self-complacence. Self-acceptance is a condition in which the individual recognizes himself for what he is; he knows his strengths and his weaknesses and accepts them for what they are. The self-complacent person may have an exaggerated idea of his own effectiveness; he demands too little of himself, settling too easily for the status quo at the expense of a truly satisfying life. The concept of self-acceptance is explored in detail in Chapter 15.

The Will to Change

We are often inclined to say "I can't do such and such," when to say "At this time in my life I don't seem to be able to . . ." would be a more realistic, appropriate statement, one which allows for the possibility of growth.

Many persons who say "I can't" are really saying "I won't." Two young people of different religions who were contemplating marriage finally decided to break off the engagement. In the days which followed, they spent much time telling friends that they *couldn't* yield on certain points of principle. Actually, each was *refusing* to move. This distinction is often a difficult one to make for ourselves. We usually reject the idea that we are willfully responsible for our inability to do something. We much prefer to place the blame elsewhere. We are then freed of the responsibility of making changes which are difficult for us.

The person who adapts creatively accepts the responsibility and knows what his inability to change comes from. Usually within a short time he is able to effect the change that is necessary. In the process he not only has changed; he has grown, as well. A new dimension of his personality has been added. A new skill has evolved and is now a functional element of his being.

Guilt and Adaptation

It is always difficult to adapt effectively when we are suffering from neurotic guilt. When we exaggerate the importance of some supposed wrongdoing beyond the point of reason, an element of neurosis has crept in. This may be the result of strong conditioning to the idea that we must always be good. Sometimes it results when we have expectations for ourselves which are beyond our capabilities. At other times it is due to failure in our efforts to compensate for limitations in other areas of life.

The person who cannot accept himself has a large measure of guilt in his makeup. Because of this he is unable to see himself clearly. His view of himself is colored by his guilt. After an action, he feels as though he should not have acted as he did, or he may feel that what he has done he has done poorly. Over a period of time the effect of this self-condemnation is cumulative. He then has a distorted image of himself, and he cannot fully appreciate what he is.

When this form of guilt is carried to an extreme, there is usually a feeling of depression when nothing we do seems to matter, we feel extremely unworthy, and our picture of life generally is distorted. It is in extreme cases of depression that suicide sometimes enters the mind as a way out. In more usual cases it seems important to us to punish ourselves for our "wrongdoing." Sometimes the depression itself serves as the punishment. Sometimes the things we do to ourselves while in the depressed state are the punishment: missing a party, isolating ourselves from friends, or forgetting to keep an appointment that would have been rewarding.

We have seen in earlier chapters that severe physiologic symptoms of response may show themselves. The psychogenic illness may often be used as a form of punishment. The sense of despair which is a part of many advanced depressions may be a forerunner of disease.

It is important to note that not all guilt is neurotic. Guilt can be a legitimate emotion. There are times when we should feel it. All of us do things which are wrong, damaging, or self-negating, and we should feel guilty about them. When we have treated another person or ourselves badly and we know it, we have cause for real guilt. However, perspective is necessary, or the feeling of wrongdoing will be exaggerated beyond the bounds of reality.

Conclusion

We have seen that adaptation is essential for well-being. If our lives are to be satisfying, it is important for us to adapt with some degree of creativity. Unless we are able to adapt creatively, there is little that is really worth living for: we merely exist. For human beings, who inevitably have expectations for themselves, existence is not enough. For health, existence is not enough. Only when we are living with satisfaction can we say that we have adapted in an appropriate manner. Only when we have moved forward in the development of our inner potential can we say that our adaptive efforts have been worth the energy spent upon them.

10.

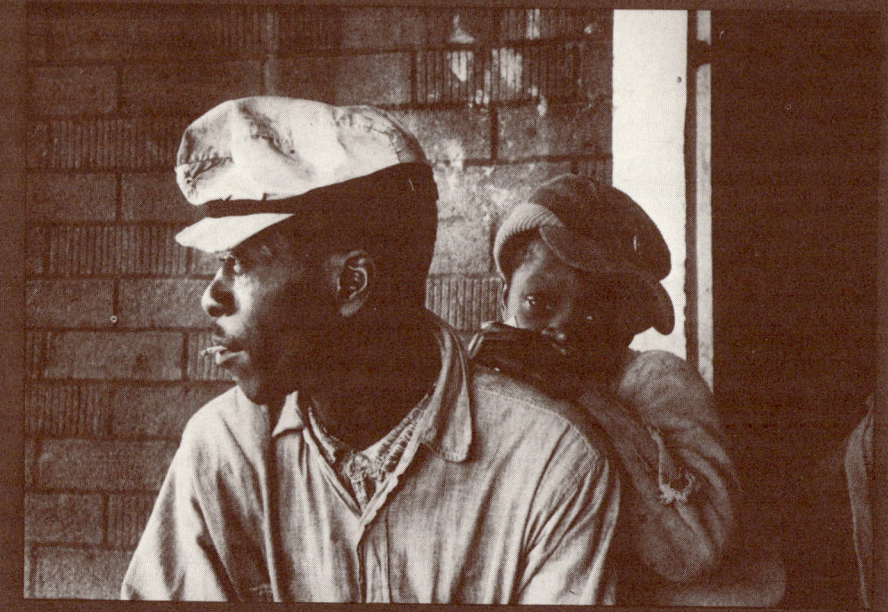

IN THE BEGINNING

This chapter is concerned with those things which contribute to the making of personality and the sense of self. The interaction of genetic heritage with one's environment in its totality constitutes experience. It is out of this interaction that the sense of self forms.

The sense of self in turn is the central factor in the process of giving meaning to the events of life. It is the core about which we make the judgments that influence our responses. In every situation we tend to evaluate the circumstances in terms of whether or not they enhance or threaten our sense of self. If we feel threatened, we make defensive responses. If we feel that the circumstances enhance our image of ourselves, another set of responses is initiated. As noted earlier, the quality of these responses shows the degree of health we possess.

Identity

When we use the word *identity*, we are referring to all those factors which collectively form our awareness of what we are, from the basic physiologic elements of our being to the values that grow out of experience. Some elements of our identity grow out of our body image.

Each of us has an awareness of what our bodies are. We are able to place our finger on any part of our body without looking. When we have an ache, we know at least approximately where it is located.

Our body image grows out of our experience with ourselves. It is the result of years of various forms of exploratory endeavor. An infant in his crib engages in these exploratory efforts. We can see the delight of the infant as his hands appear before his eyes. We share his delight as he is able to bring one hand toward the other and sense them. If we watch long enough, we learn that these explorations are thorough and continuous.

Constantine Manos, photography. Magnum Photos, Inc.

As we grow older, we become engaged in movement which further identifies for us what our physical dimensions are. We learn what we are capable of doing. A four-year-old girl in the process of play climbs about on a small complex of swings, seesaws, and ladders. As she attempts to do some things, she succeeds. In other endeavors, she fails. In the process she is developing an image of what she is and what she is capable of, a combined process of learning about herself and learning how to manipulate her environment. What she learns cumulatively comes to be known to her as part of her sense of self.

As children grow older, they have contact with a great variety of things and people constituting their environment. They learn to define themselves by watching their parents' reactions.

Sharply illustrating this, James Baldwin writes:[1]

> Long before the Negro child perceives this difference [that the world is white and he is black] and even longer before he understands it, he has begun to react to it, he has begun to be controlled by it. Every effort made by the child's elders to prepare him for a fate from which they cannot protect him causes him secretly in terror, to begin to await, without knowing that he is doing so, his mysterious and inexorable punishment. He must be "good" not only in order to please his parents and not only to avoid being punished by them; behind their authority stands another, nameless and impersonal, infinitely harder to please and bottomlessly cruel. And this filters into the child's consciousness through his parents' tone of voice as he is being exhorted, punished or loved; in the sudden, uncontrollable note of fear heard in his mother's or father's voice when he has strayed beyond some particular boundary. He does not know what the boundary is, and he can get no explanation of it, which is frightening enough, but the fear he hears in the voices of his elders is more frightening still.
>
> The fear that I heard in my father's voice, for example, when he realized that I really *believed* I could do anything a white boy could do, and have every intention of proving it, was not at all like the fear I heard when one of us was ill or had fallen down the stairs or strayed too far from the house. It was another fear, a fear that the child, in challenging the white world's assumptions, was putting himself in the path of destruction.

Among friends, children learn to expand or limit their ways of approaching them and relating to them. From friends as well as from parents and others, they learn to make value judgments about their own worth. They learn that they are "good" in some areas but not so good in others.

[1] James Baldwin, *The Fire Next Time*, Dial, New York, 1963, p. 40.

As parents begin to have expectations for their children they attempt to live up to those expectations. If they succeed, they are rewarded by their approval. If they fail, they may be punished by their rejection. Gradually, children develop expectations for themselves. They believe that they should be capable of accomplishing certain things. If these expectations are realistic, they are likely to achieve success and a consequent sense of confidence in their ability to accomplish what they want. If the expectations are unrealistic, they will experience failure with a consequent feeling of helplessness and hopelessness about themselves and their life.

All these experiences become a part of what we are. The values resulting from them are held at either the conscious or the unconscious level or both. In any case, they influence the way we respond to life's challenges.

These factors have much to do with racism, a major problem that Americans are just beginning to face. Abby Stitt, writing from the point of view of a behavioral scientist, says,[2]

> Where a child lives, how the grown-ups around him treat racial matters, his opportunities to know people from different backgrounds, his own sense of self, and even the meaning that certain colors have are all factors which can and do affect his awareness of race. Researchers working both here and abroad have explored the ways these influence a preschooler.

Many of the findings indicate that lasting values which become a part of the identity of a person are established in the early years.

Identity, then, refers to all those elements which make up the sense of self. It includes our experience with ourselves and with others. It includes the feelings and attitudes that other people have expressed toward us about ourselves and our actions. It is made up of the ideal self which we hope to bring into being. It grows out of the continuous process of evaluating ourselves in the acts of living.

Sexuality

Sexuality is a part of our larger sense of self. It permeates our identity. It is that aspect of our identity which is related to our sex, but it is more than just our sex. In any culture there are roles which are delimited for the members of each sex. Subtle directives are given to us by everyone about how we should behave as members of a particular sex.

[2] Abby Stitt, "Color-coding: Race Awareness in the Very Young," *Mothers' Manual,* May–June, 1970, p. 26.

Our sexuality includes the biologic elements of our being which produce the primary and secondary sex characteristics. It includes our sex drive and the way we learn to deal with it. The degree of success or frustration we experience in satisfying our sex drive becomes a part of our sexuality. As we are subject to the progressive influence of cultural conditioning relative to sex, we become what we are as men or women and draw conclusions about whether or not we are fulfilling our expectations for ourselves in the sex role we play.

No aspect of our identity is free of the cultural conditioning relative to sex. Everything we do we experience as a male or as a female. All our hopes for ourselves grow out of the context of our sexuality. For example, if we are failures in academic pursuits, we are not just students who have failed in school. We are also men or women who have failed in school. Since society has given a different value to success in school for men and for women, we experience this differently.

Identifying Male-Female Roles

The process of identifying our male or female role begins early in life. It is associated with the feelings our parents have about our own sex. The fact that joy is felt and exhibited more often when a boy is born is a case in point. Older children see these differences. They overhear such comments as "Better luck next time," if the new baby is a girl, or "A boy! How wonderful! I'll bet you are very proud." The residual effect of such comments becomes a factor in ascribing value to the sex with which one is endowed.

Our education, vocation, clothing, speech mannerisms, behavioral expressions, and manner of play, of walk, and of gesture are all conditioned by our sex role. The child who does not adhere closely to his prescribed role is subject to all sorts of critical and often cruel treatment by his peers and often by the adults in his life. He even builds some of these prejudices into his own value structure. As a result, he may think of himself in denigrating terms.

This is the plight of many persons today. People often have to prove their own feminity or masculinity to themselves as well as to others in our society, at the adult level as well as at the childhood level. This becomes a motivating factor in the life of every person in our culture. It becomes so much a part of the norm that it is hard to identify the influence of this factor in one's life.

It is manifest in the fact that the male child cannot readily and freely explore the range of his own emotions. He is limited in those emotions which he can express or even admit to himself. He learns early in life to repress the "less manly" feelings he has. (The implications of repressed emotions for disease have already been discussed, in Chapter 8.)

The need to demonstrate masculinity is so frequently a part of the male identity that one is led to speculate about its effect on the life expectancy of the men in our society as compared with that of women, which is seven years longer. It is a commonplace that women are more adaptable than men, that the feminine personality is far more resilient that the masculine one in our society. It is not unreasonable to suspect that this is a factor in bringing about the stress which, over a lifetime, may become devitalizing, thus causing men to be vulnerable to fatal disease far earlier than women.

The Women's Liberation movement has attempted to highlight some of the problems our society has posed for females. Although some of the points raised by the feminist movement are controversial, others are readily agreed upon by many people. For example, females soon learn that they run the risk of losing popularity with some men if they assert themselves. If they happen to be more intelligent than their male dates, they often feel compelled

Wide World Photos.

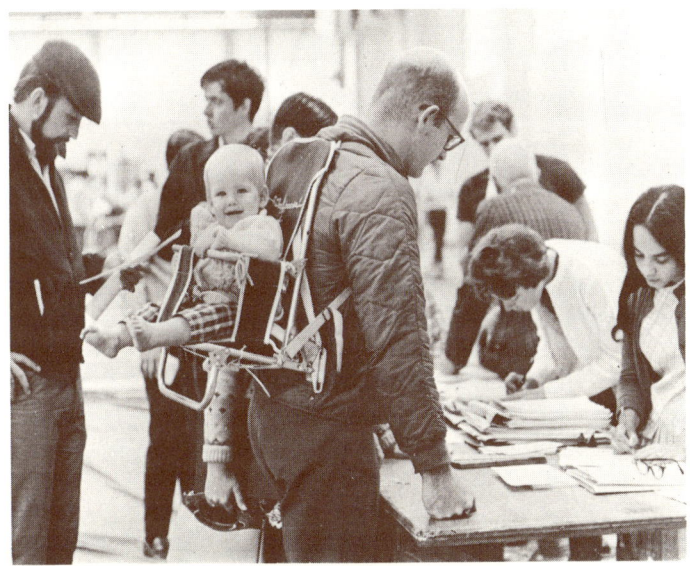

to play down this attribute for fear of offending the boyfriend. This hardly leads to self-actualization.

Another source of confusion lies in the fact that the mass media continually play up only particular aspects of the feminine face and body. The immature female often feels that unless she can conform to these standards, she is unfeminine, unappealing, and in danger of being unpopular. These standards have left the scars of anxiety and insecurity on the identities of many women.

In recent years the unmarried adult female has begun to escape being stigmatized because she is single, but many women still consider themselves failures because they are not married. This is an unhealthy position, since there are many valid reasons why a woman might not marry.

Parent-Child Relationships

Our earliest experiences with others are strongly influenced by what has happened with our parents. We determine what we are as a result of learning what our parents think of us. We come to know ourselves, in part, through the eyes of others.

We have seen that these early years strongly condition our attitude toward ourselves, toward others, and toward life. They also influence our attitude toward people who are the same sex as each of our parents. They influence our attitude toward others who stand for, or who are a part of, the same group as our parents. A female teacher in school initially represents the female authority figure in our homes—usually our mothers. We tend to ascribe to that person some of the same characteristics we have learned to ascribe ot our mothers. We may invest our teachers with the same emotional charge with which we invest our parents. Until we learn differently, this affects our relationship to these other adults. When parent-child conflicts cannot be resolved by the child at home, he may attempt to resolve them in his relationship to his teachers. If his conflicts are not successfully worked out, these hang-ups are carried forward into life, and he attempts to work out the problem in other authority-dependence relationships. The individual who is perpetually hostile to his employer is a good example of this.

Many of us carry a burden of feelings about ourselves which is primarily the result of experiences in our homes and may even hold attitudes toward ourselves which are destructive. Many of these attitudes are the product of our relationship with our parents. We may hold these destructive attitudes at the same time that we have constructive ones. These values often live side by side within us. At certain times they are activated. Depending upon the circumstances and the meaning we give to events, these attitudes have more or less influence upon our health.

It is important to recognize, however, that we are not damned by our past. If we have had unfortunate experiences in our childhood, they do not invariably cause permanent damage to our self-image. As we grow older, the influence of our homes becomes less important, and the influence of our peers and our experiences with them adds to the body of that which is built into our sense of self. Through the combination of these events many persons are strengthened.

Dominant and Idealized Personalities

The imitation of dominant and idealized personalities is essential to the process of becoming a person. Initially these personalities are one's parents. Other personalities from which children draw their identity may be a sports hero, an idolized teacher, or a friendly neighbor. Often someone who excels in an area of particular interest for the child, the idealized personality becomes a dominant factor in his life. He incorporates some feature of the idealized personality into his own value structure. It then becomes a factor in the child's evaluation of himself. His watchful self uses this value as a criterion for judging his effectiveness in the everyday acts of life.

Each of us can think back just a few years to the time when we spent large amounts of energy imitating a particular hero. We copied the behavioral mannerisms, we wore similar clothes, and we imitated facial expressions and language characteristics. This is the process of identifying. Does this mean that we will become like the individual imitated? Not necessarily. It does mean, however, that the things we do in imitating our hero will structure our experience and therefore have an influence upon the values which settle out of that experience. It does mean that these values then become built into our personality and for a time, at least, are potent factors in our lives.

Often our heroes are part of our daily lives. We have associated with these persons and have had to learn how to get along with them. We have attempted to learn what they think and how they respond to life. The total effect is to mark our lives in some considerable way. Often, the individuals we imitate are themselves unfinished persons. They may have status in the gang we belong to. They may be stronger than we and therefore compel us to imitate them in various ways. Since they themselves may be in the process of imitating other older persons, we then are in the process of imitating imitation persons—a normal process, to be sure. But if we understand, we can achieve some critical control over this process.

The "Cool" Person

On the social scene today a common image is that of the "cool" person. Who is cool? Usually he is the person who can remain emotionally detached, who never allows emotion to become a part of his life. He either carefully suppresses or naïvely represses his deeper feelings, and in effect he becomes alienated.

There are any number of idealized cool personalities in the public eye at present. Every television serial has such a hero. James Bond is the epitome of such an individual. He is an exploiter, he is tough, he is emotionally uninvolved, and he has casual, nonbinding relationships with women. The question arises —does this image have an appeal because there are so many of us who are hurting, as a result of the experiences of our lives, that we feel we would like to be like this? Or is this person a pacesetter himself who, by virtue of his being, is creating a coterie of followers who want to be like him and therefore become so? Probably both factors are at work in our society.

A more important question centers about what type of dominant idealized personalities we are incorporating into our own lives. To what extent are we doing it? To what extent is it preventing us from becoming autonomous, standing in the way of our own self-actualization? In answering these questions for ourselves we may be able to free ourselves from things we are doing which are unreasonably limiting to us, and we may thereby take a giant stride ahead in favorably influencing our health.

The Reward-Punishment System of Child Rearing

Each of us is subject to a remarkable amount of conditioning both in our homes and in the larger society. It is a system based upon the idea that values are built into people as a result of imposing a series of rewards and punishments. The basic assumption is that when we are rewarded, we will tend to incorporate a particular value into our own system, and that when we are punished, an antithetical value will be established within us. Generally speaking this is true, but it rarely works out in such a simple manner.

At the same time that we are learning what is "good" and what is "bad," we are also learning about ourselves. We tend to judge ourselves as good or bad according to the other factors which are operative within the situation wherein the conditioning takes place. For example, in one set of circumstances loaded with parental disapproval and large injections of emotion, the child learns not only that what he has done is bad but also that he himself is bad.

The phenomenon of learning has so frequently been associated with schools that we often overlook the fact that we are learning every moment of our lives. Even in sleep we are in the process of experiencing. For one thing, our dreams form a large part of this experience. From these experiences a residue of attitude and feeling settles out. This residue is the stuff of learning.

In the simple process of teaching a child to brush his teeth at appropriate occasions other things are learned as well. If the parent engages in a big scene whenever the child forgets to perform this rite, besides learning about tooth brushing, he may learn that his parents are unfair and dictatorial. He may learn that he is a forgetful scatterbrain. He may be compared unfavorably to another sibling and learn that this sibling is a threat to his own status in the family. Obviously, his sense of self is strongly influenced by these experiences.

Another aspect is that if parents continually expect things which are beyond the capability or even the inclinations of the child, he can never live up to these expectations. Through the reward-punishment system these very same expectations are adopted by the individual for himself. He then progressively sets goals for himself which are unrealistic and beyond the possibility of fulfillment. The cumulative experiences of failure to meet his own expectations for himself are devastating. He is left with the feeling that he is worthless. He may even give up about himself. We have already seen the implications of the giving-up syndrome for health.

The reward-punishment system runs throughout our society at all levels. Because it is a major factor in our early years, it remains with us and becomes the established way. It influences the way in which we see things. It marks the way we evaluate all experiences of life. Until we outgrow the ideas of good and bad which are built solidly into our identities, we are chained to these ideas.

Success and Failure

Along with our ideas about right and wrong we are subject to values about success and failure. Elsewhere in this volume we have called attention to the fact that many of us correlate "good" with "success" and "bad" with "failure." When we have been good, we have been rewarded, and we assume that we have succeeded. The problem is that often being good may run directly counter to being real. We know that if we express our real feelings of anger, we may be considered impolite or bad. The subsequent confusion creates problems in the process of self-actualization.

It has already been noted that self-actualization depends upon the individual's ability to perceive reality. Perception of reality becomes a factor in whether or not our responses are appropriate to our own best development. When they are not, we fail in self-actualization. We may even do that which is detrimental to our health.

What society, or some subculture within society, sets as good may have little to do with reality. Some principles commonly considered "good" in our society are always help others; don't feel sorry for yourself; avoid arguments; don't hurt others. None of these are suitable for all situations at all times. Take the last one, which is quite a popular concept of goodness. Hurting another could be the best solution in certain circumstances. What is more, being hurt is not necessarily a bad thing to have happen. It may be uncomfortable and unpleasant to experience, but there may be positive results. It is therefore the lot of many to devote themselves to achieving ideals of goodness which have nothing to do with the enhancement of themselves as people. We frequently find ourselves in the perplexing situation of wanting to be good and at the same time knowing that we must be real. The problem is not that conflict exists. Conflict is not inherently evil. The problem centers around the fact that many persons have been so conditioned to being good that they will find only *one* alternative open to them in resolving the conflict. If goodness depends altogether upon the number of people in society who ascribe to it, then those of us who choose to view things differently run counter to that society and must then take the consequences of being "bad" and, thus, failing.

Our concern here is not to restructure the values of society. We are concerned with evaluating the effect upon one's health of living in a society which makes it difficult, if not impossible, to do those things which are necessary for health to become a reality in one's life.

Let us add to the above confusing elements of our world the fact that success is often associated with the accumulation of material wealth. We do not here intend to decry materialism but, rather, to examine the influence of our efforts to obtain material wealth at the expense of values which are essential to human well-being. We grant that the Western penchant for materialism has done much to free man from many of the burdens of subsistence, but it has also become fatal for too many.

It would be difficult to try to ascertain the numbers of people who have fallen prey to the temptation to sacrifice human values for material ones. It is apparent that many, in the effort to acquire, have sacrificed not only others but themselves as well. This is possibly the supreme tragedy of life. When we are driven to succeed and when the standards of success can be achieved only at the sacrifice of one's health, then we have built into us the very stuff which destroys life—a thought that gives support to Freud's idea of a death wish existing within all men.

Here, then, is another of man's central problems: the fact that he is conditioned early in life to success, which is often associated with being good and with the attainment of material wealth at the expense of all else. When whole societies subscribe to this value, it becomes extremely difficult for any individual member of that society to violate it, regardless of what it means in terms of his health to follow it.

Sources of Anxiety

It is apparent that the processes of social indoctrination and personality formation work together to build in conflicting values about oneself and one's worth in the scheme of things. It is important to realize that these potential sources of anxiety are a part of our sense of self. Too often we are inclined to believe that some outside element is the sole cause of the development of anxiety. This is not so. From the very beginnings of our lives we are subject to conditioning which instills conflicting attitudes. We are taught, for example, that we should love our parents and that this love is shown through obedience. At the same time we are taught that we must think things out for ourselves. In each case we are "good" if we do what is expected. Obviously there are circumstances when thinking for ourselves runs contrary to being obedient. How is one to be good in such circumstances? It is impossible to do both without the skill which enables us to reason with our parents in working out the conflict in the situation.

Situations of this sort range throughout the whole realm of human experience. They are inherent in boy-girl relationships. They are a part of the competitive structure of materialism in the academic scene. They are woven into the very process of growing up and freeing oneself of values which may have been important in childhood but in the complexities of adulthood simply do not work.

It is not the purpose of this chapter to develop these ideas too deeply. We merely wish to point them out so that there is a recognition that these forces are at work in the process of identity formation. When we are able to identify what factors of our own sense of self are at work, we are one step toward working out the conflicts which develop. Furthermore, when we can understand what motivates us, we are freed to move forward into the unknowns of our own personal development. We are facilitated in the process of self-actualization. We stand a better chance not only of protecting but also of promoting our health.

Sources of Confidence

In the area of physiologic development there is a phenomenon known as the *demand principle,* the concept that organs and systems of the body grow according to the demand placed upon them. A muscle, for example, will grow in girth and in strength according to the amount of work it has to do. In a progressive system of exercise a muscle will increase in strength. When that activity is lessened, the muscle atrophies, or wastes away. The heart develops in the same way. If an individual runs several miles every day, his heart will develop in strength and efficiency to keep up with the task that is set for it. When that activity is lessened, the runner's heart will lose some of its size and return to the lower level of strength and efficiency demanded of it.

From all that can be determined, the same principle works in the development of human personality. The challenge of resolving reasonable conflicts develops skills which are designed to deal with the tasks at hand. But the challenges must be within the limits of the individual's capacity to deal with them. When they are too great or persistent and do not yield to the person's efforts to deal with them, he resorts to other methods of "taking the heat off."

When challenge is consistent with the ability of the individual to meet it, the management of it becomes a source of confidence. He progressively views his life as a matter which he can handle. He sees himself as a person with competence in the task of coping with life. He tends to view life optimistically. He does not have to resort to self-destruction to avoid the burdens of life. He is a healthy person.

11.

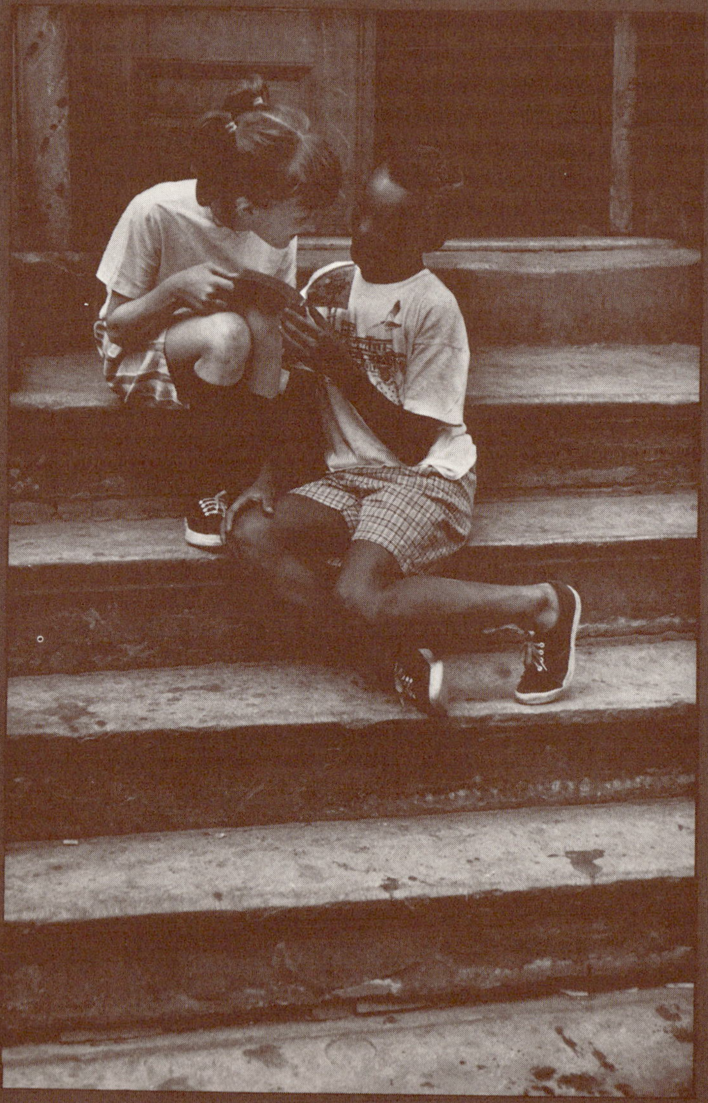

VALUE CONDITIONING

In the preceding chapters we have seen how identity develops; that man's purposefulness influences his response; how the process of purposeful response progresses toward a gradually unfolding being, a being continually in the process of becoming something that he was not before; and that, in this process of becoming, he does not automatically end up as a fully realized human being but may become something that is human to only a minor and insignificant degree or, on the other hand, may manifest many of the finest qualities we attribute to being human.

However, to establish a concept of the human organism in its fullness it is necessary to go beyond the phenomenology of observable traits. We must formulate some concept of how these traits and experiences affect us.

Man as a Value Structure

Man is a value structure. It is vital to recognize him as such if we are to understand health. We are not stating that man *has* a value structure. We are saying he *is* one.

In the functional sense, man's purposes are so inextricably intertwined with his responses that it is impossible to separate response from purpose. The athlete going into competition has as his purpose to vanquish his opponent. That he may not do so registers within him as a threat to his integrity. His body reacts in ways which ready him for the contest. Purpose and response are acting together. Without purpose the response is not the same. Function is always influenced by those purposes which are dominant in the situation. In the functional sense man's purposes and resposes are unified.

Purpose and value register within one in the same manner. In fact, it is possible to substitute the word *value* for the word *purpose* without changing the meaning of what we are discussing. In the case of the athlete, his purposes are made up of such values as

Bruce Davidson, photography. Magnum Photos, Inc.

"I am a man of skill," "I am a man of courage," "I am a man who wants to win." Together these values constitute his purposes in the athletic contest.

Substituting value for purpose in the principle stated above, in the functional sense man's *values* and his *responses* are unified. In this chapter we will attempt to discover what a value is, how it develops, and how it influences us in our living.

What Is a Value?

It is useful to think of a value as any residual belief, attitude, thought, or mind set which grows out of experience and which is carried forward into future experiences. It may be derived from any and all of the enormous range of experiential occurrences. It can be primarily physical or largely abstract.

Physical values may be the result of our becoming aware of our size, weight, and physical looks. They may also result from experiences with our bodies. We know, for example, about how far we can jump. We know what it feels like if we are touched in a particular area of our body. We know that we can throw a stone but not a feather.

Values related to the abstract are more involved. They may begin with some physical experience—the knowledge, for example, that we have a large nose. Our speculation about what this will mean in our lives produces values derived from abstractions. The concept of love is abstract, and yet we have many values about it. These values strongly influence our response when we are in a relationship which we consider to be a love relationship.

In value formation, the experiences of thought are neither more nor less important than the experiences of the body. In either case interaction between the person and his environment produces the experience.

Values are cumulative. They become part of the sense of self and influence future responses. They are held at any level of consciousness and need not be consciously recognized by us to be effective. Values either center about the self or are a projection of the way the self relates to the not-self. The idea that we are tall centers about our sense of self. The fact that a tree's bark is rough is not directly related to the self, but the roughness of the bark is a projection of how we see the bark.

In other words, values influence how the self sees the self and the perspective in which the self is seen in relation to all other things. Values dictate the function of the self and the way it projects itself into the events of life. They direct its relationship to others. They are all embracing and are a part of every aspect of life.

Our attitudes toward ourselves and others grow out of the cumulative set of values which constitute the self. Our view of life is also dependent upon this value structure, and our personality is the projection of it.

Levels of Consciousness

As we have noted, values are held at various levels of consciousness. We know some but not all of what we feel and think about ourselves. Some of the knowing which influences us is below the level of conscious recognition.

Though we know how tall we are, we are not always aware of how we feel about this fact. An adult male who is 5 feet tall in a society where the average male height is 5 feet 9 inches may have strong feelings of resentment or inferiority about his lack of height, yet he may not be aware of these feelings. Other values existing at deeper levels of consciousness may influence how he acts with girls who are taller than he, yet he may be totally unaware of the cause of these actions.

Clearly, such feelings can cause difficulty in understanding one's responses to a particular situation. At the conscious level, the reason given to support one's dislike of another person may be totally different from the real motivation stemming from values at deeper levels of consciousness. Opportunities for self-deception are inherent in unconscious motivation.

Hierarchical Structure

Some values are more important to us than others. Wherever possible, we attempt to maintain a degree of relative status among our values. However, this is not always possible. When we are unable to ascertain the relative importance between two antithetical values, we find ourselves in conflict.

Some of the most important values we hold are those which have to do with survival and meeting the basic needs for food, shelter, and warmth. Under most circumstances these take precedence over all other values. Under certain special circumstances, other values may predominate over those associated with survival. The person who surrenders his life for a cause is an example of this. The boy who "takes a rap" for a friend is another case in point.

One part of the process of maturing in life is to establish an effective, realistic hierarchy of values by which to live. When we cannot do this, we give signs of being retarded in our development. Usually this is the result of not having been able to perform some task of growing up at the right time. We have not learned to see things in perspective. We interpret them erroneously and therefore respond to them in inappropriate ways, and so we function with a limited degree of effectiveness in life.

> After Amy, a college freshman, received her driver's license, she frequently drove some of her friends to school. Amy was an outgoing girl who cared a great deal about what people thought of her. Being popular was important to Amy. To impress her friends and to cover up her inexperience in driving, she took more risks than were necessary. Her attitude about danger was "It can't happen to me." But when she had an automobile accident, the close brush with death convinced her that it could happen to her. What her friends thought of her driving ability became far less important than her concern for safety.

In Amy's hierarchy of values, people's opinions of her, at first more important to her than survival, became secondary when the accident caused her to see things in their real perspective.

How do we achieve perspective? We continually seek meaning in the events of life. We find this meaning only according to our past experience. If we have not been able to understand fully what has happened to us in the past, we can give only limited meaning to it. As a result we are ill-equipped to give value to what we are to experience in the future. If we can make no sense of the past, we cannot establish an effective hierarchy of values to help us find meanings, and consequently life becomes progressively more confusing.

Influence of Values upon Function

We have stated that values influence all that we do. Let us look more closely at the influence of values upon physiologic function. The following case illustrates the *negative* influence of values upon *physiology*.

> Don, a young man who had graduated from college four years previously, had taken a position in a relative's business. His father had been influential in obtaining the job for him and was most anxious that Don do well. Don was fully aware of this concern and worked hard to live up to the responsibility placed upon him. He had always been an extremely conscien-

tious person. He graduated cum laude, went to work five days after graduation, and had proved himself worthy of several promotions in his four years with the firm.

In the past year Don began to notice that he could not sleep well. He spent many nights awake thinking and planning his work for the next day. He often went without eating lunch in order to accomplish work assigned to him. He frequently took work home and often stayed late on the job. Many times this was because he was unwilling to trust the work to anyone else. When he began to notice that his stomach was frequently "tied up in knots," Don decided to see a doctor.

To his astonishment he was told that he had high blood pressure and there were indications that some tiny ulcers had developed in the lining of his digestive tract. He was advised to slow down and to take a vacation (his first since college days), and he was placed upon a special diet.

What values about himself were at work in Don? During his college years he had worked equally hard. He seemed driven beyond reason toward success. In spite of past successes, he felt inadequate. He believed he was not very intelligent and could succeed only by dint of hard work. He also believed that his parents did not think too much of him. He knew they liked him, but because they were continually comparing him to his cousin, he felt they were disappointed in him when he was unable to perform in school as well as his cousin could. He believed that he had to prove himself on the job, that only in this way could he recover from his feelings of inadequacy and establish himself in his father's eyes.

Because of these beliefs, or values, he felt himself to be in a state of continual emergency. Nerves and glands functioned so that he would be able to cope with the emergency, at least in a physical way. His muscles were continually tense, as though he were in combat of some sort. He expended great quantities of energy, and though he ate large amounts of carbohydrates, he did not store them up in the form of fatty tissue but burned them up in his nervous tension. As a result of the attitudes he had about himself, the physical part of his response to his life situation was qualitatively poor.

A dynamic illustration of the same kind of influence is described by James Baldwin.[1]

> I learned in New Jersey that to be a Negro meant, precisely, that one was never looked at but was simply at the mercy of the re-

[1] James Baldwin, *Notes of a Native Son*, Beacon Press, Boston, 1955, pp. 93–94.

flexes the color of one's skin caused in other people. I acted in New Jersey as I had always acted, that is, as though I thought a great deal of myself—I had to act that way—with results that were, simply, unbelievable. I had scarcely arrived before I had earned the enmity . . . of all my superiors and nearly all my coworkers. In the beginning, to make matters worse, I simply did not know what was happening. I did not know what I had done, and I shortly began to wonder what *anyone* could possibly do, to bring about such unanimous, active, and unbearably vocal hostility. . . .

It was the same all over New Jersey, in bars, bowling alleys, diners and places to live. I was always being forced to leave, silently, or with mutual imprecation. I very shortly became notorious and children giggled behind me when I passed and their elders whispered or shouted—they really believed that I was mad. And it did begin to work on my mind, of course, I began to be afraid to go anywhere and to compensate for this I went to places which I really should not have gone and where, God knows, I had no desire to be. . . .

That year in New Jersey lives in my mind as though it were the year during which, having an unsuspected predilection for it, I first contracted some dread, chronic disease, the unfailing symptom of which is a kind of blind fever, a pounding in the skull and fire in the bowels. Once this disease is contracted, one can never be really carefree again, for the fever, without an instant's warning, can recur at any moment.

Another case shows the *positive* influences of values on *health*.

Mary left college in her junior year. She married a young man from her hometown whom she had known since her high school days. She went to work and helped support her husband and herself while he went on to graduate school. A year after he finished his graduate work, they had their first child; two years later, they had another. Though she had wanted to complete her studies, she was not greatly upset that she had not. She made the transition from college to work to motherhood with ease. She enjoyed being a wife and mother and made the most of whatever came along. She slept well, enjoyed her food, maintained an attractive figure, and got the kind of exercise her body demanded. Some discipline was necessary to effect these things, but she managed to exert this discipline. She was rarely sick—in four years she had only two colds and nothing more severe than this.

What were the values at work in Mary's life? First of all she liked herself. She knew that she was not the greatest person in the world but believed that she could get along pretty well in most circumstances. She believed herself capable of working and did not think it a hardship to work as a filing clerk while her husband went to school. She felt neither superior nor inferior to him. She believed that children would be important in her life but knew they would demand a great deal from her. She believed herself capable of meeting the demand. As far as physical factors were concerned, she managed to keep stress to a minimum. Clearly the quality of her response to her life situation was good. She functioned well and had no unreasonable expectations for herself or for her husband. All this she showed in her entire being.

We may see then, from these case studies, that the interpretations a person makes in a situation are strongly influenced by the values he has about himself in relation to the situation—values that influence the unique meaning he gives to every circumstance.

The Power of Suggestion

All of us have a certain amount of suggestibility, that capacity to respond to suggestion *as though the suggestion were objectively true.* The very process of reading meaning into events has made us this way. When we are told, for example, that a tree is tall, we use our imagination to picture how tall the tree is. When someone tells us that a man is strong, we think of him as such. In other words, we allow ourselves to be led to a conclusion.

Usually, the greater the status of the suggester in the eyes of the suggestee, the more the suggestee will be influenced. Most of us are more influenced by a person of recognized authority than by a stranger in the street. When a physician tells us that we have a serious throat condition, we give greater credence to the statement than if it had been made by a shoe salesman.

The suggestee is more open to influence under some conditions than others. Emotions may be a factor. If we are already frightened and someone reports further disaster, we will be more influenced than if we were in a calmer frame of mind. Repeated exposure to an idea renders us more susceptible to it. Advertisers are aware of this. Suggestion may also take the form of linking one idea to another. When skiing is described as fun, we are ready to have fun when we go skiing.

The power of suggestion operates on many levels. It affects us not only on the attitudinal level but on the behavioral and physiologic levels as well. If a comedian has been known to be funny in the past and his reputation is well established, we are set to be entertained by him, and we behave accordingly. If most of the audience finds him entertaining, often we will be influenced to act as though we too have been amused even when in reality we are not.

We all have had the experience of thoughts which produce physiologic changes. An embarrassing thought makes us blush. Sexual feelings are often aroused with a simple succession of thoughts. Feelings of excitement are stimulated simply by thinking about a threatening situation. The student who conjures up thoughts of failing an examination can easily stimulate his heart action and changes in his blood chemistry.

Hypnosis

It is possible to place a subject in a hypnotic trance and convince him that he is to be touched with a red-hot poker. The subject is asked to look at a pencil held in the hand of the hypnotist. The hypnotist says, "You see this branding iron I hold in my hand? I am now going to touch you with it. It will be slightly painful but will do no real damage. You know how it will feel, do you not?" The subject, under the influence of the suggestion, mutters, "Yes." He is then touched with the dull end of the pencil. He will pull his hand away, rub it, and act as though it had been burned. He may even develop a redness in the area, and a blister may appear at the point of contact with the "branding iron." *Regardless of the reality, he will respond as though the suggestion were true.*

In this situation the hypnotist has used suggestion to influence the physiologic function of the individual. He has activated values closely associated with function. He has touched upon the value which, in effect, says, "I am a person who can be burned." Each of us has had the experience of being burned. Each of us knows how it feels. Under the proper circumstances we can produce in ourselves the sensations of being burned.

Preconditioning

Little is yet known about just how or why suggestion works. Preconditioning is important. The desire to cooperate with the circumstances of life is basic. As long as this cooperation exists, suggestion is effective.

Some people are more susceptible to preconditioning than others. It would seem that some are more likely to be dependent on externals than others. They are willing to give decision making over to others. They cooperate, even to the extent of doing things they would not usually do themselves. It is not that they would do things that are strongly against their personal wishes, but rather that they can readily follow the direction implicit in circumstances. Such people make better subjects for the hypnotist than others do.

Most of us can be taught to cooperate if we can see the advantage in it. The value of cooperativeness then becomes a part of us. We say to ourselves, "I am a person who cooperates." For example, when we go to a physician for the purpose of being healed, we are inclined to cooperate with his directions because we believe it is to our advantage to do so. The very fact that we have gone to him is evidence of another value which we have incorporated into our being. We have learned that physicians can help us. "I can be helped by a physician." We believe, and we act upon this belief. The healing process may begin with this belief and the suggestion of cure inherent in the visit.

There are persons, however, who can be healed by some physicians but not by others. We sometimes have not only the general value of being capable of being healed but also the value, often based upon experience, that only certain kinds of physicians can be of help to us. Usually this specificity is intangible. We cannot easily identify why we respond to one doctor but not to another. We only know that some men instill a confidence and trust in us that others do not.

If we are persons who cannot readily yield our autonomy to another, we must have confidence in the ability of a particular person to do what he says he can. We must believe, deep within us, that help is possible, and that the particular person to whom we turn is the one who can provide this help.

From this we can derive a principle: When a person, because of what he is or because of what he has learned, is able to give himself to another or to certain circumstances, he can be influenced by the suggestions inherent in that situation. This influence may be profound enough to motivate us. It can even change physiologic processes associated with purpose and value. This happens on a totally subjective basis and is little related to objective reality. Therefore, through the manipulation of the value structure that we are, both behavior and function can be altered, the initiating stimulus being suggestion.

Suggestive Influence of Situations

The process of association, that is, linking one idea to another, is effective in conditioning response. Automobile accidents, for example, are often associated with physical injury. This is evidenced by the question, "Was anyone hurt?" when we are told of an accident. If we were to see a stopped car, with a woman lying on the ground before it, in the middle of the road, we would easily assume that she had been hit and injured by the car. This assumption would probably be accompanied by physiologic fear reactions within us.

Many persons find their lives totally directed by this kind of suggestive assumption. They have never developed the skill of accurately evaluating a situation free from its suggestive influence. The responses that are linked to these assumptions are therefore often inappropriate.

Nearly every situation has inherent suggestive implications. The college scene is filled with such situations. Classrooms with their structured arrangement; interpersonal relationships, with the status hierarchy; clubs, fraternal organizations, teams, recreational pursuits—all suggest. The very role we see for ourselves in the various circumstances of life suggests response to us.

Suggestive Influence of Culture

As one's experience grows out of his culture, that culture has a potent suggestive influence upon him. In the small culture of one's home environment values are built into our lives in such a way that we learn to function according to those values.

Some children are kept for so long in a dependent relationship with their mothers that even when they grow up and are freed from this dependency by circumstances, they may find themselves falling into old patterns of responding to their mothers. This may happen even against the will of the person. It is even possible for the person to be aware of his feelings of dependence and still to be influenced when in the presence of his mother. His responses become those of his childhood. He may even produce physical symptoms associated with those times in his childhood when he used these same symptoms to gain sympathy from his mother. Asthma, for example, is frequently associated with such circumstances. An asthmatic reaction may prevail even when one comes in contact with a person who symbolically represents one's mother. Or it may happen when one finds himself in situations which are reminiscent of the emotional content in which one lived as a child.

In the larger cultural setting of our peer group, school, community, race, and nation, equally potent conditioning influences are operative. The culture which centers about the mystical foundations of religion, for example, produces many more people subject to these experiences, and the functions associated with them, than the culture which is oriented about a more impersonal and objective scientific approach.

The following case study illustrates the often subtle but potent affect of culture in the whole complex of value patterns.[2]

[2] Gordon Allport, *The Nature of Prejudice*, Addison-Wesley, Reading, Mass., 1954, p. 301. Reprinted by permission of the publisher. All rights reserved.

"I wanted to join the Congregational Church when I was 11 years old because all my friends went to that church and seemed to have such a good time. But I didn't. Why? Well, in some subtle way, which I've never been able to figure out, the family made it clear to me that there was a certain dignity in belonging to the Episcopal Church. Also, it was the old story of grandfather and great-grandfathers having sat in those same pews."

Here we see that the girl's family had established for her a value frame of reference. It would be well for her to maintain dignity, status, and a prideful design for living. Within this directional set she gradually develops her specific attitudes—pro-Episcopalian, anti-Congregational. First she begins to take a certain view of herself—one of subtle superiority. Her prejudices, such as they are, will be merely incidents in the maintenance of this self-image. Her broad values (the scheme she lives by) will form her view of outgroups. In this instance, there probably will never be hatred or unkind discrimination. Rather there will be just the slightest sense of superiority over groups that are less "dignified"!

Although Americans usually consider themselves to be scientifically oriented, many have been so conditioned to such ideas as the association between wet feet and colds that it is not unusual for a person who has got his feet wet to produce the symptoms of a cold. This phenomenon persists even though there is no scientific evidence to support a relationship between colds and wet feet.

Millions of people in our scientifically oriented society are convinced that a regular intake of pills of one sort or another is essential for good health. We believe this, and we act as though it were true. Research on the use of the placebo (a worthless sugar pill) indicates that some people are cured of carefully diagnosed disorders simply by being told to take a placebo regularly. The symptoms of the disorder disappear!

Industries have been established to capitalize on the potency of suggestive influence. It enters our buying habits. It influences how we vote. It conditions our attitudes with regard to international relations. In our scientifically oriented, well-educated society we are influenced far too often, behaviorally, physiologically, and attitudinally, by suggestion.

It is important to recognize how influential our values are on our health and how greatly the quality of our responses is influenced by values that result from suggestion, whether they be given by a person, a situation, or the culture we live in.

12.

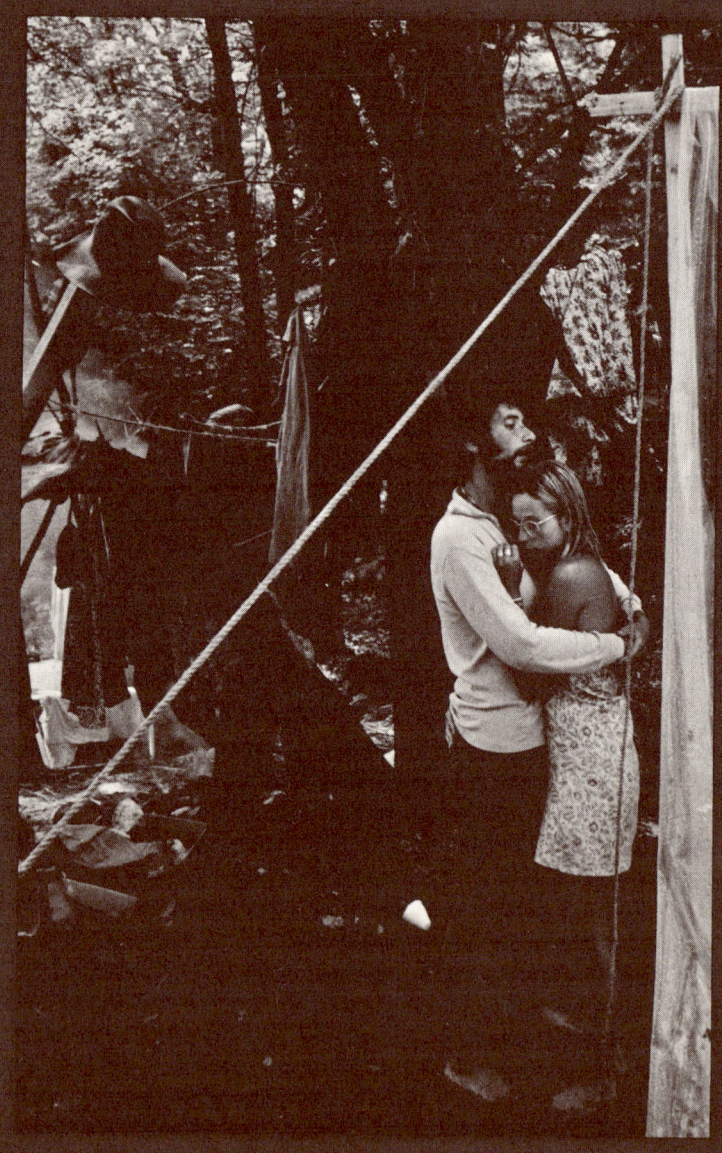

CONFLICT AND THE DEVELOPMENTAL TASK

Many people believe that conflicts lead to mental illness and emotional disturbance. This is not true. The assumption that conflict is necessarily evil often makes people try to avoid the conflicts which inevitably develop when people live intimately with one another. These conflicts are necessary. Yet, husbands and wives frequently strive for a conflict-free relationship; parents often attempt to prevent the development of conflict between themselves and their children; friends are dismayed if conflict is a part of the relationship. The concept of togetherness has no place for conflict.

The underlying assumptions in these beliefs about conflict are that the major task of life is to adjust and that the person who can adjust is healthy because his life is stress-free. Few ideas could be farther from the truth.

Conflict is a necessary part of the process of growth. It is a basic experience of life. The person who regards himself as conflict-free is unable to perceive the realities of life. He is distorting the nature of experience by a predetermined prejudice against an important aspect of life and is establishing expectations for himself which are not realistic. He has a criterion for judgment about himself which dooms him to self-condemnation. And he is likely to develop attitudes which make it almost impossible to deal with conflict when it arises. In resolving conflicts it is essential to identify the conflicting issues. When people deny that conflict can exist in the healthy person and assume, therefore, that it cannot be part of their own lives, they tend to hide the evidence of it. Hiding it, they obscure the issues at stake. The issues, then, become impossible to deal with.

Types of Conflict

Interpersonal Conflict

We deal with two broad categories of conflict in this book. The first is interpersonal conflict, which arises when individuals are

Burk Uzzle, photography. Magnum Photos, Inc.

opposed to one another in their purposes. Parents and children are frequently in conflict with one another. Each of any two individuals involved in a human relationship has purposes for himself which run counter to the purposes of the other person in the relationship.

Frequently these are little more than differences of opinion. At other times there are more important differences in which each person sees the relationship jeopardized by the other.

> Bill, a senior, and Jean, a sophomore, attended a large Eastern university and had been dating one another for several months. They thought of themselves as going steady and talked about the future. Bill planned to go on to graduate school and expected, when he finished, to go into teaching. At that time the couple would marry, and Jean would continue with her studies until graduation.
>
> Bill had never been a very popular person. He had one or two close friends whom he had not seen much since his relationship with Jean had begun. On the other hand, Jean had, from the very start, been quite popular among both men and women. She had a large circle of friends and was reluctant to give them up to spend her entire time with Bill.
>
> While there was no immutable reason for this to cause difficulty between them, the situation frequently became the source of long and involved arguments. Bill saw Jean's continued relationship with a wider circle of friends as a threat to his status with her. He felt that if she really cared for him she would gladly give up these others to be with him. On the other hand Jean felt that she would suffer as a person if she did not maintain the friends she had found upon entering the college.
>
> The conflicts focused on nothing specific. There were many occasions when their disputes would break out over something which seemed quite insignificant. If Jean wanted to go somewhere with a group of girls, Bill was upset. Often, when Bill wanted to be with Jean alone on a date, she felt it would be more fun if they went with a group. She was miffed if he insisted on his way.

Each of these young people saw themselves differently in the relationship. Each of them had different expectations for themselves in the situation, and each expected that the other would be willing to do that which would enhance his own expectations for himself. Conflict was inevitable. It was not so much that the conflict centered on specific issues. The source of the conflict lay in what each of them was. As long as each continued to see the problem in terms of what the other was denying him or her, the issue would not be resolved. Until they were able to identify just what was bothering them and to communicate it to the other, no growth could take place. The lack of growth was evident in the relationship as well as within the individuals.

Intrapersonal Conflict

The second type of conflict is that which exists within an individual himself. This is not clearly marked off from interpersonal conflict; frequently it is part and parcel of such conflict. But it is important to make the distinction in attempting to establish guidelines for a healthful resolution of conflict.

Inner conflicts usually result when external circumstances precipitate an emotional charge from two conflicting values which have long been established as a part of the value structure. This happens so often that each of us has experienced it. Girls are frequently placed on the horns of a dilemma when a young man about whom they care a great deal expects sexual intimacy. Here the values about being virtuous are in conflict with the values about giving oneself to those we love.

In the entire process of establishing a set of values, young people are frequently thrown into inner conflict. As they grow older, they find that the values by which they have been living are no longer operative. In the process of finding a new set of values, the old ones frequently must be abandoned. Conflict ensues. It is a rare individual who can move through life without facing this challenge over and over again.

The Developmental Task

The work of moving forward in life provides countless opportunities to test one's values. In an effort to describe this process, psychologists have devised the concept that, in any given culture, events are forced upon the individual which are prescribed by the circumstances of common cultural experience and that these events present the individual with what have been called *developmental tasks*. The theory suggests that unless these tasks are performed within a roughly described time block, growth is arrested. Then other tasks, which depend upon previously performed ones, cannot be accomplished. The husband who is a "mama's boy" has not performed the developmental task of separating himself from dominant emotional attachments to his mother. When he marries, he probably will remain under the domination of his mother to such an extent that it will be difficult for him to function in the new emotional relationship. He will not easily relate to his wife, because, never having successfully revolted against his mother, he is still attempting to revolt against her.

Another manifestation of this syndrome may be found in the person who has transferred his emotional dependence on his mother to his wife. He attempts to relate to her as he related to his mother. He uses the same methods of pleasing her that were successful in pleasing his mother. He attempts to fulfill his needs for affection with his wife in the same way that he attempted to do so with his mother. Usually this does not work. The issue becomes further complicated when children enter the picture.

Developmental tasks must be performed by all of us from the time we are born until the day we die. Little children must perform the task of allowing siblings to enter the picture. Older children must learn to share the attention of teachers with their classmates. Adolescents have many important developmental tasks to perform, from beginning the process of forming their own values, through the bridging of the heterosexual gap, to deciding upon a lifework. Marriage, parenthood, middle age, and old age all have developmental tasks.

These tasks are interrelated, the performance of one depending upon the successful performance of a previous one. Frequently individuals who have not been able to perform some of these tasks have a distorted view of a particular area of experience. The result is that their perceptions are progressively distorted and experience becomes increasingly confusing. The individual who has not bridged the gap from homosexuality to heterosexuality, for example, distorts subsequent experience which falls into the realm of heterosexuality.

Frustration in Developmental Tasks

The very nature of the developmental task guarantees a certain amount of frustration and anxiety. In the first place, the developmental task implies that choices be made. Before the choices are made, elements of one's existential situation must be identified. Because these elements are a part of one's inherent nature, they are exceedingly difficult to identify. For example, in performing the task of establishing a set of values for oneself, it is often necessary to identify what values exist within oneself as a result of parental conditioning. Furthermore, these values must be examined in the light of new experience. The old experience out of which they grew is no longer relevant. Parents instill values in their children for particular reasons. These reasons are not always rational. They have been established in an emotional context that becomes activated when new experience tends to refute the old values.

If the values are to be changed without subsequent guilt, the feelings must be evaluated, set apart, and placed in proper perspective. This is not accomplished easily. It necessitates self-examination, which is often painful. Protective mechanisms within us often are operating to obscure the painful factors and are often expressed as hostility. The greater the degree of obscurity, the greater the amount of frustration involved in accomplishing the task.

Even if this were all that were involved, the task would be difficult enough. But frustration is an experience itself. It has its own component of confusion and anxiety. The individual often feels that he is not doing what he should be doing. The process frequently becomes a circular one. Studies have shown that frustration and confusion tend to increase hostility in people toward others.[1]

Adolescence and early adulthood in our society are fraught with such frustration. On the one hand we are encouraged to grow up. At the same time we are coerced into being good and obeying our parents. The two demands are often inconsistent with one another. To the extent that individuals can resolve the conflicts inherent in such situations, they proceed along the path of self-actualization. To the extent that they cannot do this, they remain statically caught in the trap of their confusion, and development does not take place. The skills for resolving conflicts are dealt with in detail in the next chapter.

Self-testing

The performance of one's developmental tasks is largely a matter of self-testing. As we move forward in the process of assessing ourselves, we find that there is no blueprint to follow. We seek answers from others. If the person whose help we seek is wise, he will respond not so much by telling us what to do but by asking us questions which will help us sort the many issues involved. An adviser who is not as wise will offer answers to our questions, and they may be misleading.

Whatever the circumstances, each of us, if he grows, comes to the conclusion that he himself must make the decisions and bear the consequences of those decisions.

If we have been fortunate in performing the tasks which came earlier in our lives, the amount of anxiety is reduced. If we have not done the earlier tasks well, we do not have the skills or the confidence necessary to do what we must in the present.

[1] Harold Proshansky, "The Development of Intergroup Attitudes," Review of Child Development Research, vol. 2, Russell Sage, New York, 1966, pp. 336–339.

The Risk of Failure

In any endeavor where there is no assured path toward success, failure is a possibility. Developmental tasks require that we have a certain amount of courage. When this is lacking, we cannot move into the unknowns which face us in the process of becoming.

Usually, unless the circumstances are extremely fortuitous, there is a passage of time in performing developmental tasks. Within that period of time, many things are attempted. Many feelings are tried on, as it were. As this is done, we learn to try these things again or to reject them. Usually we reject them because they have not worked. When they have not worked, there has been a failure of some sort. This is natural and reasonable to expect. However, many of us have had the kind of experience with failure that has made us extremely cautious. It has grown out of proportion to reality. Therefore we are often unwilling to risk failing again.

Parental relationships are important in this regard. Unless we have been encouraged in spite of our failures, we may be unwilling to attempt those things in which success is not guaranteed beforehand. To some extent, this phenomenon has been used, by society and by parents, to prevent people from straying from the chosen path. It has been used to emphasize the value of conformity, to prevent the questioning of values and the challenging of tried and true elements of the established order.

For example, marriage is important in the established order of Western society. The sanctions against divorce were so strong a century ago that many people were willing to live lives of extreme and unusual suffering rather than to break the bonds of marriage. Particular religious and cultural groups at present restrict individuals in the same way. The force of these sanctions is so strong that it is a rare person who has the courage to go against them. To do so would be to risk failure and ostracism.

We often feel that failure in marriage is the worst kind. For many of us this is failure as a human being. The social sanctions too are so strong that when we violate them, we think we risk isolation. Suffering this, we feel that we will be unable to avail ourselves of the human recognition and love that is essential to us. If there is the threat of social disgrace or removal of parental love, we are often fearful and therefore do not do the things which seem important for us. The risk of failure is great in performing the developmental task.

The Developmental Task in Experiential Terms

What is the developmental task like? How do we know when it is operating in our lives? These are questions which students frequently ask. Developmental tasks are so much a part of our normal experience that we often cannot specifically identify what is happening. Some description of the experiential aspects of this phenomenon will be helpful in understanding it.

First, what does it proceed from? Undoubtedly a combination of factors are at work to precipitate a particular developmental task. For each individual, the combination may be different. But one of the first things which happens is that the person becomes aware of a need to grow.

This need may be manifest in a variety of ways. It may show in a feeling of boredom. One would like to become something other than what he is at present. Another manifestation may be one's susceptibility to being interested in new things. One may be led to try something new by an older respected peer, or he may be dared into it by his own age-mates. Fear may be another motivation. As one sees others around him moving to another stage of being, the fear of being left behind may motivate him to try something new. Curiosity, anger, or anxiety may also be motivating factors toward growth.

Events which are beyond the control of the individual often initiate growth. For example, the young adolescent has to deal with the biologic changes in his body. A girl who experiences the development of breasts, regardless of her feelings about this, must learn to see herself differently. A boy who is motivated to reach out toward girls because of the glandular changes he experiences at puberty necessarily sees himself differently. In each case an old self must be left behind, and a new self must be sought out, tried on, and developed.

Many experiences come about with the passage of time and force changes in the way an individual sees himself.

> Susan, the daughter of a physician, had entered college thinking that she would like to study medicine. While the first two years of her study were fairly well prescribed, she paid particular attention to those courses which she felt were related to her major field of interest. But during those two years she had an experience with an English professor who had a profound influence upon her. He was brilliant, inspiring, and enthusiastic about his subject and his students. She found the classes she took with him fascinating. She spent several hours discussing things with him that were of interest to her. In the process she felt a change taking place within her. She began to realize that medicine would take study and dedication that would rule out of her life some of the things she was beginning to enjoy in college.
>
> Susan was a likable girl. She had become popular with her

classmates and found that she liked the social life of the college. She also discovered that she enjoyed the free time for exploring areas of interest not directly connected with her studies. As all these things came together in her life, she began to realize that her image of herself as a physician was changing. In time her interest waned. A vague sense of dissatisfaction developed. In her relationship with the admired teacher she saw other things which were fascinating to her. With her friends she came to realize that life is more than just a matter of study and dedication. She felt it was time for a change in the direction of her life.

Problems began to develop for her. Should she give up the goal toward which she had been pointing for a number of years? Could she disappoint her father? What would her friends back home think about her if she gave up her intentions? These were just a few of the questions that bothered Susan. It meant that she had to think of herself in entirely different terms. She also asked herself the more searching question, "Am I giving this up because I am lazy?" At this point her confidence in herself was shaken, and thoughts of failure arose.

For several months she vacillated, feeling that she was wasting her time in indecision. She had not told her parents, and felt guilty about not doing so. At the same time she could not bring herself to tell them, for she feared that if she did, they would be terribly disappointed in her.

In the process, she dropped out of some school activities and did not do well in classes. She developed a cold that she could not shake. Her friends wondered what had happened to her. Clearly it was a period of distress in her life. She felt she wasn't worth the opportunity that her father was providing for her. She finally decided that she would speak with her parents and tell them what she had been going through. She thought she might take a job for a few months and then perhaps be able to decide what to do with her life.

After telling her parents, she began to see things in perspective. She could talk more freely with her friends and her favorite professor. Within a few weeks, she decided to switch her major, and with her counselor's help she reorganized her program of studies for the spring semester. She felt as though a great load had dropped from her shoulders. Once more she entered the stream of college life.

The change seemed dramatic and sudden, but it was not. It had been building for some time. Her sense of self had gone through a change. The realization of what she had to do had been clouded by the feelings which surrounded the whole experience. Unreasonable guilt had retarded the decision-making process. When she decided to tell her parents of her plan to drop out of school, she felt relieved, and the tension that had been building up within her was released. The creative flow of thought was again established, and she moved through the developmental task of selecting an area of major study which was more consistent with her real interests. In taking this step, she began to exert a degree of autonomy which heretofore she had been unable to show. It is difficult to determine just what developmental task was predominant in Susan's situation, but it is clear that the decision to discuss things with her parents freed her to do what she had to do in choosing her major subject. When this was done, she was again able to get involved with school activities and social life.

In summary, the developmental task tends to follow a general pattern, the stages of which are clearly illustrated in Susan's case. These stages can be listed as follows:

1. Horizons widened (for Susan, through college life)
2. Sense of dissatisfaction (with choice of major study)
3. Doubts (about vocational choice and about self)
4. Worry about what to do
5. Conflict (conflict between pleasing parents and pleasing self)
   a. Vacillation in feelings and on what to do
   b. Dropping out (dropping out of activities and friendships)
   c. Grades tumbled
   d. Development of cold symptoms
6. Decision on course of action
7. Release of tension
8. Clarification of thoughts and feelings
9. Restoration of perspective

While the specifics may differ from person to person, this is not an atypical case. For Susan there happened to be two tasks which were interdependent: it was important for her to declare her independence from her parents' expectations for her, and it was also important for her to choose a course of study at college which was her own. The experiential aspects were probably similar to those which most people go through when they are faced with making changes in their own lives.

As long as the conflict remained unresolved, it influenced many responses to her life situation. Clearly her behavior and her attitudes about herself and her own worth were affected. The cold she developed was evidence of her physiologic response to the situation. It should be noted that the cold symptoms disappeared shortly after she had decided upon a course of action. She had experienced a rebirth. She had been freed from an old way of being and was ready for the next tasks of her life.

The Element of Choice

In the performance of every developmental task there are a number of choices which individuals must make. In the first place one must choose between remaining at a level of existence which has become comfortably familiar and moving toward a being which is not yet established. In Susan's case the comfortable and familiar was to be her parents' daughter. In this role she had learned to do what they expected of her. She sought to please them. She did not have an identity separate from them. The being which was not yet established was that of independent thought and action. She had not yet learned to move out on her own, make decisions for herself, take responsibility for those decisions. The self that could do this was not clearly identified. The lack of clarity was frightening, for she felt motivated to reach toward a self with which she had no experience. It was a self which might fail and which might bring down her parents' displeasure and disappointment.

Another level of choice often presents itself in the need to decide between two clearly stated alternatives. In the choice of a career one may have interests and talents equally divided between two or more areas of endeavor. One may, for example, be equally equipped to teach and to be an artist. The choices may seem simple in such a situation. The artist has an unstable future before him. The teacher affiliates with a vocation which has much inherent stability. The artist, if he succeeds, can expect financial rewards which are quite tempting. The teacher, however, looks forward to remuneration which is limited though assured.

Even though the choices seem simple, they usually are not. Each alternative requires the individual to relinquish some aspect of his being which he cherishes. It is never easy to give up a part of oneself which is of value to him. In some cases it might be easier to give up a limb than to lose a part of one's identity. In fact, the two are not dissimilar. In each case an amputation must be performed. Whether the amputation is physical or psychological, the experience is painful.

Danger arises when the individual deceives himself into believing that he has suffered no loss and attempts to deny the feelings he has. In such cases there is an alienation from the inner core of one's being. If the feelings which demand expression are not expressed in direct ways, they become subtly disguised and are projected in ways that are both confusing and distressing. These feelings frequently manifest themselves in forms of illness which cannot easily be identified.

The element of choice, then, is important in performing the developmental task. When one is unable to make decisions or when he cannot clearly identify what the choices are, the process of growth is retarded. The subsequent confusion precipitated into the individual's life has a marked influence upon the quality of his response to life.

Identity and the Developmental Task

One's image of oneself grows from successfully performing developmental tasks. If Susan had failed to "do her thing," she would undoubtedly have developed a sense of self which was not acceptable to her. She would have felt a vague but persistent sense of failure.

Most of us have experienced failing to do what we felt we should have done. These experiences are frequently the outgrowth of relationships with our parents or other authority figures but may be associated with our peers. Usually they have moral overtones. As a result of the sense of failure, we devalue ourselves in our own eyes.

Fitting in with the mass of society can be a form of failure to perform one's own unique developmental tasks. Since society tends to reward those who conform, the failure is masked. However, the inner sense of dissatisfaction with onself is ever present. One's confidence in oneself is limited. The subsequent distortion of reality renders one incapable of responding in the most appropriate manner to the challenges of life. The long-term effects on one's health are damaging.

When we have experienced more failure than success, we project ourselves as uncertain and inadequate. We often compensate for these feelings of uncertainty with efforts that serve to fool ourselves but not others. Some common compensatory efforts are aggressive behavior, daring, boastfulness, and driving measures to succeed at all costs. Too often these efforts serve only to make others distrustful of us. When people cannot trust us, they shield themselves from us. A barrier is set up, and we thus feel isolated from others.

Sometimes, however, compensatory efforts succeed in creating experiences with success. The boy who feels inadequate in academic circles achieves success in athletics. The girl who cannot get along with friends finds success in schoolwork. In many cases the compensatory efforts succeed in bringing the person a sense of worth he would not otherwise feel.

The complexity of establishing a sense of self that is worthy of being is enormous. When we realize the number of experiences to which we are subject and when we understand the impact of these experiences on us, we recognize what a wonderfully adaptive organism the human personality is. We should be awed that we have turned out as well as we have.

13.

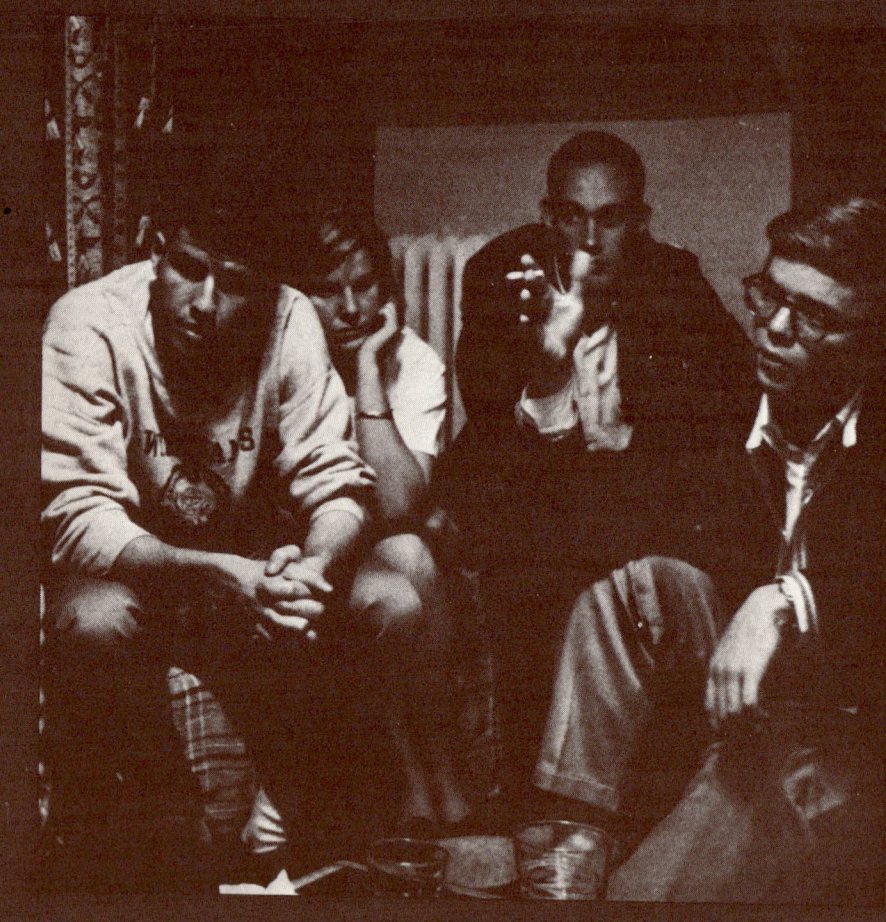

THE SKILLS FOR RESOLVING CONFLICTS

We must learn how to deal with the recurring challenges in our life. The quality of our response to life depends largely upon how well we handle the conflicts before us. Each age group has specific sources of conflict. In order to deal with conflict we must identify what within us is in conflict, evaluate its importance, and choose a path which will lead toward growth and self-actualization. The other alternative is self-destruction, despair, and nonbeing.

Conflict and Age Levels

Each age group makes an effort to withdraw from the zone of conflict. This is a natural process. The steady pattern of withdrawal and reemergence is essential in the process of growth, just as the cyclic pattern of waking and sleeping gives us a chance to recoup from the devitalizing strains of life.

What is tragic and unfortunate is that too many of us, of all ages, have interrupted the rhythm of withdrawal and emergence and attempted to insulate ourselves altogther from the challenges of growth. Youth today accuses those over thirty and hurls the indictment, "You have failed. You are copouts. You seek protection in the establishment. You never get on the firing line." The older generation views the youth of today with alarm and says with equal vigor, and sometimes with hysteria, "You are dropping out. You will never amount to anything. How can you be like me if you don't get out and work, climb the ladder of success, face up to the tasks of life?"

The issue appears to be that the older generation wants its youth to emulate them, whereas the youth see no value in this. They are not sure what they want, but they know that they don't want to be like their parents. Both sides seem to miss one of the central issues involved: In each case they are avoiding the task of facing conflicts which inevitably grow out of life.

George Zimbel, photography. Monkmeyer Press Photo Service.

The older generation structures its life so that conflict is minimized. The housewife whose "bag" is children, shopping, housework, and socializing has reduced her existence to a dependable, familiar, unchallenging routine. When children upset the routine, she objects. When her husband fails to bring in the necessary money, she feels threatened. When friends do something out of the ordinary, she drops them. The rough spots are soothed with aspirin, Compoz, "ups," "downs," liquor, gossip, and luxuries. Husbands have similar routines: the rituals of rising and starting the day, the familiarity of the job, supper, television, newspaper, and bed. They have their own sporifics: rationalization, liquor, a little sex on the sly, and the passive observance of sports on TV.

No doubt their life seems hard and earnest. But life becomes difficult largely as a result of what we expect of it. If our expectation is that it should be easy, free of conflict, pain-free, and perpetually tranquil, we are being unrealistic. When boredom, anxiety, and frustration arise within the context of these expectations, we conclude that something must be wrong.

The older generation has passed these carefree expectations on to its youth. At one and the same time parents have been instilling both a sense of responsibility and an idealized concept of life. It would seem that neurosis is almost guaranteed for future generations. Under the circumstances, it is essential for the individual to assess his way of life honestly. No real answer will be found in hurling accusations at others. Young people cannot solve the problems of life by accusing their parents of doing a poor job of bringing them up. Regardless of cultural conditions, regardless of the values of other people, regardless of influences others seek to exert upon us, we can work things out for ourselves.

Constancy of Conflict

We must recognize that conflict is constant in a life where growth is valued. The preceding chapter deals with the developmental tasks which continually unfold in the process of growing. We have seen that growth remains a possibility throughout life and that it is possible to arrest one's growth by avoiding developmental tasks.

Many of us fail to recognize that even when we avoid the challenges of growth, we do not avoid the conflicts which accompany it. Within all of us lies the drive to develop, to bring our potential for living creatively into being. Its very existence is a precursor for conflict whether we perform the developmental tasks or not.

The sooner we recognize that conflict is basic to life, the sooner we will stop trying to avoid it. This recognition must be more than a simple intellectual affirmation—it must be an acceptance at an emotional level. Most of us have experienced the discrepancy which exists when we know something intellectually but not emotionally. The intellectual affirmation of a fact does not change one's way of reacting to it when the occasion arises. The same error may be made again unless there is a basic change in the value structure that each person is.

Simple recognition that conflict is ever present is not enough to eliminate the fear of it. We must affect the internal changes which make it possible for us to be different. These changes will usually come about through time and the constant reminding of ourselves that conflict is to be expected and cannot be avoided. In this process we look for conflict, identify it, and name it for what it is. We should become aware of the evasive tactics we have customarily used to avoid conflict.

To sensitize ourselves to what is happening within us, we must develop our capacity for introspection. For many Americans this has been a difficult thing to do. The gregarious, outgoing qualities which mark so many Americans tend to keep us from becoming introspective. In fact, many of us have devalued this as a personal characteristic. One of the major efforts of many young people is to be a part of the crowd, to be in. In order to get in, one must attend to the superficialities of the group and adopt the values it holds. The result is that many of the unique qualities characterizing an individual are covered up. If a person is introspective, he tends to suppress it and perhaps concentrate on developing a facility for snappy patter that so often seems to be valued by the group.

Unhealthy Handling of Conflicts

In the preceding chapter we saw that conflict is not bad in and of itself. What makes it good or bad is what we do with it, how long it lasts, and what it leads to in our lives. If it lowers the quality of our response to life, then we can assume, for the time being anyway, that it is having a negative effect upon us. If it produces excessive distress or if it renders us incapable of properly assessing the events of our lives, it has impaired our health.

The following case history illustrates an unhealthy way of solving a conflict.

> Shortly after Phil arrived at college, he met a girl in whom he became very interested. Within a few months he found him-

self spending every spare moment in her company. As a result his studies suffered. After the first semester he was put on probation, which meant he had to have a B— average in the second semester. He was torn between doing well academically and maintaining his love relationship. He began to view his professors as threats to his comfort. From this exaggerated and distorted point of view, he began to do things in class which his friends and acquaintances could not understand. He would make disrespectful remarks, be inattentive, challenge every statement of his teachers. He became increasingly difficult to get along with. His friends began to avoid him, his girlfriend couldn't understand him. He couldn't really understand himself.

He fell into the habit of telling anyone who would listen that "This is a jerkwater school." He went into long dissertations about the "lousy" faculty the college had. He was able to prove this, he believed, because of the way he had been treated by his teachers when he had "spoken up, which is my right."

Paul Burlin, "Young Man Alone with His Face," 1944. Oil on canvas. Collection, The Whitney Museum of American Art, New York. Peter A. Juley & Son, photography.

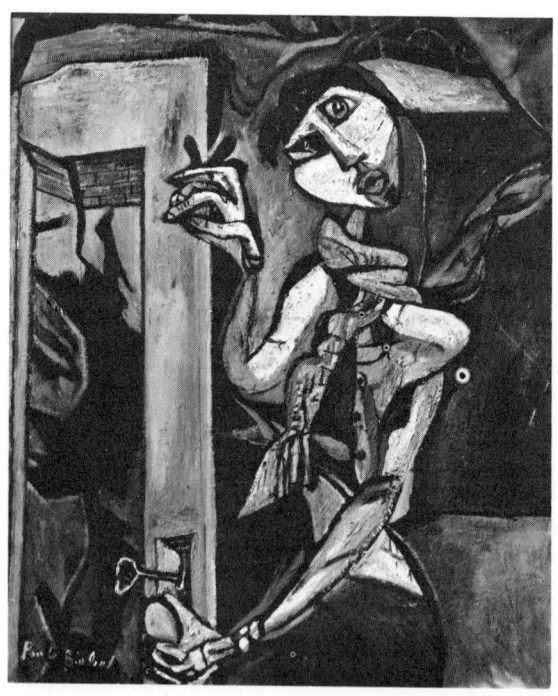

Anyone who knew Phil and who understood some principles of human motivation could see that he was justifying his bizarre behavior by reasoning that the school and the teachers were no good. What was more difficult to understand was that he was establishing a case for busting out of school. Even if no one else would believe the case, he could himself. For him this was a safer course than to fail without reason.

Many attitudes Phil had held about himself, about others, and about his education and career were changed. Even though he tended to believe the case he had created for himself, he could not feel very good about himself for following the path he had chosen. A slow, insidious self-hate, a creeping sense of guilt, and a subsequent sense of depression pervaded his being. He moved farther and farther away from the central conflict. Life seemed to mean less and less. Because things did not seem to matter, he could see no reason for trying to maintain the old attitude of cooperation with the establishment. He saw little value in continuing, and thus he was going to drop out.

We need apply only several of the criteria for judging health to determine that the quality of Phil's response was low. First, *What did the response proceed from?* His decision to drop out grew from efforts to justify behavior, which was not geared to reality. More than this, his dropping out did not resolve the original conflict: it simply avoided it. Another criterion: *What is the future of the response?* Phil's behavior led him nowhere. He became isolated from his friends, he cut himself off from educational opportunities which he valued. He made the relationship between himself and his girlfriend difficult. And, perhaps most serious, his response resulted in his devaluing himself. *Was it consistent with past performance?* No. *Was it consistent with cultural mores?* No. *Was it self-affirming?* No; it merely denigrated others. The response did not show a *reasonable perception of reality*; it developed from a fear of others, and it lacked *creativity*. Neither did it *restore homeostasis*, because he became increasingly threatened by the results of his own behavior.

The only conclusion we come to is that, in Phil's case, the way in which he handled this particular conflict did little for his health during the period of time we have considered. Because conflict sometimes does lead toward such destructive results, we frequently assume that it is damaging to health. The truth is, however, that conflict does not have to produce destructive response. As we have seen in the previous chapter, it frequently leads toward growth.

Unresolved Conflict

The foregoing section clearly illustrates a conflict which was not resolved. In fact, Phil never realized that a conflict existed. He was not clearly aware that he was being pulled in two different directions at once. Almost from the outset he began to establish a case to justify his reactions. The more he did this, the more serious the conflict became. He was diverted from the real issues. His energy was expended in fruitless efforts to avoid the real source of the conflict. With each statement to the effect that the school was no good, he took one more step away from the basic issue. The conflict was not resolved; it was merely avoided.

At one time or another each of us has attempted to deal with conflict through avoidance. Some of us have been fortunate enough to recognize the limitations and even the hazards of such behavior. As a result we have developed the skills for resolving conflicts, albeit in a happenstance way. We have performed the developmental tasks of life. We may even have launched ourselves on the path toward self-actualization.

The dangers of not resolving conflict are not that we do not take care of the particular issue involved. The real hazards are that we do not accomplish the central tasks of life: identifying ourselves, finding a purpose in our lives, and becoming self-actualized.

When this does not happen, our lives are unrewarding. We can see no value in exerting ourselves for anything. The will to live and to grow diminishes, and we are then open to any force which would move us toward death and destruction. There is no standstill point in the process of being human. When we are not being, we are in a state of nonbeing. In a state of nonbeing, our vitality, energy, hope, and faith are progressively depleted. When a serious enough challenge arises, we do not have the stuff to deal with it. To exist in the zone of nonbeing is the hazard of not resolving the conflicts of life.

This does not mean that we are mortally endangered if we fail to deal with one or even with several important issues of life. But if we develop a pattern of refusing to accept the challenges of life, we fail as human beings. We may continue to function fairly effectively on the biologic and animal level for a time. But because we are driven to relate in a creative manner to all that is around us, including other human beings, we create problems which are insurmountable as they accumulate.

Sources of Conflict

If we attempted to list all the sources of conflict for people, we could fill volumes. Conflict originates in every conceivable situation. In these pages we shall deal with the major sources of conflict for only one age group: college students.

A conflict should not be confused with its source. For example, a student may have a conflict between his desire to live with a girl and his desire to conform to his parents' wishes. This conflict has its roots in three different sources: (1) The student is concerned about developing a set of values of his own. (2) He has the need to remain acceptable to his parents; he has not entirely grown away from them. (3) It is necessary for him to deal effectively with his drive toward sexual satisfaction. These three sources of conflict are operating in one situation and thus cause the conflict which divides him against himself.

The sources of conflict for college students can be categorized in a number of ways. In this volume, five categories of conflict source are dealt with: (1) establishing an identity, (2) determining how much to conform to society's demands, (3) dealing with competition and academic pressure, (4) using drugs, and (5) coping with the problems of sex and sexuality. Some of these categories are broad enough frames of reference that most of the difficulties which young people face may be lumped together within them. They are not uniquely those of college students, but they come more sharply into focus during the years of later adolescence and early adulthood than at most other times.

Identifying Problems

Even if we confine ourselves to the categories of conflict listed above, it is not feasible to discuss all the possibilities inherent in those categories. When discussing phenomena of human experience, it is always useful to establish the specific areas of concern under discussion. Virtually every existential situation precipitates some form of conflict, because it activates values which are in opposition to one another. An element of conflict is inherent in the experience of going from a dark house into a sunlit day. The organism desires to remain in the steady state to which it has adjusted in the house, but at the same time it is motivated to accommodate to the new conditions into which it has moved. This demands a decision, which in this case is made for us by our biologic structure. When our eyes are confronted with increased amounts of light, they automatically change to close out excessive light. Whatever conflict exists is only momentary. An interpersonal exchange, however, continually demands decisions of us, because we must choose between at least two possible alternatives of response.

The person who has had many experiences that demanded

accommodation and who has been encouraged to accommodate without unreasonable penalty is equipped to handle the varying challenges of life. He has developed the skill of finding resources for accommodation, which have become progressively more useful to him. He is also familiar with the experience of responding spontaneously. He has, in fact, developed one of the qualities necessary for actualization and is able to identify his problems clearly. The spontaneous individual is able to size up what is happening as it happens. He recognizes (1) what is at work, (2) how it developed, and (3) where it is apt to lead him.

What Is at Work?

The totality of every existential situation includes the past, the present, and the future, all of which come together in one instant. Other components are the physical features of the situation (including their influence on the persons involved) and the interpersonal features which are continually in flux.

Conflict may be initiated by any one of these elements. If the individual can deal with the events as they arise and if he can derive satisfaction from his manner of adapting, there is little chance that lasting conflict will develop within him. But it is probably impossible to deal with all aspects of life as they arise. If this were possible, there would be no conflict worth mentioning. Problems develop when one is not able to respond immediately and with finality to a situation. He then internalizes what is happening and attempts to deal with it at a later time. When two potent values have been activated and cannot be reconciled in the moment, the struggle between them lasts for some time. When a person is able to identify these values and can understand where they have come from, he stands a better chance of shortening the time of conflict. But when he cannot identify them, the resultant confusion causes him to invest many subsequent events of his life with some of this conflict. To dispel the tension generated by the conflicting attitudes within him, he must first discover what it is that is troubling him.

A major task, then, in minimizing long-range conflict is to be able to identify what is happening within oneself. The discussion in these pages will be mainly concerned with conflicts which become internalized rather than with those between one person and another.

How Did the Conflict Develop?

Another skill of the spontaneous person is that he can readily determine how a conflict developed. He is able to spot with little difficulty what in the existential situation and what in him are at work to produce the conflict. He knows where in his own background a conflicting attitude developed. Threatened by a particular situation, he knows that he is threatened. And he knows what in the situation threatens him. When one is taking an important examination, there is real cause to feel threatened. However, when one feels so threatened that he cannot perform well on the examination, there is an unreasonable element in his feeling. It would be important for him to discover what in his past has caused this unreasonable reaction. The chances are that he will discover that his parents have had unusually high expectations for him, that he feels he is always under the burden of doing peak-level work, and that he too expects this kind of performance from himself. At the same time he knows that he may not be able to perform up to this level, and anxiety immobilizes him.

In a conflict-producing situation, then, it helps if one is able to recognize where the values in conflict originated. This principle applies to the origin of the values in one's past and also to the origin of the conflict in the existential moment.

Where Is It Apt to Lead?

Another skill in identifying the conflict lies in the ability of the individual to determine where his responses are apt to lead him. A prior question to this is where are the *feelings* that are activated going to lead? On the basis of past performance one can usually tell what his feelings are apt to produce in him. When one has seen himself cope successfully with anger in the past, he can reasonably assume that he will cope with it well at present. If he has been unable to deal with feelings of jealousy, for instance, he knows that he can expect trouble when those feelings are aroused. Unless he can bring some new element, some new resource, into play, his feelings of jealousy can be expected to bring about the same reactions they have in the past.

With this knowledge one stands a better chance of modifying his reaction and, thus, alleviating the difficulties of the past. He is equipped to evaluate what is happening to him. He can then establish the perspective necessary and search for other alternatives open to him.

Signs of Conflict

The mature healthy individual has the ability to observe himself in action in such a way that he is able to start from any point of the experience cycle and trace the conflict back to its origin. He can start with a feeling, a bit of behavior, or a physiologic change and recognize its meaning by discovering its origin.

What are some signs of conflict? One set of signs operates at the physiologic level; they range all the way from mild neuromuscular tension to serious physical dysfunction. Circulatory, digestive, respiratory, metabolic, and endocrine dysfunction, among others, may result from long-range unresolved conflict. This does not mean that every time one manifests these symptoms he is necessarily in conflict. But when these symptoms appear, it is helpful to consider the possibility of intrapersonal conflict. Usually when it has gone this far, the problem is serious and cannot be dealt with by the individual himself. He should seek professional help in working out the causes.

Other, less serious signs of conflict in the physical realm are the vague feelings of uneasiness one has. Usually he cannot fully describe them. They produce a sense of restlessness, of disquiet, of the need to do something. One may pace back and forth or take a walk in order to relieve the tension. Many a busy executive has found that walking alleviates the tension of a conflict-producing job. Often, with the tension gone, one can attend to the real issues. Some people use walking as a means of solving the problems. By walking they express their need to move and thus bleed off the tension of the unresolved conflict. Sports and hobbies provide a ready means of relieving unneeded physical tension. It is not unusual for some persons to invest the competitive contest of sports with meaning which in itself symbolically resolves the conflicts of his life.

Many a young person has found himself in a life situation which evokes a good deal of hostility. He may be angry for a number of reasons: because he has a problem, because he can do little about it, and/or because he can't identify the problem. For whatever reason he is angry, he can get a lot of the feeling out of his system in contact sports. Through the contest he is able to transfer the feelings of anger from the problem he has to the enemy (opponent). He is able to deal with the secondary sources of his anger and gain a great deal of satisfaction from the task.

Work serves a similar purpose. A young man's mother asked him to chop down several trees to make room for a garden. She asked him to do this on his only day off, and he was furious with her. Nevertheless, he recognized that the request was not unreasonable, and he held back from expressing his anger toward her. Chopping down the trees was easier because of his anger. He was able to put into the swing of the ax all that he would have liked to have put into a swing at his mother. Each blow was satisfying as it bit deep into the wood. By the time the job was done, his anger was dissipated and satisfaction had replaced it.

Another level at which symptoms of conflict manifest themselves is the feeling level. Fear, anxiety, jealousy, anger, guilt, hate, and confusion are all potential signs of conflict. Usually, when these manifest themselves in unreasonable amounts or when there is no explainable cause for them, one can suspect that some conflict has been activated within.

Because of the tendency to justify our feelings and our behavior, it is important to avoid being misled by our own rationalizations about these emotions. A student, finding himself in a group situation in which he was called upon to evaluate some of his behavior, flew into a rage. In one grand explosion he indicated that the group was no good, the class was a waste of time, and the teacher didn't know what he was talking about. The emotions were excessive, and the reasons given for them were incorrect. They were clearly justifications. The student believed them at the time and to this day is not entirely convinced that his reactions were for reasons other than the ones he expressed. An objective observer could see that this young man, through the group process, had come very close to surfacing a conflict which he had harbored for a long time but had not been able to resolve. He made extremely uneasy by this turn of events. Rather than examine the internal developments taking place within himself, he reacted blindly to the sense of threat he experienced. Immediately this covered the truth which was about to be bared. His attention was focused on the group, the teacher, and the class as the cause of his discomfort. He successfully avoided the painful task of dealing with the conflict.

This illustrates the third symptomatic level of conflict—the level of behavior. If we know enough and are able to be honest with ourselves, we can usually tell from our behavior that conflict is present. In the case above, the excited behavior, the unreasonable remonstrances, and the other defensive mannerisms shown were clues that some careful introspection was needed.

Because feelings, physiologic change, and behavior are so intricately intertwined, it is often difficult to identify which is which and which one produces the others. However, when we are engaged in an internal search for the meaning of our feelings, our behavior, or our physiologic condition, we can usually tell when we have hit on the truth. We say that "something clicks." As we rummage around in our storeroom of experience and meaning, we can try out several different ideas. As we "try them on for size" and remain open to signs of recognition, we know truth when we hit on it. We also know what is off target. When we hit on the truth, a definite change in our attitudinal frame of reference takes place. A degree of order replaces confusion. This may have two effects: On the one hand, a slightly heightened sense of excitement occurs. At the same time, because we have got closer but not close enough, there may be a corresponding increase in anxiety or frustration. In any event we are aware of a change.

This change is different from the steady state of frustration which accompanies a fruitless search. If we continue in this state, a sense of boredom develops. We are inclined to put the whole thing aside for the time being. The search should not be given up, although it may be wise to put it aside for the time being.

In all, the search for the true conflict is not unlike the search of the scientist or the artist. The scientist attempts to work out a theory and establish the proofs of it. The artist searches for the line, the movement, or the sound which will adequately symbolize what he feels. Not entirely sure what the answer is, the artist or scientist must search sensitively for it and attend to all the clues that reach his consciousness. So it is with the person who would identify what it is that is bothering him.

Sensitivity to oneself is one key to spotting the sign that will lead us closer to the truth. Much in our way of life diverts us from this. We are not a people who are used to looking within. We have tended to emphasize the obvious, the concrete, and the easily noted. In our extrovertive tendency we have been so boisterous that we often overlook the insights which can only come through sensitive, watchful waiting. Often the answers come when we least expect them. Unless we are ready to receive them, we pass them by, and though they manifest themselves over and over again, we may never notice.

Calmness and Confidence

Each of us knows the pitfalls of dealing with situations under crisis conditions. There is an enormous tendency to see things out of perspective. Every threat is exaggerated. Even things which are not threats are taken to be. We function on the basis of our distorted interpretation of things and not on the basis of reality. Our responses are not appropriate. We do things we later wish we hadn't, and we create an image of our own capability from which we can derive little confidence.

"Don't blow your cool" is the cry of thousands of young people today. The sentiment is to be admired, but some examination of its meaning is necessary. Does it mean we should remain calm and be confident that most things will work out all right in the long run? Or does it mean that nothing is worth caring about?

To say there are things worth caring about is to state the obvious. Above all, we ourselves are worth all the investment of time and energy that we can put into developing our resources for full and rich living. In fact, we are worth so much that it is often worth risking our security, our status, and even our safety to achieve certain elements of self-actualization. This is not a pitch for martyrdom or for a Kamikaze dive into the thick of things without a reasonably cautious look at them. The importance of risking some things is that, unless we do, often we do not define what we are. If we play it cozy, we may never find out what is worthwhile and what we do care about. We will not discover that we have the courage to be, which is so important in the actualizing process of life.

Swimming instructors who work with adult nonswimmers are aware of this phenomenon. Most people who have not learned to swim in childhood have built up a series of unrealistic fears about the water and their own inability to survive in it. Their fears have become so exaggerated that they are unable to function in the water. Not only do they believe they are unsafe, but they are immobilized by their fear. An instructor must spend several weeks establishing a reasonable degree of calmness in his pupil before the job of teaching him to swim can begin. Then, step by step, skills are taught which not only are related to swimming but are designed to establish confidence in the learner.

So it is with other areas of life. Unless people are willing to move toward those things which threaten them, they will remain in fear of them, and their general confidence in themselves will remain limited.

The important conflicts in life often grow out of circumstances in which the individual has experienced significant feelings of threat. The whole realm of self-testing for some people may have elements of threat about it. Self-testing refers to any endeavor in which one pits himself against some force which works against him. This force may come from parents, other people, physical laws (like the law of gravity), or other sources of resistance against which one works in developing himself. A person who has had much frustration and many threats to himself in establishing his own ways of behaving, in contrast to what his parents wish for him, will probably feel threatened in a situation when it is necessary for him to buck authority. A person who has been encouraged by his parents to experiment and who has been assisted in his efforts will feel little threat in challenging authority. This particular realm is not usually a source of great conflict for him.

Calmness and confidence are linked in the process of resolving conflict. Each depends upon the degree of perspective. If a student is able to recognize that failure is not the worst thing that could happen to him, he is able to approach it with some equanimity. He knows that he will survive in spite of a momentary setback. Knowing this, he is able to accomplish the tasks of conflict resolution more readily than one who is fearful beyond the bounds of reality.

Categorizing

Once we have identified what it is that is bothering us, it helps if we can assign it to some conceptual category. Here we see man's symbolizing nature at work. For many of us it is impossible to deal with life unless we have some means of naming what it is that is happening. For example, it would be impossible for us to think about throwing a ball without having words to attach to the act and the objects involved. How would we think about ball, for instance, if we could not name it? What would we think about it if we could not link the concept of ball to some previous experience with a ball-like object? Could we discuss it with another person without some mutually acceptable descriptive category for reference?

So it is with our emotions, our attitudes, our feelings—all elements of our experience. Unless we have some way of categorizing the experience, we cannot adequately evaluate it. The more refined our categories, the greater mastery we can gain over it through understanding. In discussing our problems with another person, it helps if we can describe them in terms that are understandable to him. We ourselves gain greater understanding when we attempt to make some complicated series of feelings clear to another. Alcoholics Anonymous uses this principle frequently. Every member of the group is encouraged to accept the fact that he has a problem. He is further encouraged to discuss his problem with his fellow alcoholics. Frequently they are able to assist one another because they have had similar experiences and can thus help in the mutual task of providing categories for critical examination of the problems.

Simply to know that we have a conflict helps little. Although recognition is the first step, the labeling of its parts is also necessary for understanding. With this step, the conflict becomes a little more manageable, and we approach the next phase of the resolving process.

Analysis

Analysis is the phase of conflict resolution in which the person attempts to break down into manageable segments what has happened to him. In this phase he seeks to determine what is in conflict, what influence it is having upon him, and where it will lead him. While it is important to know the origins of the values in conflict, it is probably more important to ask oneself if what he is doing is what he wants. William Glasser poses the idea that one of our basic needs is to feel that we are worthwhile.[1] This can come about, he says, only if we are willing to correct ourselves when we are wrong and credit ourselves when we do right.

Granted that to determine right and wrong when we are in conflict is an extremely difficult task. Sometimes, both directions in which we are pulled have equal value in terms of right and wrong. It is at this point that analyzing is needed. Rightness and wrongness need not be determined by standards external to ourselves. Glasser indicates that "morals, standards, values, or right and wrong behavior are all intimately related to the fulfillment of our need for self worth." The inner need to fulfill ourselves is as important as conforming to the mores of our society.

One clue to evaluating the rightness or wrongness of our feelings or our behavior is to determine whether or not what we wish is consistent with fulfilling our basic needs. If it is not, then we must reject the feeling and find some substitute for it which is more in accord with what we really want for ourselves. This means that in the analytical phase of conflict resolution we carefully examine what is at work.

Learning to ask the right question of ourselves is an important aspect of the analytical task before us. How do we know what is the right question? Often we can never know with total satisfaction, but we will never learn to ask "righter" questions until we ask the less-than-right ones and *evaluate as we go along*. The risk of being wrong will always exist. Mature people know that life offers no guarantees of rightness simply because we undertake a particular task. Even when we undertake it in good faith, the cause-and-effectness of life exacts consequences for whatever we do. The risk of being wrong and suffering the consequences must be undertaken, or we will be helpless in the face of events, and we

---

[1] William Glasser, *Reality Therapy*, Harper & Row, New York, 1965.

will exist in the no man's land of nonbeing—a consequence of not doing what we must to effect growth.

Reorganization

The steps outlined above lead to the next important job in conflict resolution: to reorganize the values which are in conflict. It is difficult to separate analysis from reorganization. In fact, it is impossible to separate clearly any of the steps outlined so far. The breakdown proposed here is arbitrary, merely a semantic device to categorize what is under examination. It is doubtful if anyone goes through the same steps as any other person. However, the process is roughly similar in all people, and to that extent these categories are useful.

In part, the reorganization of values will result from establishing a hierarchy of their importance. The person in conflict must determine how relatively important his motivations are. He must rank the possible outcomes of his behavior and assess the basic needs associated with the conflict. As he does so, they fall into a different order. In effect, he has become a different person. Some of the old hang-ups are gone. New horizons have opened up. He probably views himself differently. If the conflict has truly been resolved, he now sees himself with a greater degree of confidence in his ability to deal with life.

The guilt, depression, and despair which ultimately creep into one's being when important conflicts have not been resolved insidiously undermine us in all aspects of life. We lose our sense of worth and zest for living. We desperately seek satisfaction in progressively less and less satisfying endeavors. The quality of our response to life is markedly poorer.

The road to self-actualization is paved with conflicts. The very fact that we have a need to grow counterposed by a need for safety is a source of continual emergence of conflict. Abraham Maslow points out:[2]

> Every human being has both sets of forces within him. One set clings to safety and defensiveness out of fear, tending to regress backward, hanging on to the past, afraid to grow away from the primitive communion with the mother's uterus and breast, afraid to take chances, afraid to jeopardize what he already has, afraid of independence, freedom and separateness. The other set of forces impels him forward toward wholeness of Self and uniqueness of Self, toward full functioning of all his capacities, toward confidence

[2] Abraham H. Maslow, *Toward a Psychology of Being*, Van Nostrand, Princeton, N.J., 1962, p. 44.

in the face of the external world at the same time that he can accept his deepest, real, unconscious Self.

This is our nature. This is the "agony and the ecstasy" of man. His own being presents him with the task for life. He can accept the challenge and move forward to reap the rewards of his inherent greatness, or he can surrender in the name of security, adjustment, and mediocrity.

SUGGESTED READINGS FOR PART 2

Allport, Gordon W.: *Pattern and Growth of Personality*, Holt, New York, 1961.
────── et al.: *A Study of Values: A Scale for Measuring the Dominant Interests in Personality*, 3d ed., Houghton Mifflin, Boston, 1961.
Bennis, W. G., et al.: *The Planning of Change*, Holt, New York, 1961.
Bois, Samuel J.: *The Art of Awareness*, Wm. C. Brown, Dubuque, Iowa, 1966.
Cantril, Hadley: *Politics of Despair*, Basic Books, New York, 1958.
──────: "A Study of Aspirations," *Scientific American*, vol. 208, February, 1963.
Clough, Shepherd B.: *Basic Values in Western Civilization*, Columbia, New York, 1960.
Coon, Carelton S.: *The Story of Man*, rev. ed., Knopf, New York, 1962.
Conrad, Jack: *The Many Worlds of Man*, Thomas Y. Crowell, New York, 1964.
Doll, Ronald, and Robert S. Flemming: *Children under Pressure*, Charles E. Merril, Columbus, Ohio, 1966.
Ellis, Albert, and Robert Harper: *A Guide for Rational Living*, Prentice-Hall, Englewood Cliffs, N.J., 1961.
Farber, Seymour M., and R. H. L. Wilson (eds.): *Creativity and Conflict: Control of the Mind, Part II*, McGraw-Hill, New York, 1963.
Fletcher, J. H.: *Situation Ethics*, Westminister, Philadelphia, 1966.
Friedman, Maurice: *Problematic Rebel*, Random House, New York, 1963.
Gardner, John W.: *Self-Renewal*, Harper & Row, New York, 1964.
Jourard, Sidney: *Personal Adjustment*, Macmillan, New York, 1963.
Kluckhohn, Florence R., and Fred L. Strodbeck: *Variations in Value Orientations*, Row, Peterson, Evanston, Ill., 1961.
Mann, John H.: *Changing Human Behavior*, Scribner, New York, 1965.
Montagu, Ashley: *Human Heredity*, Signet, New York, 1963.
Morris, Charles: *Varieties of Human Values*, University of Chicago Press, Chicago, 1956.
Moustakas, Clark: *Individuality and Encounter*, Doyle, Cambridge, Mass., 1968.

Murphy, Gardner: *Human Potentialities*, Basic Books, New York, 1958.
Sanford, Nevitt: *Self and Society: Social Change and Individual Development*, Atherton, New York, 1966.
Shostrom, Everett: *Man, the Manipulator*, Abingdon, Nashville, Tenn., 1967.
Sorokin, Pitirim A.: *Ways and Power of Love*, Beacon Press, Boston, 1954.
Stein, Maurice, et al. (eds.): *Identity and Anxiety*, Free Press, New York, 1960.
Strecker, Edward A., et al.: *Discovering Ourselves*, Macmillan, New York, 1958.
Tillich, Paul: *The Courage to Be*, Yale, New Haven, Conn., 1952.
Whitehead, Alfred North: *Adventures of Ideas*, Macmillan, New York, 1948.
Whyte, Lancelot Law: *The Next Development in Man*, Mentor, New York, 1962.

3. SOURCES OF CONFLICT FOR COLLEGE STUDENTS

14.

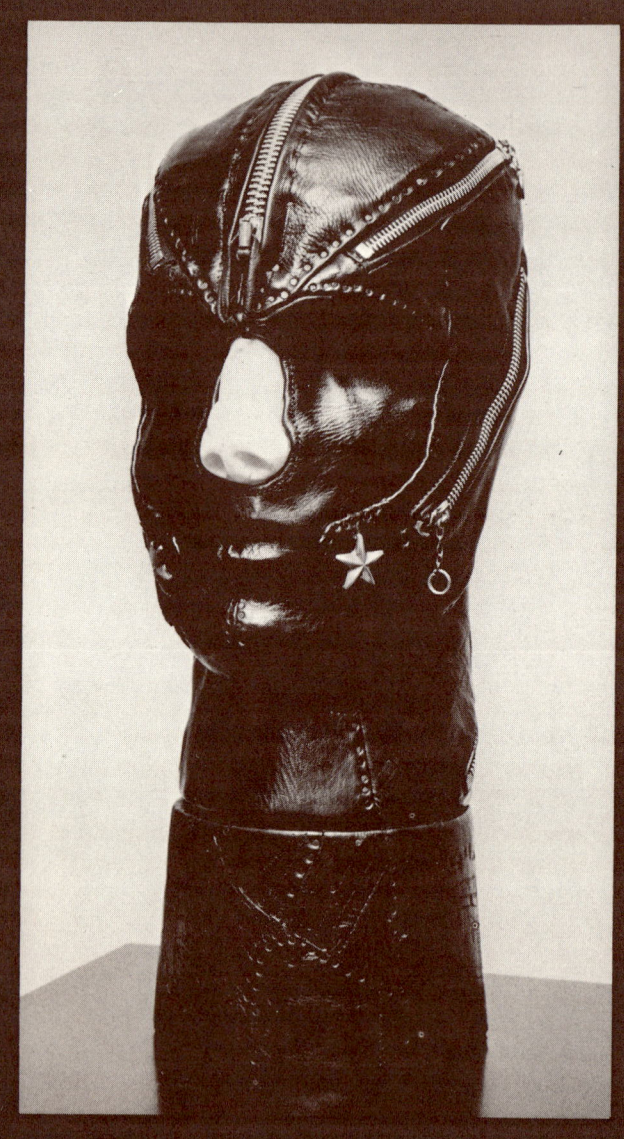

ESTABLISHING AN IDENTITY

No single area is more loaded with conflict than that of establishing our own identity. Our identity, our sense of self, is central to every experience of life. It is the hub around which all other aspects of our lives revolve, the standard by which we judge all other values, and the central motivating factor in determining our response. As we have seen in Chapter 10, our sense of self is in the process of forming from the moment of conception. The process of becoming ourselves never ceases but goes on to the end of our days. The self is the seat of all conflict, for, as the two previous chapters point out, the only real conflicts are those which we internalize, those which become, for a time, at least, a part of our identity. They are painful and frightening because they cause a rending of the self.

Aside from physical change, there is no characteristic which marks the period from puberty to young adulthood more strongly than the search for an identity. Until that time we have lived in a state of semiconsciousness. We have been content to exist within the framework of our parents' values. We have submitted our wills to theirs. But *if they have been successful as parents,* they have made us discontent with this state of affairs. They have made us restless in our desire to find what we mean to ourselves.

The manifestations of our discontent usually burst upon the scene with alarming suddenness. All at once we seem to display a variety of signs that indicate we are not happy with things as they are. But the real search comes on more slowly and, as a controlled intellectual process, hits its peak in the early college years. (Some psychologists may differ with the specific timing mentioned here and say that the process tapers off in the college years.)

In this chapter we focus on the young adult's effort to determine seriously who he is. Some of this search is carried on below the level of conscious cognition; some of it takes place in the realm of obvious knowing. At the conscious level we see what we are doing, we know we are doing it, and we can control what is

Nancy Grossman, "Head," 1968. Leather, wood, and epoxy. Collection, The Whitney Museum of American Art, New York. Gift of the Howard and Jean Lipman Foundation, Inc. Geoffrey Clements, photography.

being done. But because this phenomenon takes place at all levels of consciousness at the same time, the individual often experiences confusion.

No effort will be made in this chapter to resolve the conflicts which develop about the process of establishing our own identity. That would be an unreasonable goal. The reader's attention will be called to the general factors involved. This should help him to spot conflicts as they arise and deal with them with a greater degree of knowledgeable thought.

Characteristics of the Search

The effort to establish our own identity ranges from freeing ourselves from our parents' values (a negating effort) to creating a set of values for ourselves (an affirmative effort). Although the effort to free ourselves from our parents' values is a negating one, it is a necessary piece of work. We cannot manage the job of growing into adulthood unless it is done. Too often we become aware of the negative aspects of the process and tend to blame ourselves for being "bad." Our parents confirm us in this belief. Because in the process of rejecting the old and trying the new we do things which parents and the establishment tend to frown upon, we are judged bad, recalcitrant, headstrong, or just plain ornery. It is not easy to avoid believing these things about ourselves. In fact, there are times when we *are* everything the older generation calls us. All the same, we must go through such phases of belief and behavior.

There may be times when members of the older generation support the changes that the young members of society are trying to effect. Many parents of black students recognize the need for change in the attitudes of the white society toward them. They support their youngsters' actions, even though they may be fearful of the consequences. Many members of the establishment can recognize the need for improvement within the established structure and respect the effort being made to change these negative aspects. With or without our parents' support, it is a difficult task to confront those who resist change and settle for the status quo.

The period of early adulthood includes wide experimentation in behavior, dress, thought, and even looks. In the past few years these manifestations of the search for a specific identity have been more overtly displayed than at any time in the preceding one hundred years in the United States. This is a tribute to people of all generations today. It reflects a greater degree of acceptance among the older generation and a greater imagination among the younger members of our society.

An interesting phenomenon is taking place today with regard to the specific area of testing to find our identity. At the same time that the range of what is acceptable in dress, manner, and mores is broadening and thus providing all people with a greater opportunity to use their imaginations, another force is being felt by young people. In order to define ourselves it is necessary to push against something. We need counterforces to our wishes if we are to develop any strong sense of our own meaning or our own worth. We cannot accomplish these things in a vacuum. When the walls against which we have traditionally pushed for this purpose come tumbling down, we are not only surprised but sometimes dismayed as well. Then the task becomes one of finding new walls to push against.

This has been markedly manifest since the late 1960s. The old standards against which students have traditionally fought have disappeared. Very soon, for example, it will be no big thing for a young man to wear his hair in any style and at any length he wants. The clichés of frightened oldsters (people over thirty) to the effect that "I don't mind his long hair, if he would only keep it clean" will soon disappear. For many, these comments are old hat now. The beads, chains, and outlandish (to the establishment) clothes will no longer have the shock value that they have today.

The effect of this change seems to be that young people are attempting to define their identity in more meaningful ways. It means far more to all concerned when a band of students takes over the administrative office of a college in an effort to force change on the institution than when a group affects an unusual appearance. In other words a new area for confrontation has been chosen. The mode of contact between the generations has changed from one of violating customs to one in which there is far more at stake. One's status, one's protection by the law, and even the safety of one's head are being risked. All this is for a cause. But the cause is not only academic freedom or civil rights or social justice. It is also the cause of self-assertion, autonomy, and self-definition.

It is interesting that this is developing in a period when some of our youth are being called upon by the establishment to risk their lives in a military contest in which there is no clearly established right or wrong. Does this mean that those young people who somehow manage to escape the "call to duty" feel impelled to risk something more important at home? Does this mean that the spirit of the times demands risks for fulfillment and self-definition? If so, then we have some understanding of the motives behind student revolt and the specific path it is taking.

It seems only right that we should move toward testing ourselves in risk once again. It was present in the early days of our nation's history. It existed in the period when our frontiers were being pushed back. It is inherent in the assumption that freedom and liberty are important for human development. It is possible that many young people today feel that the only way they can establish an identity for themselves is to involve themselves in some risk-taking enterprise. To function in a zone where it really counts is what many young people believe is necessary.

If this is so, conflicts are posed for those who are unable to pick up the gauntlet. They are confronted with two opposing theses: On the one hand they feel they should stand up and be counted. At the same time they are fearful of doing so. No amount of rationalization is really satisfactory, because it doesn't establish an identity *which is satisfying.* Self-condemnation, self-doubt, and self-hate are inevitable outcomes of the failure to do it "like it should be done."

On the contemporary social scene this challenge to risk is not confined to men alone. At one time it was the sole prerogative of the male to find his worth in ventures of courage. Today, more and more members of both sexes have become involved in risk-taking ventures. Coeds man the ramparts with their brothers. Female as well as male heads are bloodied in the melees which result. Women risk jail with the same enthusiasm as men. Rather than being a path to manhood social protests and personal risk taking are now a path to personhood.

The Lonely Years

It is a favorite pastime of many older people to relive the halcyon days of their college years. The flush-faced, well-dressed old grad is a popular figure of our time. In his effort to recreate the glory of the past, he gives us the impression that something is missing from the present. When we observe him, we wonder about the real meaning of his past. Something must have been missing there as well, or he would not today be searching for kicks by rummaging around in experiences which should, for him, be best left to their time-consigned resting place.

The emptiness that youth see in so many of their elders is not the result of making concessions to the establishment. It is an outgrowth of a way of life that has been followed for a lifetime. Probably the same emptiness existed for these people in their youth. It is worth speculating on the meaning of the times in which we live and on the life styles we are following. It is important to ask ourselves what our life styles will produce for the future, how what we are doing now is going to influence us later.

Because establishing our own identity is a highly personal job, it is also a lonely one. The young person who doesn't find it a lonely task is probably not doing what he should toward self-actualization.

When one is creating an identity, he faces the same challenge the artist faces in producing an outstanding work. If the artist is really creative, he dare not be a copier. He may have to imitate in his early years, but there comes a time when he must develop a style of his own. He must give his unique statement to the world. To the extent that it is not unique, he has contributed little that the world needs. Doing his separate thing is a lonely task. His work may not be understood. It may be condemned by the authorities of the day. He may be reviled and rejected by the public, but he must have the courage to be himself in the face of all this.

Our identities too are potentially works of art. If we are copiers, our lives will have little meaning to ourselves or to anyone else. This thought flies in the face of all accepted social standards. The tremendous emphasis upon being like others tends to belie the importance of autonomy and self-actualization. The dominant health problems of our society stem from the fact that we are unable to make an effective and satisfying response to the demands of life because we are afraid to be ourselves.

Because structuring our own identities is a lonely job, we tend to seek comfort and solace among others. In addition, we *need* to interact with others to find out who we are. In many cases the group gives the support necessary for a new identity to be internalized. Evidence of this need is found in the behavior of most minority groups. Immigrants from Western Europe settled in self-styled ghettos. They socialized, worked, played together. From this cohesiveness they gathered inner strength and security until they were able to make it on their own in the larger community. The long-reaching effects of slavery, and the racist attitudes of white people, have caused black people to feel negatively about their culture. Black Americans are now accepting their blackness as a vital and positive aspect of their identities. The group has a powerful influence and gives the security that is necessary for identity to be established.

While social groups, ethnic groups, religious groups, etc., have a hand in contributing to the search for self, ultimately each of us must search for that which is uniquely ours. If we are fortunate enough to become a part of a group that encourages individuality (not necessarily being different), we carry on the search in a creative way. But when we imitate simply for the value of being in or because of the fear of being different and the fear of rejection, we do ourselves a disservice, sacrificing growth for security. After we have some security, we should be encouraged to be bolder in our search. We may then attempt to experiment with those life styles and means of expression which will be most relevant and rewarding. What does this mean in practical terms?

Simply being different is not the real measure of value in living creatively. Persons may be different and at the same time be destroying themselves instead of actualizing themselves. In one setting it may be *different* to be a cynical dropout. For the moment this adds little to life. It is a negation from which the individual must eventually recover or die. Obviously, he cannot remain *out* for long and still be in touch with what is going on. Yet dropping out appears to be extremely popular today. The effort, if indeed it does require an effort, to drop out not only is a negation of our culture but may be a negating of the self as well. When this act says that nothing is worth anything, it is patently false. If we consider the potential of any human being, we can realize that he is worth more than even our wildest flights of imagination. The unfolding of his potential is worth all the effort it requires, and the enjoyment of it is worth all the risks he can take.

Lonely or not, the discovery of self is worth all we must do to find it. We must have the faith to follow the paths dictated by the inner voice. If we can hold out long enough, we will find that which is worth cherishing. We need not, then, fill our lives with the empty reminiscences of the hollow men. We need not be copiers of other life styles or resort to destructive means to find kicks in life. The kicks will be found in being ourselves.

The ultimate question each person faces is, "What is the self for which I am searching?" The definition of oneself is determined only with the passage of time. One cannot say, as he sorts over those elements of his being, "This is me, this is not," as if plucking the petals of a daisy. What is the alternative?

Some philosophies would have us superimpose upon ourselves certain basic tenets. The supposition is that once we have incorporated these values into our lives, we not only live the good life but also have found ourselves. Some religions support this belief.

Other philosophies uphold the idea that the self is unique with every individual. Each of us has a basic inner nature which continually pushes toward expression. As we give tentative affirmation to that inner self, we observe it in action. An evaluation of this action in the context of our lives enables us to become more fully cognizant of what we are. The process is one of slow, gradual unfolding which results from continual experimental efforts.

The difference between the two philosophical points of view is represented in the life which is inner-directed versus the life which is other-directed. The inner-directed person receives his motivation from within. The other-directed person functions according to strictures imposed upon him by his environment.

The discovery of one's own uniqueness is a matter of personal choice, and the choice is rarely easy. Making a choice frequently has penalties, but there are rewards too. Presumably the greatest reward will be found with the passage of time: it is probably better to have come to the end of one's days with the knowledge that one had the courage to be than to suffer the guilt of never having been.

The struggle to establish an acceptable identity is frequently devitalizing. Young people often feel that they are one against the world. They believe that they are daring and pioneering and that only as a result of persistent effort will they be able to accomplish what they believe is essential to their own lives.

In many ways these attitudes are well-founded. Self-discovery is an intensely personal task. The lonesome feelings are experienced by oneself alone. The fears, hates, and disturbances are only known by the self. They can be talked about to others, but nothing can dispel the lonely hours that must be spent in isolation. This is devitalizing. The price in terms of personal energy is high.

The Desert-island Syndrome

Frequently young people are led to cherish visions of retreat from what they are experiencing now. The desert island is a favorite dream. Presumably it would be shared by a mate and perhaps a few sympathetic peers. The rat race would be left behind, the establishment kissed goodbye. For all but the very few this kind of escape is impossible. Therefore, other forms of escape, frequently symbolic, are sought.

Although escape is an essential factor in the recovery process, it should not be used as a means of avoiding that which should be faced. The effort to discover an identity cannot be avoided without unfortunate consequences. It has been estimated that 1,000 students will kill themselves each year, another 9,000 will try and will fail, and 90,000 more will threaten suicide.

Most psychologists believe this to be the result of "the identity crisis" of late adolescence. In the late 1960s there was an increase in the number of students with this particular problem. It seems to be difficult to find an identity in an affluent society; apparently the avenues for self-determination have been narrowed and lessened.

Talking It Over

What is to be done for students with emotional ups and downs? The girl with suicidal tendencies who says, "I don't have any friends. Each day is the same. I feel all alone. I don't know anybody," needs help. Suicide threats are often a desperate plea for help. If young people can recognize the signs which they themselves manifest in the critical circumstances of identity formation, they *can* do something to help themselves.

The thing for the student to do is to make known his needs to faculty personnel. Help is available on most campuses for those who want to be helped. While many students cannot afford a private psychiatrist, most colleges have at least one trained counselor available for work with students. Many colleges have whole staffs employed for this purpose. There is always someone with whom the student can talk, and talking it out can make a great deal of difference.

A frequent problem is that students consider it a matter of personal failure to be unable to work out the conflicts they experience by themselves. Shame is associated with the sense of failure. They are unwilling to expose themselves to another person for fear of what may be thought about them. But most people employed by colleges for the purpose of helping students with personal problems have had extensive training in dealing with these problems. They understand what is involved and are sympathetic to the student. They have skills which have been designed to help students identify the problem and to work out alternative solutions to them.

There are guideposts for assessing the worth of the counsel one seeks; this is implied in the phrase *ask him through*. A good counselor, be he a teacher, an older friend, or a trained psychiatrist, usually helps one think his way through the problem he faces by asking pertinent questions *without offering advice*. Although there may be some temporary frustration when a counselor does not immediately offer solutions, a questioning approach probably pays off in the long run in terms of the personal insight gained.

The first advantage is that the questioning approach sets the student on the path of asking appropriate questions of himself. There is carry-over value in this. The process can be used in other circumstances which demand a searching approach. Second, the questions raised should help the student narrow down the alternatives open to him. Third, he is forced to look within to answer the questions. He may have been avoiding the inner look all along and for that reason been unable to solve the problem of developing a satisfying sense of self.

Most psychologists agree that the worst thing a student can do is keep the problem hidden. The student mustn't mistake brooding about a problem for thinking things out. Furthermore the escapist tendencies serve little purpose in the process of identity formation except to confirm, in the mind of the student, that he is incapable of dealing with the central issues of his life.

The Commuter College

The student who attends college while living at home with his parents has special problems in establishing his own identity. First, we must question why he is at home. Is it for economic reasons? Even if he believes it is, we may question further. Few parents of college students do not feel the pinch of sending their children to college, but it is no longer a rich man's luxury. College is within the economic reach of nearly all who do not have dependents. At most colleges today elaborate state and federal subsidies are available for the aid of students in financial need. Between loans, grants, and part-time jobs nearly every person who is willing to work can attend an out-of-town college of some sort.

The real reason for remaining at home may have to do with the inability of either the child or the parent to separate themselves from one another. If this is the case, the problem of establishing an independent identity is severely complicated. As we have seen, the parent-child relationship is tremendously important in establishing an identity. When this relationship is one in which the parents cannot free their child to be himself, they have subtly undermined his confidence in his ability to undertake the difficult task of finding himself. Such problems begin quite early in the child's life. The values about self that were established in the very beginning undoubtedly included such beliefs as "I am a person who is dependent upon my parents," "I am a person who cannot think for myself," "I am a person who does not want to be independent." When these values become a part of the value structure, it is virtually impossible to assert independence from parents.

Parents have a variety of ways of binding children to them. One way is to produce a sense of guilt in the child. For example, when a child does something of which his parents do not approve, punishment is meted out in the form of "How could you do this to me?" from his mother. This may be reinforced by constant reminders of how much the mother is doing for the child. "I cook for you, I clean house for you, I sew your clothes, and how do you treat me?" What child can stand up under that?

Loyalty to home and family is another theme whereby children have been kept from going away to college. Loyalty is a noble sentiment and should be encouraged, but when it is emphasized at the expense of freedom and growth, it is crippling. In our society many adults have not been able to establish an identity independent of family. Successful in business they may be, but as persons they are flops.

Some young people manage to free themselves at marriage from the encircling clutches of their parents. Often, however, they simply transfer their dependence upon their parents to a dependence upon their mates. This may make for a cozy feeling for a while, but unless one of the two is extremely strong, the marriage will be rocked when children come along. Even in the event that one of the couple is strong enough to support the other's dependence, things go well only as long as the strong one is willing to play parent to the other person's child role.

Until recent times people have been able to take shelter in institutions like the home, religion, law, occupation, and parenthood. However, the coming age has all the signs of reducing the importance of these once-reliable establishments. The need to be autonomous, to be ourselves, to stand on our own is increasing with every passing year. Social change is placing too many strains on the old institutions, and the ultimate source of strength must be found in the marvelous endowment with which we are born. If we cannot discover this, the consequence will be boredom with life at best, and at worst little less than personal disaster.

Living with one's parents during the college years makes the process of determining one's identity confusing. The young person picks up behavior, modes of dress, sayings, thoughts, and practices from his friends which seem bizarre to his parents. The parents, in their own insecurity, wonder what they did to produce such weird customs in their child. Feeling responsible, they sometimes feel guilty. Being the deceptive emotion that it is, guilt is then manifest in the attitude of the parents toward their child, and neither understands what is happening. Each begins to react to the other in an increasingly confusing manner. Feelings are rubbed raw. Ultimatums are issued. Both the parent and the young person then believe it is a matter of personal integrity that these ultimatums are upheld.

The student may be asked to leave home, or the student himself may feel that he can no longer live under the same roof with his parents. Male students often feel that they do not want to take any more support from their fathers. They then begin to cast about to find some means of supporting themselves.

Another manifestation of the conflict with parents is the relationship between the student and brothers or sisters also living at home. Often problems not worked out at home are projected into the college scene. The president of a large municipal college in the United States once commented that his faculty must change the intellectual diapers of its students without being able to care for them at home.

The consequences of remaining at home in the important college years are not all bad. A marvelous opportunity for the mutual education of both parents and children is provided. The stresses that each will bring to bear on the other create a demand for learning the skills of communication that is unequaled. In a time when communication is frequently nonexistent between parents and children, the students living at home and their parents have the opportunity to deal with crises as they arise. They can enlarge the scope of their understanding of one another. They can evaluate the impact they have upon one another.

A Creative Approach

Interesting results are coming from research on creative persons. The creative individual has been encouraged to be adventurous for most of his life. Parents have supported these persons in the tasks of identity formation. Recently, two psychologists from the National Institute of Mental Health (NIMH), Dr. Lois-Ellen Datta and Dr. Morris Parloff, reported on a survey of over one thousand teenage boys who had scored high in the Westinghouse Science Talent Search. The boys, as a result of the findings, were divided into two groups—the more and the less creative—according to how the judges rated the originality of their science projects.

Replies to the NIMH questionnaires showed that "the more creative boys . . . had been given much more latitude and subjected to considerably less discipline than the less creative teenagers." One boy said, "They allowed me as much responsibility as they felt I could handle . . . I felt I was trusted." Another said, "Rules, what rules? I was treated as a responsible adult." A third remarked, "I was simply allowed to make my own decisions."

It is assumed that creativity in solving life's problems is also related to this kind of experience. Usually the person who is treated as responsible believes himself to be responsible. He then functions as a responsible individual, with a high degree of autonomy which he projects into the way he meets challenges. The less creative boys in the NIMH survey complained, for example, that "My father has a set of rules that makes the penal code look like a picnic." This suggests that a rigid home experience tends to undermine the ability to deal with challenges *in a creative manner*. It may be assumed that these students had not been treated in their homes as responsible persons. They did not think of themselves this way. Their sense of self was reflected in the amount of creativity they were able to bring to the scientific endeavors in which they were engaged. Datta emphasized that "creative behavior may be significantly related to expectations communicated in ways that the child sees as trust in his ability to choose rationally, thus enhancing his ability and desire to achieve by independence."

What conclusions can be drawn which will be helpful to young people in the process of discovering the self? The person from a home where authority has been markedly exercised by parents must go through critical stages of identity formation during the college years. Although the student who has been encouraged to be independent throughout his life has different battles to fight, he does not have as much difficulty in developing an identity which functions with creativity.

If we can recognize what the experiences of our early years

have been and then identify *how they are operative now*, we are well on the road toward solving the sticky problems in identity formation. If we have not had developmental experiences of the type which tend to motivate us to be creative, it need not prevent us from becoming creative in adapting to life. We can learn to become more creative than we have been. As we have seen, a large part of the task is accomplished if we are willing to experiment.

We should not, however, throw caution to the winds simply because we have decided to experiment with a life style or with particular ways of solving problems. To do so may be just another way of avoiding responsibility.

Experiments in how we relate to others, the kinds of relationships we establish, and the means of communication we use with others are significant areas for exploration. A questioning approach is often helpful. What kinds of people do we seek out? Are they aggressive, domineering, submissive, dependent, self-destructive, self-affirming, happy, optimistic, gloomy, pessimistic? By sensitizing ourselves to these things, we can learn more about ourselves. We can ask ourselves how we project ourselves to others. It is often useful to find out from other people how we come across to them. Do we seem to them to be friendly, hostile, enthusiastic, controlled? When we are in a group situation, do we take the leadership role? Are we quiet, do we feel a part of the group, do we believe that others like us? All this information is useful to us in our efforts to experiment with our relationships.

A general life style may be more difficult to modify. Such changes may come about without our knowledge, or they may result from a careful examination of the values we hold about ourselves, about others, and about life. Some of the values by which we have lived may be inhibiting to us. We should ask ourselves if these values are really important to us as persons. When we find that they are not, some efforts may be undertaken to relinquish them. Often parent-induced values have an inhibiting influence. If we can substitute values of our own, we take a step toward potential growth.

Proshansky points out[1] that

> ethnic prejudice . . . may develop because it provides satisfaction for the high value placed by the person on power over others or on

[1] Harold Proshansky, "The Development of Intergroup Attitudes," *Review of Child Development Research*, vol. 2, Russell Sage, New York, 1966, p. 348.

private property and its protection. On the other hand, to the extent that he can be made to perceive that his ethnic prejudice blocks the attainment of other more significant value satisfactions, or that a more tolerant attitude will lead to such satisfactions, attitude change should occur.

Research studies have shown that such attitude changes do take place.

To some extent this is like the old carnival game: "You pays your money and you takes your choice." If we follow this principle, it is axiomatic that we must be prepared for the consequences. When we are able to do this, we begin to establish useful patterns for living. It is important to remember that there is a price to be paid for any change we make in ourselves. We rarely give up old ways of living without some anxiety. But this may be a small price to pay for growth.

When we recognize that the conflicts inherent in finding an identity are faced by all people, we are less inclined to think that something is wrong with us because we have them. Conflicts about identity are signs of growth; when we accept this, we move closer to perceiving the reality of our own self.

One of the biggest challenges we face is to accept the reality of our own lives. This is often a painful process. It is never easy to relinquish old ideas about ourselves, but it is often necessary in order for change to take place. As long as the old ideas remain intact, there may be no need to change. It is only when the established values about self are shaken in one area or another that we are moved to grow, to accept what must be accepted. The case of Joan illustrates the foregoing principles.

> Joan, a college freshman, was an extremely attractive girl. In high school she had been much sought after by boys. She never wanted for dates, but she rarely was able to attract one boy for any length of time. Her self-centeredness drove them away. Her good looks and surface charm made her popular in campus life for the first few months. Within a short time the word got around that she was a conceited so-and-so. The time between dates grew longer and longer. After the first semester had passed, Joan had very few dates. She was not rushed by a sorority and found herself with very few friends. For Joan this was a frightening experience. It was something she had never known in her entire life.

Her parents were the only ones who had mentioned her selfishness. Many times they indicated that she had exploited them for her own purposes. They believed that she used situations to her advantage and that she played upon their inability to deny her things which they thought were not in her own best interest. But in spite of this insight they were unable to act in any other way. Hence, even when they spoke of their resentment about these things to her, she saw no need to accept what they said. She saw no need to accept the realities of her own identity and therefore was incapable of changing.

It was not until she experienced the isolation at college that she found it necessary to question why. Only after she began, with the help of her roommate, to evaluate some of these things was she able to accept the fact that she was self-centered. Though she fought for some months against accepting this, she finally was able to do so. That was when growth began. She approached others with a greater degree of humility and was pleasant to be with. She sought to discover other values that needed developing in her personality, and she made progress.

Hiding Places

One reason that discovering our identity is not easy is that our society provides many corners for hiding from ourselves. We can hide in academic striving. We can lose ourselves in social endeavors. We can avoid the tasks of self-definition in all kinds of escapist endeavors. Many of these endeavors are socially acceptable, and thus we are able to justify being what we seem to be. Because we obtain some approval for performing in these areas, we have no obvious need to evaluate what we are.

We can fall into the trap of thinking that because our lives are reasonably comfortable, we are all right. The person whose life is pain-free often feels that he must be doing what is important for him to do. And yet, as we have pointed out, comfort is not necessarily a sign of effective living. We have seen that one of the signs of self-actualization is a greater richness of emotional reaction. This means a richness in the experience of *all* emotions, not just those which are pleasant. Only when we are able to recognize all our emotions do we experience this richness.

The unemotional life probably presents sufficient symptomatology in that aspect alone for us to examine more closely the nature of such a life. When people are not aware of a wide range of emotional reaction, they are probably hiding important feelings from themselves. Man is not unemotional by nature. He only becomes so as a result of his particular enculturation. Many persons who have undergone psychotherapy find that one of the greatest values of the experience is that they are able to let go and allow their emotions to show. Much energy goes into suppressing our emotions, energy that could be used more creatively in personal growth.

We can hide from the challenges of *being* by accumulating material wealth. This endeavor is one of the major hiding places our society provides. Erich Fromm makes an interesting distinction between *having* and *being*.[2]

> In the use of the verbs "to have" and "to be," people talk in terms of "I have." For instance, people say "I have insomnia," instead of saying, "I cannot sleep." "I have a problem," instead of saying, "I am unhappy." And they have, of course, a car and children and a house and a psychoanalyst; but everything is expressed in terms of "I have" connected with a noun and not in terms of "to be" connected with a verb.

The heavy emphasis which our society has placed upon *having* has made it possible for us to avoid *being*. Although having makes sense in terms of things, it makes no sense in terms of people. The diversion from being to having is one of the most profound distortions of our nature. The deception serves only to confuse us, and because our society tends to weight it heavily, we have settled for this rather than address ourselves to the more difficult and often more painful task of being. The result is a desperate sense of emptiness about the meaning of our lives.

An identity cannot be found in terms of what we have. It is only defined with satisfaction in terms of what we are. To reverse the direction of our lives from "have" orientation to "be" orientation requires an enormous effort for many of us. It means denying much to which we have been conditioned in our own homes. It means denying what our formal education, with its emphasis on grades, has taught us. It necessitates searching for that which is not clearly defined and which will only be known when we have it. Because the search is fraught with anxiety, with risks, and with frustrations, many of us, in spite of good intentions, abandon it.

---

[2] Interview with Erich Fromm, R. Heffner (ed.), *McCall's*, vol. 93, October, 1965.

In abandoning this search, we imperil our health. The life situation, as it has been presented in this book, includes the necessity of being. When we avoid this, the quality of our response to the life situation is poor. In some cases, it is not only poor but destructive.

This need not be the case. We have control over these responses. We can learn to use our creative potential and develop our resources for courage. By doing so, we find a purpose for being which is rewarding in itself. Our lives are richer, and we become the kind of people we want to be.

15.

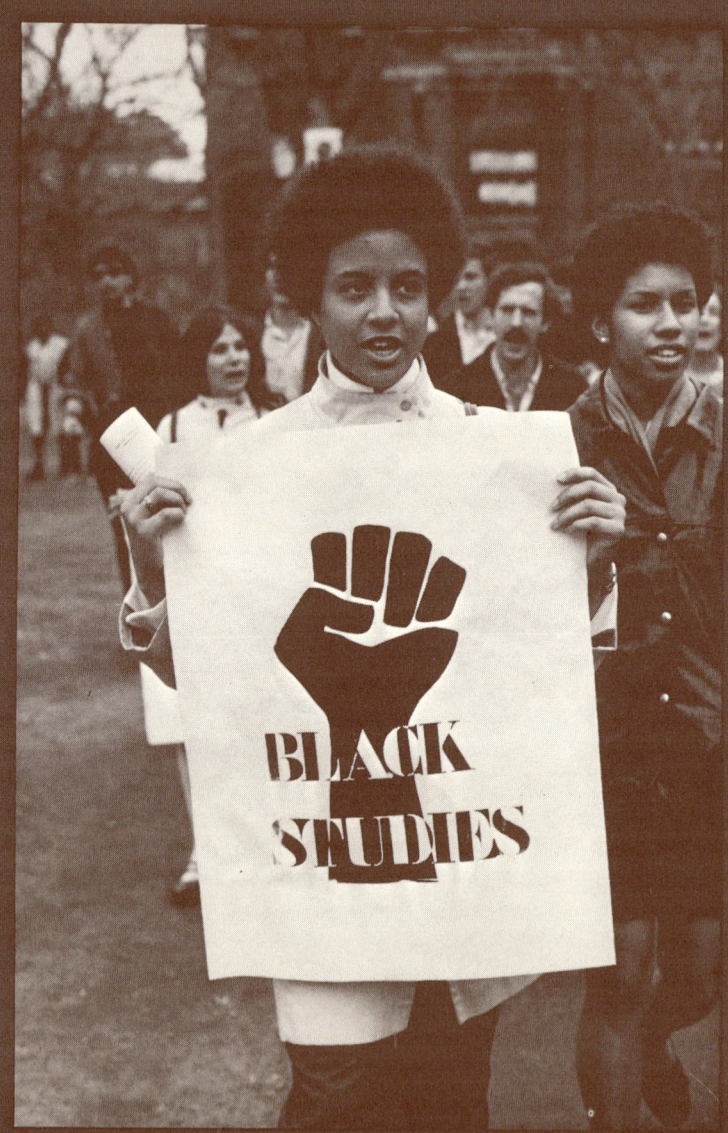

TO CONFORM OR NOT TO CONFORM

Too often we attempt to don an identity simply because it is approved by others and we hope it will make us acceptable to them. As we have seen in the previous chapters, this does not work. When we attempt to be something that we are not, we confuse, frighten, and frustrate ourselves. In our attempt to conform to some standard of being established in the past and copied by millions of our fellowmen we deny our own basic nature.

In one sensitivity training group a young coed was "rapping" to her fellow group members about her parents. With a pained and angry expression on her face she fumblingly tried to express her feelings about them. "I don't know, it seems that they don't really care about me at all. All they want is, like, for me to be what they think I should be. They don't know where I'm at, and they don't care."

"You're right," one of the men replied. "I love my parents, and all that, but they really don't want me to be me—at least, not the me that I want to be."

Again the girl spoke. "But what can I do? I have to do my thing, but my mother makes me feel so damn guilty about it when I do."

Here is the basic problem of conformity. No group of young people, when talking about the things which concern them most, is long free of the topic of conformity. The need to conform and the need to be themselves continually grate within them. Finding an outlet for their sexual drives is tinged with the problem of conformity. Finding a set of values of their own is related to it. The challenge of being themselves is intricately interwoven with it. In short, one of the basic developmental tasks of early adulthood is to resolve the conflict of whether and to what degree we should conform.

Constantine Manos, photography. Magnum Photos, Inc.

What Does Conformity Mean?

Like every real conflict, the problems which center around the issue of conformity are painful, anxiety producing, and frustrating. They hurt because they produce anxiety. They are frightening because we are frustrated in finding the answers we are seeking. They frustrate us because we cannot identify what is wrong. All we know is that we are not comfortable in one or more areas of our life.

One young man in a health education class professed to having found a solution for himself. He told his classmates, "When I first got here, I tried to make it socially the same way I had in high school. I tried to fit in with the crowd, but I found I couldn't. So I stopped trying. I was lucky. I had a girlfriend. We just spent all our time with each other. But I guess that isn't right, either. We never see anybody else." He thought he had found a solution, but he felt it wasn't quite right. In a society which emphasizes gregariousness, we tend to blame ourselves if we are loners. He hadn't really solved the problem. He had merely withdrawn from the zone of pain.

Another young man said, "I'm one of those guys who's always the center of the crowd. I can make the right crack at the right time. I don't know—I guess I learned that in high school. But, you know, I always knock myself afterwards. It's like they all want me to be that way, and so I am. I guess I really don't like myself for doing it. I don't feel like I'm being myself, whatever that is."

Here we have two young people each dealing with the situation in different ways. And yet, neither of them feels that what he is doing is right. One condemns himself for being an isolate. The other dislikes himself because he fits in at the expense of being himself. In fact, the second man is not even certain what he is. Probably the reason he doesn't know is that he is merely being what others want him to be.

At the moment of speaking each of the young people found himself locked in a way of being which did not bring satisfaction. Why was this so? It would seem to be a fairly simple thing to break a pattern of behavior if it causes so much distress. Yet there are few among us who are able to do this easily. The task is difficult even for those who are older. A graduate student in her late twenties in a similar kind of sensitivity session admitted her inability to break a relationship she was having with a married man even though she recognized that it was "sick." She was fed up with it and with herself. She even hated herself because of what she was doing and yet had been unable, for two long years, to break out of the trap in which she found herself.

In actuality it is foolish to speculate about whether or not we have the willpower to do the job we have to do. If we had it, there would be no conflict. We could draw upon this source of strength to control whatever we needed to in ourselves, and because we had the power to free ourselves from the enculturation of our society, we would be more able to act autonomously and, thus, be ourselves.

Self-acceptance

Most of us have a conscience which operates with varying degrees of strength in different areas. A conscience, the watchful self, can be a valuable asset. It enables us to see ourselves in action. It provides guidelines for behavior. It tells us when we are not performing up to expectations. But when it is so overbearing that we continually condemn ourselves, no matter what we do, our conscience has made it impossible for us to live with ourselves. We are then ill equipped to resolve the conflicts of our lives.

For every effectively functioning individual a strong measure of healthful self-acceptance is essential. The comic strip character Popeye had the right idea when he said, "I am what I am and that's all that I am." He had no unreasonable expectations of himself, and he valued what he was able to do. If we assume that the only way we will be acceptable to ourselves is by doing what others expect of us, we are doomed. Our adaptive responses to life will be continually geared to what others expect. No adequate or autonomous identity will grow out of the experiences created from this motivation.

We must be able to convince ourselves that we are acceptable persons in our own right. No one else can do it for us. Each of us has a responsibility to ourselves to find elements within ourselves which are worth valuing and which we must put to work so that we can value ourselves more. One such quality may be that we are sensitive to another's feelings. In other words we can listen intelligently and know what others feel. The basis for empathic ability is not yet clear, but social scientists have found that it seems to be a prominent feature of personalities possessing ethnic tolerance. Through this power to empathize we are able to render great service to others.

One person may have the ability to be an excellent conversationalist. He handles words well, can articulate his ideas, and knows the skills of communication. It would be foolish for him to damn himself because he happens to be inadequate in athletics. It would be as foolish for the good listener to assume that he must also be a central person in a group that values joking, kidding, and witty banter. As a listener he can fit in well and be a valued group member.

Most of us are not comfortable in a stereotype. Not all men are endowed with the stereotyped manly qualities. Not all women are comfortable in the stereotyped pattern of femininity. A generally useful principle of human relations is to reject the stereotypes of ourselves and of others as well. They add little to the human experience. They contribute nothing to the ability to be autonomous.

A basic task of becoming mature is to learn to accept ourselves with all our faults and foibles. Even the best of persons is not without faults. A personal fault, itself, may make other qualities we possess of greater value by contrast. Many professions are made up entirely of people who chose their line of endeavor because of some "weakness." Many execellent teachers started in their work because of their sense of inadequacy. As a result of this they have chosen a field which offers a degree of stability. Psychiatrists often study psychology in an effort to understand themselves better. Many persons with outstanding analytical ability have gone into lines of work which enable them to use this skill, rather than try to use qualities in which they are deficient and which may initially render them inept in the social graces. In the process of becoming skilled in their chosen field, they have poured their energies into their work, have found success, and thus have been able to begin a slower process of unfolding in the realms where they originally felt themselves to be deficient. In the long run they have become useful individuals. They have also moved ahead toward self-actualization.

Self-acceptance is vital. When it is accomplished, we no longer feel eompelled to be like others. We are then free to allow our inner, hidden self to unfold. Enormous quantities of energy are conserved when we reject the temptation to conform to the expectations of others.

The Revolt against Self

Discontented people usually articulate some measure of resentment against others. A student in a large metropolitan university complained about the treatment she received in a gynecologist's office. She had gone there to obtain a prescription for birth-control pills. As a matter of policy the physician had his nurse-receptionist obtain a medical history of all new patients, and in the course of routine questioning the college student revealed why she was there. The nurse-receptionist, noting the student was not married, asked when the wedding would take place. The student squirmed uncomfortably and lied. She was not, in fact, contemplating marriage at all. The truth was that she did not even have anyone about whom she cared a great deal.

Her complaint was that "they" seemed to feel that the only acceptable sexual experience took place within marriage. She went on at great length about the narrow-mindedness of society and proclaimed that she was not about to conform to such idiotic conventions. If she had not protested so strongly, she would not have been suspect, but an older friend, overhearing the conversation, realized that this young woman had been making inferences from her interview with the nurse-receptionist which were simply unfounded. The student assumed, from the line of questioning, that her request for the Pill was being challenged. No such intention was in the interview. The student's own sense of guilt was at work. In effect, she was condemning herself and using the interview as a means of doing so.

This is a familiar technique. All of us have done it. What we recognize as a weakness in ourselves, we assume is something which is imposed upon us by society. We then proceed to blame society for ideas we have dreamed up ourselves or which have been *a part of our own value structure.* Young people in the midst of conflicts about satisfying their sexual drives blame society for its rigid moral standards. Young women, fearful of yielding to the advances of their dates, blame the men for causing problems. Students caught in the academic rat race blame the institution for expecting so much from them.

The things about which we complain most bitterly are usually those which have been established within us. No young person of college age can truthfully say that they are really restricted in expressing their sexual drives. Nor can they say that colleges expect too much of them. The problem really is an internal one. What most of us are most strongly in revolt against are the values which we ourselves hold. We have expectations for ourselves which are inconsistent with other desires we have. If any person is willing to accept the consequences of his behavior, he is free to do most of the things necessary for growth into full humanness.

When we have begun to accept responsibility for our own feelings, we increase the chances of upgrading the quality of our response to life. We are not totally freed from problems, but we have learned some of the skills of dealing with them. Our reserves of energy are used for more productive efforts. We are not then in revolt against ourselves.

Why Do We Conform?

Basically, conformity results when we are fearful of another mode of behavior. When we lack the inner conviction of our own ideas, we tend to follow those of other people. This phenomenon can be observed in a wide range of contexts. It is natural that this should be so in the earliest years of our lives.

During the years of late adolescence and early adulthood we substitute one set of values for another. For many this is scary. Whenever we shuck off an old identity and grow a new one, we are made uneasy. We have seen how the developmental task is accomplished, and we have followed the step-by-step emotional influences. Within the context of the developmental task there is the pull toward a new self and a corresponding attachment to the old. It is a tug-of-war, in which we are torn between two forces: we want to go ahead, but we are fearful of doing so.

Conformity often takes place in the social scene at the college level of development. Usually there has been an obvious break from an old context of living. Students have left home in a symbolic sense if not in a real sense. They feel cut off from the comfortable and familiar identity of the home. Because of the drive to belong, they are almost compelled to seek acceptance in the new environment. If the efforts they have used previously (in high school) do not accomplish this, they then attempt to adopt the attitudes and behavior of those to whom they wish to relate—the in group. Dress, speech patterns, ideas, political beliefs, social attitudes—all tend to be similar.

The reasons center largely around the safety in being a part of a group. This is not an unreasonable motivation. It can be expected that when people are breaking away from one style of life, the home style, they will seek some form of safety in other relationships. The person who cannot become an in person suffers real anxiety and pain. His sense of self-doubt is apt to be exaggerated. He has left the old but has not made it in the new. He wonders where he is. He assumes something is wrong with him.

Because the assumption of worthlessness is extremely painful, the individual tends to project this sense of wrongness to others. As one young man said, "I don't give a damn about them. They aren't worth my time." He then proceeded to construct an elaborate rationale to explain to his faculty-member "friend" just why he had rejected "them." The "them" in this case was the fraternity group that had not bothered to rush him.

So it is that in the process of growth, as we are compelled to leave the old and familiar, we are driven toward another context of conformity. When we are not able to make the transition, we scramble desperately to find meaning in almost any context that presents itself. Some of us are fortunate in that we happen to relate to circumstances and situations which have developmental outcomes. Those of us who are less fortunate relate to circumstances which can result only in creating further self-doubt.

The extreme, but not uncommon, situation is that of a person who becomes involved in behavior and practices which tend to destroy his well-being. This indicates a lack of integrity and also leads to further disintegration within him. Clearly, the quality of his response to the existential situation is poor.

Resisting Growth

We stand a better chance of moving through the transitions of life effectively when we know that our ultimate goal is one of self-actualization. So many times young people have no clear perception of where they are going. Neither can they see themselves in perspective. The resulting anxiety is often devastating, and many are led to do almost anything to escape it. It is well, however, to remember that some degree of anxiety is inescapable in the process of growth. The movement inherent in growth causes anxiety to arise. Without it there is no need to grow.

A very real danger lies in the fact that many people attempt to arrest growth simply to avoid the pain it entails. The symptoms of this are all around us. Often this is more easily seen in others than in ourselves. How, then, can we know when we ourselves are resisting growth?

The first step is *recognizing that it is possible* that we are resisting growth. This presumes an honesty with oneself which may be unprecedented. To some degree all people tend to resist growth. The resistance is stronger at some times than at others.

Second, we must be capable of *recognizing a sense of threat* when it arises in us. When we are open to growth, we are less inclined to feel threatened by new experiences. We listen to suggestions of friends or associates and are willing to take some risks in encountering the unfamiliar, from trying new foods or a new dance step to entering into new relationships with people.

When, instead of accepting responsibility for what happens in our lives, we are in the habit of *blaming others*, we are showing a sign of resisting growth. When we experience frustration, those of us who resist growth are inclined to seek an explanation in circumstances outside ourselves. If we fail a course, we may blame it on poor teaching. The breakdown of a relationship is often blamed on the other person. A rejected suitor tends to blame the person who rejected him.

Another sign of resistance to growth is *refusal to affirm oneself* in a group situation. This self-negation shows itself in a wide variety of ways. The person who dresses to be like others, the person who adopts the opinions of others, the person who gives up his own beliefs for fear of being different—all are resisting growth.

Antithetical to this, but equally a sign of refusal to grow, is the practice of so *strongly dominating others* that they have no opportunity to initiate events which would cause change to occur—the young man, for example, who dominates his fiancé to such an extent that she cannot make decisions of her own, or the girl who, through her temper tantrums, manipulates her boyfriend. The person who refuses to associate with others unless he has his way is also resisting growth.

Unusually aggressive behavior is related to domination of others and has the same purposes. It may often be a sign of resistance to growth. By being continually on the offensive we keep others from attacking us or even from reaching us.

General withdrawal is another clue to our unwillingness to grow. When we avoid issues, commitment, or confrontations with others or with the circumstances of our own decision making, we are exhibiting a refusal to put ourselves in growth-promoting situations.

Inability to be spontaneous is an avoidance to growth. When we must resort to regular patterns of response that have worked for us in the past, we are not growing.

The *lack of an adventurous spirit* about life shows limited confidence and usually eliminates participating in those circumstances out of which growth proceeds.

Lack of creativity in solving life's problems is another sign that we are rejecting growth. When we cannot be creative in finding our own resources, we are not unfolding the potential inherent within us.

Mature Self-control

When persons are able to assume responsibility for their own actions, they are on the path toward freedom from the need to conform to any set of values other than their own. They have developed the autonomy which enables them to function independently of what others think. If they experience failure, they can assess the reasons for it, knowing whether they have been responsible for the failure or whether it was inherent in the task they undertook. They are not concerned with self-blame but are able to develop a sense of perspective about what happened. The experience is taken in stride without undue stress.

For many of us, self-control has connotations of holding back. If, in our homes, we have learned that expressions of certain emotions are "bad," we learn to disguise these emotions. It is possible that we ourselves will not recognize them for what they are. This is not what is meant by self-control. Quite the contrary, the individual who possesses it is able to express those emotions which are appropriate to the situation at hand. If anger is indicated, it can be shown without undue guilt. If love, or joy, or pain is felt, it can be expressed. The person with mature self-control is aware of what he is feeling. If confusion exists, he can recognize it as such. From this point he is able to introspect to discover what feelings are producing the confusion. He then knows what to do about the feelings.

The person with mature self-control has greater freedom to be himself. He is not compelled to conform for the sake of security, for he has found security where it is most important—within himself. As he learns more and more to express himself, he moves further toward discovering his inner self. More and more he becomes himself as time goes by.

He has greater freedom from guilt when he makes mistakes. Stress becomes less important in his life. Conservation of his resources is possible, and adaptive energy is not needlessly expended in recovering from neurotic feelings of threat.

The mature individual is able to tolerate differences in others. More than this, he welcomes this difference, because it adds savor to his own life where it touches him. He is inclined even to seek out those people who can add variety to his life. He is freed from the monotonous sameness of a relationship with others who differ little from him in background or life style. When he reaches this stage of existence, his whole life opens up before him, and he discovers experiences he did not dream of before.

The person who has gained control over his own feelings is better equipped to withstand expressions of anger and displeasure by others. He can assess the context in which the anger is shown and knows when it relates to him and when it is a problem of the other person. He may even develop the skills of helping others deal with their anger when it arises. Since anger is an emotion which many cannot handle with ease, he can render a great service in this respect.

Finally, when challenge arises, the mature individual can keep things in perspective. He does not "blow his cool." However, this is not mere covering up of feelings. By maintaining his cool he allows his feelings to flow freely and reaps the rewards of the energy mobilized from them.

Intelligent Cooperation

It is important to make a distinction between conformity and intelligent cooperation. There is little to be gained in the overall scheme of things when we conform for conformity's sake alone, but there are many occasions when cooperation is important.

One may ask what the difference is between cooperation and conformity. Often there is no difference in motivation. One may cooperate for fear that if he does not, he will be subject to discrimination or ostracism. But other elements in cooperation take it beyond the limits of conformity. Cooperation is associated with a goal which is not mere acceptance. It is usually associated with getting a job done. One cooperates with another in order to bring some degree of mutual benefit. Conformity, on the other hand, smacks of exploitation—a use of a relationship for selfish gain.

In a cooperative effort it is not necesary to give up or obscure one's basic identity. Cooperation does not cause one to deny what he is. To be sure one must often surrender temporarily some of his own personal desires. For example, one may cooperate with a friend in order to get an unpleasant job done. In the process he may have to get himself dirty, tire himself out, and perhaps even risk injuring himself. Another example of cooperation is seen in the effort to help another person work out a personal problem. There may have to be an investment of time, effort, and comfort to accomplish the task. In each case there is a voluntary effort of the will to commit oneself to working together with another person. In conformity the voluntary element of the task is absent. One is much more apt to be compelled by an inner drive toward security when he conforms.

Cooperation may, however, take the form of conformity. When one agrees to conform to the mores of his culture for the reason of protecting another person's feelings, he is acting unselfishly. When one agrees to behave in a conventional manner because this facilitates the human relations of the situation, he acts with intelligence. Good manners often fall in this category. They make it possible for people to work together in difficult situations without unnecessary friction which would serve only to exaggerate the differences involved.

Cooperation and conformity are not opposites, nor are they mutually exclusive. The big difference is in the element of conscious and voluntary choice and in the goals involved. When there is an element of mutuality of concern in the act, then it can be described as cooperation. When we are solely concerned with our own well-being and are fearful of acting in a self-affirming way, conformity is in effect. Growth results from cooperation. No growth results from unquestioning conformity.

When we are free from the need to conform, we are able to tolerate difference in others. More than this, we are able to welcome difference in others and enjoy the richness it adds to our own lives. Through all this we become bigger people. We are also more effective. We are able to enter into cooperative efforts with others without sacrificing our own identity. We become more individual, and our value to ourselves is enhanced.

16.

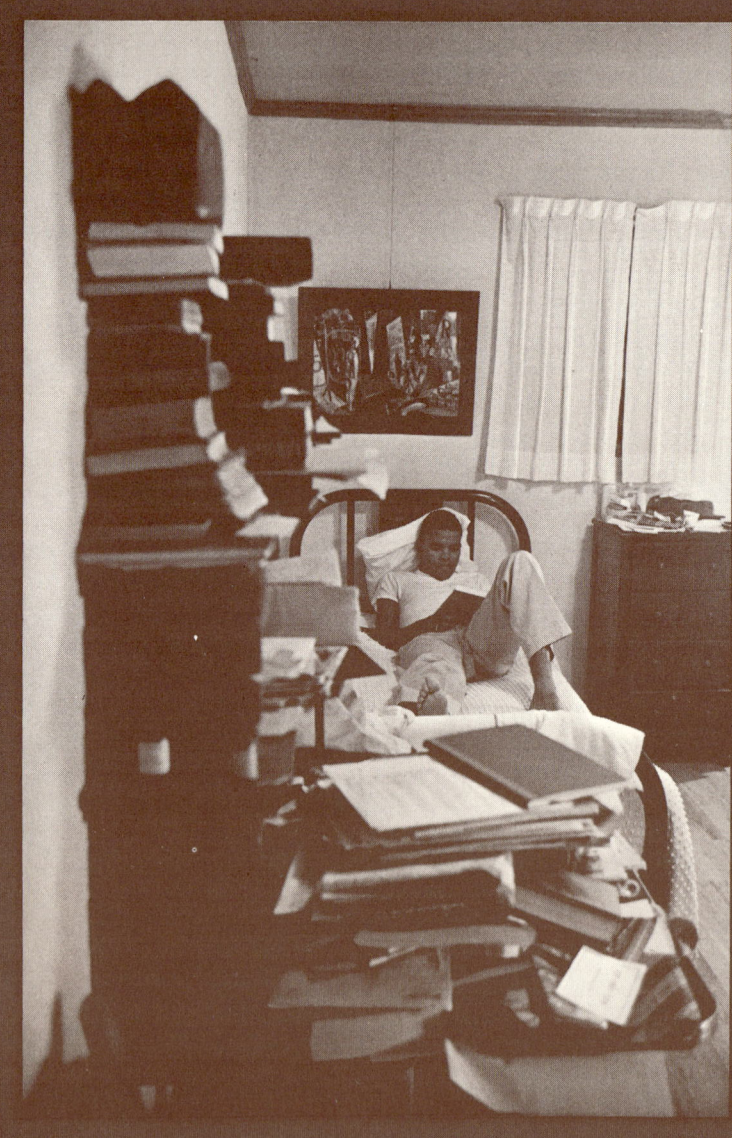

COMPETITION AND ACADEMIC PRESSURE

At the time of this writing one of the authors spent much time in discussion with students at Brooklyn College who were involved in a vigorous confrontation with the administration. Three words came into the discussion frequently: *dehumanization, impersonal,* and *irrelevant.* The students were giving voice to a loud and lusty wail of protest against practices of academia. Because of its massive size and its effort to produce large numbers of degree-bearing graduates, the institution, they said, was impersonal, which contributed to the dehumanizing experience. Because of the concern of the academic establishment with numbers and its consequent lack of concern for the specific interests of individual students, much of the educational material to which the students were exposed, they claimed, was irrelevant to their lives. On a broader basis, they said, the whole society was engaged in similar dehumanizing practices.

The Extent of Student Protest

As one listened to what these students were saying, one could not help but recognize the legitimacy of their claims. Much of the student revolt across our nation has been of a similar nature. The specific issues differ on individual college campuses, but the students' basic concern is with obtaining a greater voice in what happens to them in the important years of transition from youth to adulthood.

What is interesting, and perhaps tragic, is that many young people are not engaged in vigorous protest. To the thoughtful observer the high incidence of escapist endeavors—the use of pot, the increase in drinking, the incidence of suicide—all indicate that something is wrong somewhere, something so painful that for many life as it is isn't worth living. Yet the percentage of college students directly involved in active participation in events aimed at bringing about change is relatively small. It is often difficult to say

Magnum Photos, Inc.

where student sympathies lie, but it is not hard to count heads among the activists. An estimate of 20 percent of the student body of any particular campus engaged in active protest would be high.

What does this mean? Are the vast majority so bound up in the need to conform that they are unwilling to risk the consequence of promoting change? Do they actually believe that the established order, rigid and alienated, is really better than anything else? Are they already so alienated that they are not aware of the potential hazards of conformity? Are they so bemused by dates, parties, studies, and athletic spectacles that they see no need to change? Or are they engaged in personal change to such a degree that they are not capable of rocking the boat?

The Nature of Academic Pressure

What is the nature of academic pressure? The term suggests the sense of oppression which results from being forced to produce at a high rate and in extreme competition with fellow students. While this is a part of the problem, it is by no means all. If students use this label to describe all the problems associated with college life, they deceive themselves and make it difficult to identify the elements of conflict. Establishing their own identity, integrating successfully into the college scene, and dealing with the problems of sex and sexuality (discussed in Chapter 18) are also involved.

If students could separate out the tasks involved in meeting the demands of study imposed upon them by professors, most students would have little to worry about. They have enough intelligence and aptitude and the goals necessary to accomplish the tasks. But there is a basic conflict: Many young people have been conditioned to the idea that they are a success *as a person* only if they produce material evidence in the form of good grades. At the same time they are driven toward identifying themselves as persons by developing their unique and individual potentialities.

When seeking his identity in endeavors as narrowly defined as traditional academic study, the student is often apt to experience frustration in large doses. It is true that a sense of worth may be developed through academic excellence, but for most students this is not a broad enough context to provide complete satisfaction. The ensuing frustration becomes a stressor. The frustrating situation demands a response which will release the tensions generated. But too many students are unequal to defending themselves against the threat they feel in the frustration and can only seek some form of escape.

Generally speaking, students accept the academic situation which places each student in competition with his fellows and creates conditions which call for maximum effort most of the time. Therefore, when they do not perform at maximum levels, they feel guilty and unworthy of the faith which their parents have placed in them, and of whatever belief they have had in themselves.

Since most students do not think of themselves solely as intellectual, they desire to seek fulfillment in other areas of life as well. This necessarily takes time from the effort to achieve academic excellence. The student who does give a large portion of his energies to other endeavors may actually be succeeding *as a person* more than the one who devotes himself wholly to his studies, but he often believes that what he is doing is not right, whereas the student who confines himself to the narrow world of study believes himself to be a success.

For the many students who, faced with this personally paradoxical situation, feel they must resort to escapes, as heretofore mentioned, this becomes the ultimate in producing anxiety, frustration, and an excruciating sense of the meaninglessness of life. No wonder so many intelligent students are eager to reorganize the system that, they believe, places them in this uncomfortable situation.

Success of Others

The college student often sees others around him who are "succeeding" when he believes he is not. Every campus has its quota of eager beavers who are willing to spend much of their time getting the grades. Most students believe that it is against these individuals that they should measure themselves. Even if they reject the idea that study is important to the exclusion of other things, they find it difficult to overcome the insidious influence of comparison.

The norm then, becomes willingness to forgo some of the important elements of living to achieve excellence in studies. This is fine for some students but not for all. In an effort to establish himself in the scheme of things, the individual conforms to an ideal established by those who have different inclinations from his and then measures his worth in terms of other people's values instead of his own.

Parents and teachers work together to reinforce values about the importance of academic excellence. Many teachers measure themselves in terms of whether or not they are able to get large numbers of students to give evidence of having remembered large amounts of information. The "good student," then, is one who has demonstrated his ability to remember this information at least long enough to record it on examinations designed for the purpose of testing memory. If the institution is a large one and has many large classes, the teacher is tempted to reduce the time spent in marking such tests by making them short-answer tests. Many colleges have computers which will grade such papers for the teacher.

The result is one more experience in the dehumanization of which so many students complain. Each one feels that he has been reduced to a memory machine. Serious questions can be raised about the morality of such practices.

In order to survive in such situations, many students resort to cheating on an examination. From files of "successful" term papers, maintained by various student organizations, the same material is used over and over again. In most cases this kind of dishonesty adds little to the cheating student's self-valuation. Brought up in the context of being honest, it is difficult for him to think highly of himself when he violates the values which have been established within him by his parents. The student then wonders at the purposes of his entire life. In his loss of innocence he frequently becomes, at least temporarily, disillusioned, convinced that the establishment and his life as a part of it are meaningless.

Some colleges are apt to be anxiety mills. Both students and faculty contribute to this. It is important for the student to assess accurately the nature of the school he attends before he condemns himself for not living up to the norm. Once he has done this, he should become aware of his part in producing the anxiety he feels.

Once again, when we can get things in perspective, they do not bother us so much. We see the total person; we are not trapped into believing that academic success is the *sine qua non* of the successful life; and we are able to free ourselves from the unreasonable sense of oppression we sometimes feel in the academic setting.

The following letter, written anonymously and appearing in a number of college newspapers, gives a humorous touch to the problem of keeping things in perspective.

Dear Mom and Dad,

It has now been five months since I left for college. I have been remiss in writing, and I am very sorry for my thoughtlessness in not having written before. I will bring you up to date now, but before you read on, please sit down. You are not to read any further unless you are sitting down. Ok?

Well, then, I am getting along pretty well now. The skull fracture and the concussion I got when I jumped out of the window of my dormitory when it caught fire shortly after my arrival are pretty well healed. I only spent two weeks in the hospital, and now I can see almost normally and only get those sick headaches once a day!

Fortunately the fire in the domitory and my jump was witnessed by an attendant at the gas station near the dorm, and he was the one who called the fire department and the ambulance. He also visited me at the hospital, and since I had nowhere to live because of the burnt-out dormitory, he was kind enough to invite me to share his apartment with him. It's really a basement room, but it's kind of cute. He is a very fine boy, and we have fallen deeply in love and are planning to get married. We haven't set the exact date yet, but it will be before my pregnancy begins to show.

Yes, truly, I am pregnant, I know how much you are looking forward to being grandparents, and I know you will welcome the baby and give it the same love and devotion and tender care you gave me when I was a child. The reason for the delay in our marriage is that my boyfriend has some minor infection which prevents us from passing our premarital blood tests, and I carelessly caught it from him. This will soon clear up with the penicillin injections I am now taking daily.

Now that I have brought you up to date, I want to tell you that there was no dormitory fire, I did not have a concussion or skull fracture, I was not engaged, I do not have syphilis, and there is no man in my life. However, I am getting a D in history and an F in science, and I wanted you to see those marks in their proper perspective.

Your loving daughter,

Burdens from the Past

Most American universities are diversified enough for students of varying degrees of intelligence to achieve an education. Every high school graduate should be able to get through college. If he is unable to do so, he is probably carrying burdens from the past which are crippling him. He may lack confidence, be disturbed by his inability to crack the social scene, or have left a girlfriend behind, or he may be failing because his failure serves a purpose in his life. For one student, failure may be a means of self-punishment. For another, it may serve as the best means he has of retaliating against his parents for real or imagined hurts they have inflicted upon him.

Persons engaged in such tactics may thoroughly believe and protest loudly that self-punishment is not a factor with them. But any student of average intelligence who has produced the high school marks necessary to be admitted to college and who is failing must examine his motives. His failure cannot be laid to lack of intelligence. Unless he has been ill, has missed work, or is distracted, he can assume that his failure is serving a purpose for him. This is a dogmatic statement, but in a middle-class society in which success and failure are loaded with symbolic significance, it is virtually a truism.

What are the burdens of that past which contribute so much to academic pressure? There are so many and they vary so much that only a few of them can be indicated here to illustrate what is meant:

1. Parental expectations
2. Value conditioning
3. Attitudes about self
4. Attitudes about education
5. Give-up-itis
6. Judging self-worth by grades
7. Unrealistic expectations
8. Compensation for social ineptitude
9. Loss of perspective
10. Need for self-punishment
11. Need for status
12. Need to compete

Concerns about the Future

Academic pressure is often complicated by students' concerns about the future. Both men and women are influenced by these concerns. Both have important stakes in the future which are directly related to their attendance at college. These concerns tend to be exaggerated in the mind of the student. Young people often feel themselves to be in a bind if they are in college primarily to prepare themselves to be wage earners. Most of them are concerned with more than just self-support. For them, identity will depend on the amount of success they achieve in the professional or business world, and therefore they believe that what happens in the college years is critically important to their future.

Both men and women want to prepare themselves for a future that will be satisfying and productive. One distinction between the male and female experience should be made, however: The male has an additional pressure, because his job usually will be the primary source of income after he has established a permanent relationship with a female. More often than not, especially during child-rearing years, his income supports the entire family. While women are more apt to think of their wage-earning potential as temporary or as supplementary to the household, men assume that their wage potential is crucial.

In recent years, both men and women have recognized the need for more flexible patterns of life. Marriage is no longer the measure of social success that it once was. Women can choose a career, home, or both. Some couples have moved toward a style of life that rejects materialistic standards of success. They look upon work as merely a way to provide for basic survival needs. It is a healthy sign that these many alternatives exist in our society.

Another source of concern centers about graduate school. A frequently used rationale is that unless one gets good grades, he cannot go on to graduate school. For some the necessity for graduate training is essential. For others, however, graduate school has become essential only because it postpones facing the realities of the workaday world. Facing this challenge squarely might really be a salutary thing for many persons. The avoidance of the task simply prolongs the anxiety.

As long as our country maintains its need for large numbers of young men to man its military establishment, the draft continues to be a source of anxiety. At present the need to maintain full-time status as a student haunts many young men. This creates pressure not only to succeed but often to remain in courses which are totally unsuited to the interests of the student. Few college men are willing to accept the possibility of being drafted lightly. For most there is a desperate sense of urgency associated with remaining in college. This is so even when they feel they are not getting anything worthwhile out of their studies. Most men students believe they have no choice open to them but to remain in college. It is not strange that they feel the pinch of "academic pressure."

Whenever our concerns for the future bear heavily on what happens in the present, a sense of urgency arises in us. This stimulates some people to work well and produce better than if the pressure were not there. For others, the anxiety may impair performance and, when coupled with other immediate concerns, may be a load that is too great. Unless the student has a strong constitution, some breakdown is inevitable.

Reduction of Anxiety

When this combination of pressures is felt, it is often necessary to seek some kind of out. Some outs are constructive and developmental. Other forms of escape are destructive. For some persons active participation in athletic endeavors is an effective means of relieving the pressures they feel. Contact sports such as football, soccer, lacrosse, and hockey allow a release of large amounts of tension and aggression. Individual sports such as skiing, archery, bowling, and swimming appeal to those who can transfer their feelings about other things into movement. Combative sports such as wrestling, boxing, and judo allow the participant to test himself against an opponent in feats where safety is risked and where skill is at a premium.

Many other areas of endeavors are open to college students for the kind of escape that is necessary to break the tension of academic pressure. Student organizations provide a change of pace. Campus politics open the door to those who need to feel that they have an influence upon their social environment. To the extent that these activities provide a symbolic outlet for otherwise unexpressed feelings, they are constructive. When they also lead to the development of skills and talents heretofore unused, they are developmental.

However, when an activity, whatever its nature, diverts one's life energies from the tasks of self-actualization, it is destructive. It is customary to condemn such activities as drinking, pot smoking, and the like. But there are times when these escapes provide a respite for persons which can be experienced in no other endeavor. Many a soldier in combat has found that a roaring drunken escapade is a salutary thing. Even though he feels depleted, exhausted, and dissipated afterward, it has served a purpose in breaking the tension in which he existed prior to the binge. He is then able to return to the demanding circumstances of his daily existence. Tension has been released, anxiety reduced.

To determine the effectiveness of an escape it is important that we recognize what we are doing and the reasons for which we are doing it. If we deceive ourselves, we are unable to evaluate the quality of our response. Furthermore, it leaves us helpless to influence that response constructively.

The Lost Self

In the crucible of academic pressure, young people frequently find themselves lost. Usually the young person feels himself pulled in many different directions at the same time. He is incapable of responding adequately to all these pulls. Since he tends to give credence to the validity of these pulls, when he cannot respond to them, he thinks of himself as a failure.

He tries to protect himself by saying that nothing matters, but deep within he knows that it all matters a great deal. These conflicting attitudes are a very real part of all of us. As time goes on, the diversion may become deeper. A sense of desperation sets in.

At this point of desperation, the young person is apt to venture into areas of experimentation that he has never known before. In the words of the straight society, he "goes off the deep end"—and there may be several deep ends at one time. He seems to be saying, "If I can't find myself within the establishment, maybe I can outside it."

The events of such a period are scary indeed. Those who love the person most are often frightened by his bizarre behavior. Because parental values have been well established within the young person, he may even scare himself with his own exploits.

The interesting thing is that most young people grow through this period of experimentation and are often better people for it. As we have seen in the previous chapter, often the people who do not go through a period of wild experimentation do not become self-actualized. They play it safe at the expense of their own development. The period of lostness is usually a period of transition from one way of being to another, leading to something more constructive and ultimately much more satisfying. If this stage could be recognized by those in it as a preliminary to growth, it would be less frightening, and thus less devitalizing.

College Is Not for Everybody

College is probably not for all people. Some individuals might benefit a great deal if they went to work for a few years before entering college. Others, already in college, would benefit if they dropped out and went to work or entered the military. The rationalization for not doing this is that it becomes that much more difficult to get back into the study routine once one has left it. Nothing could be further from the truth. When there is solid motivation, the academic studies entered after a few years of maturing are immeasurably more valuable. This fact is attested to by countless numbers of students who have had the experience. Some students have taken on the responsibilities of families that they must support. The task of doing this and working toward a degree is a hard one. Even so, studying is often far more rewarding at such a time than when a person enters college directly from high school.

Making a Choice

Academic pressure is more or less real according to the way in which we see it. If it is our choice to become so involved in it that it dominates our lives to the exclusion of all else, one set of consequences will ensue, whereas if we recognize that the college years are only a short span of time and that we have many more years before us, our choices will be different.

If we assume that academic excellence is paramount to making ourselves more effective persons, then we must give ourselves sufficiently to this endeavor to get satisfaction. If we assume that we will become better persons by following another path, then this is what we must do. Something in between may be the choice for others. Whatever we do should be done with zest. In spite of what many people feel, life in the United States is not like life in a jungle. One of the values of living in a society like ours is that few mistakes are irrevocable.

The only really irrevocable decision is to play it safe. When this is followed to the end of our days, the life lived will be wanting in many areas. The rich life, the healthy life, can rarely be found by playing it safe. Self-actualization does not come to those who are not willing to take risks. The very process of unfolding one's potential necessitates moving into areas of being which are unfamiliar. One must risk being wrong; one must risk failure; one must risk the potential hazards of self-induced growth.

Academic pressure, if one chooses to identify the college scene in these terms, does not need to be defeating. If one can sort out the many factors which lead him to believe that he is under pressure, he will recognize that it is not pressure at all. Academic pressure is usually of one's own making. Like all potential sources of conflict, it is good or bad, not by virtue of what exists, but by virtue of how we feel about it and how we respond to it. We have some degree of control over this. We can have increasing measures of control over it as we learn the skills of identifying what it is that bothers us.

17.

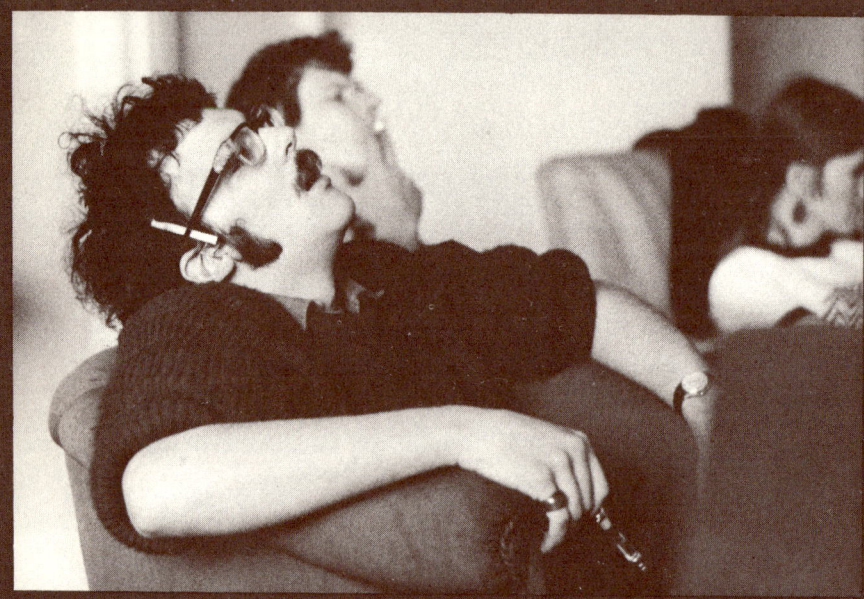

THE DYNAMICS OF ADDICTION AND DEPENDENCY

One source of conflict for college students has to do with the use of drugs. The large numbers of young people who are using drugs of one kind or another have created a climate of opinion in which the nonuser of drugs feels unable to make an effective decision. The decision is a personal one, but unfortunately many students in their need to conform to the values of their peers make their decision to use dope entirely on the basis of social pressure.

The primary purpose of this chapter is to enable students to think about what they are doing so that their decisions about drug use will be a result of their own examination of themselves. The views expressed here may not agree with those held by the reader. They are expressed to provide a basis for thought and discussion and should be read in that spirit. They are not the views of any one group, nor do they preclude ideas which may not be in agreement. They are the convictions of the authors and result from discussions held with people of all ages who use or have used mind-altering substances enough to recognize some of the influences the substances have had upon them. The focus in these next pages is upon the person who uses drugs rather than the drugs themselves.

The Drug Problem

A graduate student reflecting on his experiences with psychedelic drugs came to the conclusion that these drugs no longer served a purpose for him:

> I have stopped taking drugs. . . . It became too easy to "grove" on something . . . without ever coming to terms with real problems, without ever really thinking. The borders of illusion and reality became hazy.
>
> I consider it now a part of the growing-up process. It was an answer. It no longer is. I am still overwhelmed by the mad-

Ian Berry, photography. Magnum Photos, Inc.

ness that is my country, but I must find another way of coming to terms with it.

For the student who made this statement, these were important words, and they are equally important for those who attempt to understand the college drug scene. The statement tells us a lot about why young people become involved in using drugs. For many they appear to be an answer to some of the difficult and painful tasks which youth and young adults must face as they come of age in the United States. The older generation has tried to accomplish the same thing by eroding sensitivity and the awareness of reality, by dulling the cutting edge of life, and by anesthetizing the painful stab of conscience.

In neither case has the appropriate response been found. Closing one's eyes, dulling one's senses, and refusing to face reality do not work. Only the steady, often painful process of moving toward maturity and self-actualization enables one to cope effectively with life no matter how unpleasant its challenges may be.

The increasing frequency with which young adults are using drugs of various kinds has put panic in the hearts of the straight society and has become a problem of national proportions. Statistics indicate an enormous increase in the numbers of young people using drugs on a more or less regular basis. In the first half of 1970, in New York City alone about five hundred people died from an overdose of heroin.

Any person, young or old, who has never used any of the mind-altering substances, is in a state of confusion about what to believe. Research, being incomplete, only stirs up controversy. The laws vary from state to state, and enforcement is inconsistent. Newspapers refer to a bust of four or five young people as a drug raid of major proportions. Innuendos of sex orgies accompanied by drug use scare many parents, and they are thus unable to discuss the topic of drugs with their children except in moralistic terms. The regular users of mind-altering substances promote their own brand of propaganda. A large amount of energy is dissipated in the fight over whether or not to legalize marijuana.

What is one to believe?

Agencies concerned with the rehabilitation of drug addicts are in conflict with each other. Few agree on what method should be used, and each claims for itself the one true method. There is a religious fervor among these people which reminds one of the sin and salvation preachers of the early American frontier. Great heat is generated, but very little light is shed.

Political figures, seeing the American panic, have entered the scene. Each candidate is eager to capitalize on the fears of his constituency. He promises to solve the problems by establishing programs, and he proposes the expenditure of various sums of money for this purpose. In the meantime, in order to create public backing for his programs, he highlights the worst aspects of the problem.

Social Factors

The attempt to solve problems through the use of drugs has become a part of the life style of millions of Americans. We take pills for everything from nutritional deficiency to anxiety to muscle aches and pains. The person who takes a pill to go to sleep is not, however, doing anything to discover what it is that is keeping him awake.

A diet pill is an easy answer to the problem of overeating; it is much harder to exert personal controls over one's eating habits. Aspirin cures headaches for many people, but it does not enable them to discover the cause of the headache. If we ignore the cause, we have done nothing to prevent recurrence. The phenomenon is cyclic: symptom–pill–relief–return-to-symptom.

Some people are able to use drugs to relieve a symptom but at the same time do the work that is necessary to prevent the symptom from arising again. They can recognize what causes the symptom and act to correct the condition from which it grew. Headaches, for example, are frequently the result of repressed anger. It is important for people who often experience headaches to examine the circumstances which precede the onset of the headache. If they find that anger has been repressed, they may learn to express their anger so that the headache does not occur again.

Using inappropriate patterns of dealing with life, many people have become addicted to, or dependent upon, a great variety of devices which create an allusion of doing things the easy and painless way. In addition to the various pills with which they avoid accomplishing basic tasks, some people use reading, for example, as an escape from working out difficult problems; others use TV. Most devices of this kind are socially acceptable, and often their use is even encouraged, but people frequently become dependent upon them to avoid reality. Whenever they become dependent upon an area of their life style for security, that part of their life style should be questioned.

Seeing Drugs in Perspective

The increasing use of drugs must be seen in relation to what is happening throughout our country and in relation to the many other devices on which we are dependent but which are socially acceptable. *Social acceptability is not the criterion of whether a practice is worthwhile.* As we have noted, many practices which have achieved social acceptability are damaging. The use of drugs must be seen in perspective.

The occasional user of marijuana is in no greater danger than the occasional social drinker. In truth, he may be in less danger than the inveterate smoker of cigarettes or the person who depends upon laxatives to perform a basic function of nature. Overeating, a problem for many Americans, is more damaging in the long run than an occasional puff of pot.

On the other hand, the person who has found that the only way he can find any enjoyment in other people or in himself is by using a mind-altering substance is in trouble. Somehow, he has not developed his natural capacity to enjoy life. He has become so inhibited that he is unable to see things with a naïve sense of wonder. Apparently he is unable voluntarily to let his mind become involved with ideas or things so that they have fresh meaning for him. He believes that to accomplish this he must depend upon some artificially induced state.

We need to recognize that we are dependent upon, and addicted to, many practices, drug use included, which are at the least nondevelopmental and at the worst destructive. Within this frame of reference we have allowed ourselves the luxury of avoiding a critical look at what we live by, regardless of the consequences to ourselves.

What Motivates the Drug User?

The Search for Kicks

Apparently some people's motivation in trying drugs for the first time is the search for new and more exciting experiences. The very fact that taking a mind-altering substance is against the laws of most states provides something of a thrill. The illusion of excitement and daring creates a sense of unity among those who use legally forbidden substances. It accounts for the sense of in-ness which the pothead or the acidhead experiences. This camaraderie may be totally new to the individual. Perhaps for the first time in his life he feels himself to be a part of a group the members of which are sharing something outside parental control. This in itself provides a thrill, and the compelling force of the in feeling often renders the individual incapable of objectively deciding against the practices of the group, even when it is in his own best interests to do so. Furthermore, the first-time experience with mind-altering substances may add a dimension to life which is equally compelling (see "The Search for Deeper Meaning," below). The temptation to try it again and again is great.

Escaping Reality

That the drug user is trying to escape reality has become a cliché. All the same, there are unquestionably many persons who use drugs because it enables them to avoid the pain or the boredom of their everyday existence.

> While Tom had never got into the hard drugs like heroin, he had been psychologically dependent upon pot, LSD, mescaline, and peyote. For him, no day had been complete without turning on. No insight, he believed, was real unless it was induced under the influence of dope.
>
> Now, in his early twenties, he has rejected dope as a means of filling the void in his personality. He testifies to the futility of drugs as an answer to life's problems. He says, "Whatever the original motivation for taking the stuff, whether it is kicks, a search for personal insight, or the desire to appreciate things more, I believe that the basic and ultimate reason for using dope is to cop out. As a college radio commentator on drugs, I have never interviewed a drug user who was not fundamentally avoiding personal responsibility for his own life."

The Search for Deeper Meaning

Some people who use marijuana find that the world and life seem more meaningful. The gist of their message appears to be that everything is seen in a new dimension. Music has new meaning, color is richer, persons are comprehended in a different light than ever before. Insights into oneself become more meaningful, and one may learn to cope more effectively with his hang-ups by focusing on them in a manner never before attempted. Qualities of courage, lovingness, humor, and freedom are experienced as they have never been when the individual was straight.

Some people who have used dope extensively are skeptical of the validity of these experiences *as they apply to the challenges of daily life.* One former drug user says, "Yes, the claims are valid.

You do experience things you have never known before, but while you're in one kind of world of reality [*a highly subjective concept*] under the influence of the drugs, it is a mistake to assume that the insights you gain when you're in that condition can be applied to the reality of the straight world."

Major Drugs

We are mainly concerned here with those drugs on which some form of dependence develops. It is important to recognize that while some drugs do not establish a physiologic dependency, they nevertheless produce in the habitual user a need to continue using them. The use of the drug becomes a part of his life style, and he cannot imagine living without it.

Many users of the "soft" drugs (those which do not produce a physiologic dependency) fail to recognize that a substance which interferes with the normal process of cognition, evaluation, and decision making can, when regularly used, limit the kinds of experience necessary for growth. They uncritically assume that they are in control, that they are not doing anything which is harmful to the body and are, therefore, safe. This assumption should be carefully examined, for it is not unquestionably true.

Psychedelic Drugs

The most widely used psychedelic drugs are marijuana, hashish, and LSD ("acid"). Along with the other psychedelic drugs, like STP, peyote, mescaline, and morning glory seeds, these hallucinogenic substances commonly produce a high in which the user feels that he sees things with a greater intensity than under normal circumstances. Most users take these substances for their purported value in producing personal insight and a mystical relationship to one's environment.

Unquestionably there are changes brought about in the way in which the user sees things and in the way in which he sees himself in relation to what is around him. However, these two questions arise: (1) What are the physiologic and psychologic effects of these substances on the user? (2) Are the "mind-expanding" claims realistic?

Although research on the effects of these substances is inconclusive, it is known that LSD is a powerful drug. Microscopic amounts can produce effects upon the user. It is therefore extremely easy for the novice to overdose himself, not only producing a bad trip but possibly with profound and prolonged effects upon his psyche. Nearly every type of personality disorder has been noted among persons who have undergone a bad trip. An exaggerated sense of anxiety is frequently characteristic of an overdose of LSD and sometimes leads to behavior in which the individual attempts to drop out of everything.

With marijuana the story is different. Its effect is much milder. It does not produce the marked changes experienced while under the influence of LSD. For the infrequent user there are probably no more damaging effects than those experienced by the infrequent drinker. The danger appears to be that the person who has serious work to do, as everyone has, in dealing with his life problems may feel that he does not need to take care of this work if he can escape into the euphoria that marijuana produces.

Marijuana, unlike LSD and most other hallucinogens, acts as both a stimulant and a depressant. It tends to accentuate whatever the user's mood is at the time of use. However, it often results in a sense of depression as its effects wear off. Some former users of marijuana report that there was a tendency to experience paranoid feelings during the entire period of time when they were using the stuff, including periods when they were not under the influence of marijuana.

Opiates

Opiates are drugs derived from opium, the most common being morphine, codeine, and heroin. These drugs have a profound narcotic or depressant effect upon the habitual user. Initially "hard" drugs may produce a kick, or thrill, but the tolerance one develops to the drug soon necessitates larger and larger doses to produce this effect. Eventually the kick is gone, but the pain-deadening effect and the physiologic dependency remain. The habitual user finds himself more concerned with getting his fix to avoid the painful and sickening effects of the absence of the drug, once the body has formed a dependency upon it, than he is with achieving a sense of euphoria.

Some users of heroin may mainline the drug for long periods of time with a once- or twice-a-week frequency without developing a physiologic dependence on it. This is probably due to the fact that most of the heroin available today is so cut with other substances that its potency is limited. If it were purer in content, this freedom from physiologic dependency would probably not last for long.

Most persons using the drug, however, soon find themselves dependent upon it. Once this occurs, the risk of overdosing is ever-present. It is difficult to determine whether the deaths from an overdose are the result of the depressant effect of the drugs upon the vital organs of the body or of the impurities injected into the system along with the drug. Individual variability is also probably a factor in these deaths.

Sedatives

The effect of a sedative is to quiet one's reaction to anxiety-creating thoughts or events. Sedatives have a wide usage among people of all walks of life. Barbiturates are frequently prescribed by physicians for patients who have difficulty in managing the anxieties of their lives. Even within the medical profession there is some controversy about the value of their use for some patients. Either side of the argument may be supported. The patient with a bleeding ulcer needs sedation. On the other hand, the person who is having difficulty with the events of his life may not be benefited in the long run by the administration of a depressant drug. It may be more important for him to receive help in learning how to deal with his problems than it is for him to deaden the impact of these problems upon him. This is one of the dangers of the use of sedatives on a habitual basis.

Furthermore, barbiturates may become addictive. Another danger lies in the fact that it is possible to ingest excessive amounts of a sedative. Hundreds of suicides in recent years have been accomplished through the use of sedatives in large amounts. These deaths are usually the result of respiratory arrest due to the action of excessive amounts of the drug.

Among the sedative drugs are bromides, barbiturates, tranquilizers, and alcohol. All these have a depressing effect upon the person and his system.

Alcohol

Few people recognize that alcohol has some of the same properties as the other depressant drugs. Jones, Shainberg, and Byer[1] indicate that "alcohol, when consumed in abusive amounts, is truly addictive, and the sudden withdrawal of alcohol from an addicted person produces serious disturbances." In other words,

---

[1] Kenneth Jones et al., *Drugs and Alcohol*, Harper & Row, New York, 1969, p. 42.

dependency on alcohol develops in the heavy user, as with other addictive drugs. His drinking becomes a part of his life style. He drinks in times of crisis, and even an evening with friends must be accompanied by heavy drinking.

It should be of interest to every "social drinker" to assess his drinking habits. When he gets together with friends, does he feel that a drink of alcohol is necessary to make the evening complete? Even people whose drinking goes no farther than a couple of drinks an evening find this amount essential to conviviality. While this amount of drinking can hardly be considered a problem, the fact that it is felt to be necessary and is missed if not available bears examination. Perhaps it is only a habit, but perhaps there are other reasons. Does this social drinker need to receive a little courage from a few drinks to free himself from the inhibitions he feels when sober? Can he be himself only when high on alcohol? If this is so, probably a large amount of his capacity to enjoy life is locked up most of the time. This is a tragedy of contemporary life. Millions have lost the ability to enjoy themselves without additives.

The tragedy is multiplied when one becomes dependent upon the additive, for if he does not learn to develop his innate ability to enjoy life and deal with his feelings, the skills of recognizing and releasing them are never used.

The social drinker, and even the heavy drinker, is not to be confused with the person who is classified as an alcoholic. Theories and definitions of the alcoholic vary, but all authorities agree that he has personality disorders, social problems, and physiologic dysfunctions.

Once started on a drinking spree, the alcoholic finds it impossible to control his drinking. Frequently, once he is a confirmed alcoholic, he will begin with the intention of having one drink and then will continue drinking heavily until he is no longer able to lift a glass. This ordeal may continue for days, weeks, or months. The interest in food is lost; his preoccupation is solely with where the next drink is coming from. Family, friends, and other responsibilities are totally neglected in the pursuit of alcohol. Nutritional deficits are created, and damage is frequently done to the body.

It is important to note that alchoholism does not manifest itself in this full-blown stage overnight. There is a stagelike progression toward these circumstances. The alcoholic consistently rationalizes his drinking. Many an alcoholic, even when completely unable to stop drinking, will argue that he can stop any time he wants to.

He refuses to recognize his own dependence upon drink. Others may be suspicious of the compulsive nature of their drinking but not be far enough along in it to realize that they are in its grip.

Some alcoholics may consume less alcohol than other persons who are only heavy drinkers. This knowledge clearly enables the alcoholic personality to convince himself that he is not in any real danger of becoming lost in drink.

The early stages of alcoholism are similar to the kinds of drinking experienced by many social drinkers. The process moves from controlled social drinking to escape drinking, in which the individual drinks to get away from things that bother him. The incidence of escape drinking increases until the individual one day experiences his first blackout. He returns to consciousness after some period of hours or even days of total lack of awareness of where he has been or what he has experienced. From this point on he moves toward an increasing loss of control of his drinking, until he has periods of prolonged intoxication and finally total addiction to alcohol.

The complete cycle varies in time span among individuals. Some may reach addiction in a matter of months. Others may find the cycle spanning a number of years. Simply that one is not in the final stages of the cycle is no indication that he is not on the way. Wherever alcohol is a definite and important part of one's life style, the user should be alert to his motivations and the direction this element of his life is taking.

Amphetamines

Amphetamines stimulate the body, producing some degree of euphoria and providing a pickup for the user. The drugs in this classification have been used for some time by physicians in cases where it is necessary to speed up certain body processes.

They are frequently used by persons who suffer from minor periods of depression, for they are effective in snapping one out of these states. However, they are not effective in cases of chronic depression. The habitual user of amphetamines will develop a tolerance for them that will necessitate his taking larger and larger doses in order to provide the kick he experienced when he first started using them.

The habitual user of amphetamines readily develops an emotional dependency upon the drug. As he increases his daily dose, he tends to suffer loss of appetite, experiences a marked increase of irritability, and as a result loses sleep. He becomes aggressive and difficult to get along with, and thus isolates himself from others simply because they cannot stand to have him around.

This combination of events produces a sense of being alone. Paranoid feelings multiply, and living becomes intolerable. The habitual amphetamine user is a sctup for heroin. With the depressant effects of heroin and its eventual production of oblivion, the anxieties of life are gone.

Another danger in the prolonged use of amphetamines is that the excitation it produces pushes the user to expend his reserves of energy without replenishing them. The result is physical exhaustion and the accompanying psychic disturbance that such exhaustion produces.

Phoenix House

To become more familiar with the dynamics of drug use, we spent several days discussing this phenomenon with residents of Phoenix House, a therapeutic community under the direction of New York City Addiction Services Agency for the rehabilitation of drug addicts. Each of the discussants had been a resident in the community for at least a year, and all of them had been heavily addicted to hard drugs for several years. They had broken the habit and were engaged in a rigorous program of self-evaluation which caused them to face up to the "character disorders"—*their words* —that had led them toward addiction.

We asked if they thought there was a basic element common to the lives of all persons who become addicted to drugs. Ira, a man of about fifty who had spent nearly half of his life in prisons and who had been on drugs for 32 years, ventured an answer. His face showed the depth of his thought as he hesitantly said, "I would say that deprivation, a sense of deprivation, was the common factor."

"Do you mean deprivation of love?" asked Bren, a twenty-two-year-old who had been on drugs for 10 years.

"Yes, but not just that," Ira replied. "I mean the deprivation that comes from whatever keeps you from being yourself."

"For instance?"

"Well, religion, for instance. Not believing, but being forced to go to church. Not having what you want. Not being able to think what you want—parents often prevent this. Not having a sense of freedom. Or feeling that the world is all against you. All these things make you feel deprived."

As we continued to explore this idea, it developed that all eight of the participants, who ranged in age from fifty to eighteen, some black, some white, both men and women, and members of various religious backgrounds, had had experiences which left them feeling a basic sense of loss. They all felt that life had shortchanged them, and all admitted to feeling hurt by the experience.

The discussion eventually revealed that there was a definite pattern in the life of the addictive person. For each of them, there had been a steady progression from feeling deprived to becoming an addict. The only thing that differed was the time span.

First there was the sense of deprivation. It is interesting to note that all people experience this. Every one of us, if we review our own lives, can find circumstances which left us with the feeling of being deprived of what we needed to fulfill ourselves. Accompanying the deprivation there was a deep hurt which was carried through months or years of life. This too is an experience common to all people. We have all felt hurt by life or by persons close to us. The pain surrounding a sense of deprivation is more intense and more lasting than any physical pain we can experience. It becomes a part of our personality.

Our natural tendency is to try to eliminate the source of the hurt. When this cannot be done, other defense mechanisms are brought into play. It is possible to suppress the feeling of pain. We can say that what we want really doesn't matter, or we can deny the existence of the pain and convince ourselves through attitudinal adaptation that we really aren't hurting. But often when we do this, the effort is so great that all other feelings are suppressed along with the pain. The ability to experience fear or anger or love is also dampened, and as a result we turn off many of the satisfying experiences of life which would do much to counteract the sense of deprivation.

Anger often overlies pain. Many people have incorporated anger into their life styles. This also results in turning off the satisfying experiences of life. An angry person cannot feel pain; neither can he fully feel love or friendship, and he thus deprives himself of those experiences which are really necessary for him to mature.

The result of the turned-off existence is that life becomes flat and uninteresting. Each of the Phoenix House discussants admitted to having dull lives before they began to use drugs. For them drugs were a way of changing the experience of their lives. "I was fed up with school and the silly things the other kids were doing," said Barbara, a woman of thirty who had resorted to prostitution to support her increasingly expensive habit. Wayne, a sensitive young black man, put it this way: "I was so damn disgusted with my parents, my friends, and my whole race that I was willing to do anything to get away from it all. Reefers seemed to be the answer, for a while."

In one way or another every one of these former addicts indicated that they just didn't give a damn about their lives or anything in them. All they wanted was to be able to get away, even if for just a little while. For most of them marijuana created the illusion of being able to escape. Most of them used alcohol too. But it didn't work for long. While under the influence of dope, they became introspective and aware once again of the pain they were feeling. Life became unbearable for them. Feelings of paranoia overwhelmed some of them. They felt that everything was stacked against them.

"Man, I felt I couldn't get anywhere." "Nobody really cared what happened to me." "I felt my boss was out to get me." This was the way they put this phase of their experience. As time went on each of them felt an increasing desire to get away from it all. Heroin provided the answer. With it they would feel nothing. Life could be endured. No more pain; no more anger; no more need to care what happened to them or what other people did or felt. Nothing.

The rest of the story is familiar to most of us through the news items that appear in the mass media about addicted persons. The desperate search for the next fix or the money to pay for it, the lack of sleep when the next day's supply is not on hand, the focus on drugs to the exclusion of anything else, and the progressive deterioration of personality.

The person moving toward addiction is unwilling and perhaps even incapable of admitting the fact that he is dependent upon whatever he is using. Throughout the experience leading to heavy addiction not one of the former adicts had been able to respond to the warnings of others. It did not matter if the person was one who had been through the experience or not. When he was on marijuana, he believed that he could stop any time he wanted to. It did not occur to him that this was his only hold on an interesting life. This is the nature of the psychological dependency that may develop in the user of the "harmless" soft drugs.

What conclusion may we draw from these observations made by the former addicts of Phoenix House? Should we assume that pot, LSD, mescaline, and the other psychedelic drugs inevitably lead toward addiction to the harder stuff? Definitely not. There is no evidence to lead us to believe this is so. Can we say that all drugs are dangerous and that the solution to the problem of drug abuse is to ban all drugs? Again the answer must emphatically be no. Drug use is symptomatic of more fundamental problems. The individual who needs dope is unable to develop innate resources for living satisfyingly. He places the blame for his lack of enthusiasm in life outside himself and avoids personal responsibility for the development of these resources.

Risks of Trying Drugs

There are risks involved in experimenting with dope. One is that the person who depends upon drugs to lift himself out of despair, who turns on to find relief from pain, who gets high to be in with the crowd may not be facing the reality of his own personality. He needs to look more, not less, at what he is and where he is going.

Another hazard lies in the fact that whereas not long ago there was a sharp line between those who used soft drugs and those who used the physiologically addictive substances, now more and more young people are moving across this line. Heroin use is beginning to assume epidemic proportions. Many times heroin is easier to obtain than marijuana. The social acceptability among many drug-using groups includes a ready acceptance of heroin.

Perhaps another reason for this is that the hysteria with which the establishment has viewed all drug use has created the impression that there is really no difference in the effect of the different drugs. Reaction to this hysteria may well cause many young people to become involved in heroin use simply to indicate their disdain for the irrationality of the establishment.

Furthermore, the straight society has issued such dire predictions about the use of all drugs that the person experienced in the use of the psychedelic drugs is skeptical and does not believe what squares say about any of the drugs. Thus, he may assume that heroin is no worse than the marijuana or LSD that he has experienced.

It is impossible to draw sharp conclusions about the risks involved in experimenting with any of the agents which can alter one's consciousness. Individual variability of reaction is one factor which presently makes conclusions difficult. Another is that the grade of marijuana varies in its influence. Since the drugs used, the use of them, and the experiences resulting from them are highly subjective, current research studies are always open to question.

The social mystique which surrounds the use of hallucinogens also presents a problem. Probably most of the users of pot, hash, and acid are in an age group ranging from sixteen to thirty. This age range is widening every day. Most of these persons share a disillusionment with the established order of things. They feel bonded together in a common plight and powerless to change society.

The young in this age group feel that the use of the soft drugs is their thing. They feel a sense of unity in the experimentation with these agents. It provides an opportunity to exercise autonomy in their lives, and they therefore tend to believe that anyone who "smokes" or "trips" is really into things in an important way. The indiscriminate acceptance by some people of any person who does these things is startling.

This social mystique, as mentioned at the beginning of this chapter, creates a climate in which the social pressure to experiment is heavy and which encourages many persons who should really leave the stuff alone to try it. Their need to be accepted by others compels them to join in the group's practices. They are not in control of what motivates them, nor do they understand what is happening to them.

Some users of marijuana avow that they have, indeed, learned to see life with a renewed appreciation. The question remains, Is this true, or does it only seem that way to them? From one point of view it does not matter if life really does become richer under the influence of drugs. The danger lies in the self-deception which may take place about the influence of the drug. Responding to life fully is developmental. Depending upon a chemical agent for this purpose is not.

Another risk is one already discussed—that marijuana tends to heighten whatever mood the user is in when he smokes. The person who is chronically depressed does himself no favor when he smokes pot or hash. The fearful person often experiences a heightened anxiety under the influence of these drugs. Paranoid attitudes are accentuated. The sense of being an outsider becomes intense. A rationale about the cruelty and inhumanity of society is exaggerated. The individual is then further separated from other human contact necessary for his continued growth.

One risk which former addicts emphasize is that persons in the early stages of addiction, while still on the "soft stuff," refuse to recognize that they are becoming emotionally dependent on these drugs. Nearly every reformed addict recognizes that it was impossible for him to accept the fact that whatever he was using had become necessary for him, that he used all kinds of rationalizations to avoid facing the truth of his dependency.

At that time he probably could have stopped using drugs. Knowing this, he took no account of what was staring him in the face—that even though he could stop if he wanted to, he somehow *did not stop*. It takes a lot of courage to face the truth. It takes the courage to deprive oneself of that which appears to make life bearable. Few people can do this easily. Usually only those with some inner strength are able to make this kind of decision.

This leads to speculation that the potential addict, once on the path toward the use of drugs of any sort, because he is so dependent, hurting, and incapable of self-discipline, is caught in the momentum of his acts. Only one thing can help him: the discovery and utilization of sources of personal strength that heretofore have not been operative in his life.

How Can the Potential Addict Be Helped?

The necessary strength is found when the void of deprivation begins to be filled through success in interpersonal relationships or in personal undertakings in his own life. The young person who finds a relationship with another which makes him feel worthwhile develops inner strength. Success in academic pursuits may begin to fill the void. The person who commits himself to something and in the commitment overcomes his sense of worthlessness no longer feels deprived.

Even more important, recognizing one's sense of deprivation, facing it, and expressing the pain involved frees one from the crippling effects it has upon him. He recognizes what his feelings are; often he is able to define the source of them. He finds that if he expresses these feelings, they will not dominate him. In effect he learns to exorcise a demon from his life.

He may from time to time feel deprived again, but if he can work his way through it by releasing the feeling, it need not interfere with his life. This, however, is no simple task in a culture which, as we have seen, makes little room for a rewarding emotional life.

Can We Know?

Is it possible for us to know if we are potentially addictive? Probably it is, within some limitations. The key to this knowledge is honesty with ourselves. Some questions honestly answered may give us the clues.

Members of Synanon, a California group founded for the purpose of rehabilitating drug addicts, believe that each person must learn to state "the utmost syllable of their conviction regardless of the consequences." Underlying this is the assumption that only through this kind of honesty can people learn to live as they were meant to, given the human nature.

Members of Synanon are so convinced that a lack of honesty is at the base of most of society's difficulty today that they are attempting to establish themselves as a self-sustaining community. Their relationships with one another, their business practices, their educational beliefs—all are permeated with the belief in the importance of honesty. Only on this basis, they assert, can people save themselves from the morass into which they have sunk.

Most of us would balk at the exercise of complete honesty with one another. We have been taught that we must be concerned with not hurting the feelings of others. This mistaken concept assumes that other people are so weak that they will be destroyed by the expression of what we feel or believe about them. When examined, this is patently false. The development of honesty in direct communication with others is essential to the health of individuals and to the improvement of our society. To the extent that persons can bring this honesty into their lives, they will enhance their development toward full humanity.

If we can, then, answer such questions as the following with honesty, we can know if we are subject to dependency and addiction.

Do we feel deprived? On what asumptions do we feel this?
Are we often depressed? For what reasons?
Can we express our feelings? How do we do it?
Are we working toward autonomy? How?

Conclusion

The college scene, for many people, creates a strong sense of worthlessness. Coupled with the disillusionment many young people feel about the world they live in, there is powerful motivation to escape from it. We can understand the enormous appeal of the mind-expanding drugs. The devotee of psychedelic drugs believes that he has never seen life more clearly than when on a trip. He believes himself to be, often for the first time in his life, in touch with the basic realities of life, with the extraneous elements reduced. At the same time he is able to see into all things as he has never done before. He is a part of all around him, he is in and of all things that come into his range of perception.

When this experience is contrasted with the pain and confusion of his daily life, it is no wonder that he seeks to renew the experience frequently and that he is led to believe that the psychedelic way is the only way to achieve personhood. In spite of this, these questions must be raised: Is this the answer? Does it really make one a better person? Does it truly upgrade the quality of one's response to the existential situation of life? Does it prepare one to deal more effectively with the challenges inherent in achieving personhood?

These words from *Psychology Today*[2] serve as a fitting conclusion to our thoughts about drugs and the people who use them:

> Whatever the case as far as addiction is concerned, it remains true that all drugs constitute a kind of psychological crutch and that any form of real dependence upon such drugs can lead to severe personality problems.
>
> We know that many serious persons have reported some transient or long-term value in the use of certain drugs, especially the psychedelics. They say that their aesthetic appreciation has been enhanced, and there is some hard evidence for a slight shift of this sort for part of a group of normal subjects. If, however, we search for major productions of art, letters, music, or visionary insight, exceedingly few clear-cut and lasting monuments to drugs are available. Effects of drugs simply do not seem to have compelled creativity. Aldous Huxley's greatest output, for example, preceded his experimentation with drugs; thereafter, he tended to write *about* drugs, not to *create with* them.
>
> Numerous cultures through the ages have used drugs that induced the sort of experience garnered through LSD, but none of these cultures eradicated mental disorders and disease. In fact, the use of such drugs is often associated with some form of psychosocial deprivation on the part of the user or on occasion with marked privilege (as in Brahmins in India and college students in the United States and Canada). That private satisfactions might have been achieved by the individuals and that groups may have achieved some spiritual equilibrium seem apparent, but whether such drugs have been an overall palliative in the general titre of human misery is another question. . . .
>
> In general, we have been more awed than aided by our experience with many drugs. Here undoubtedly are agents that reveal previously hidden consciousness and modes of thought, but revelation, although perhaps instructive, is not tantamount to understanding. For that we must employ our mental faculties in the undrugged state. This is the lesson of civilization.

[2] *Psychology Today: An Introduction*, CRM Books, Delmar, Calif., 1970, p. 421.

SUGGESTED READINGS FOR PART 3

Anderson, Harold (ed.): *Creativity and Its Cultivation,* Harper, New York, 1959.
Armstrong, William H.: *Study Is Hard Work,* Harper, New York, 1956.
Bugenthal, James F.: *The Search for Authenticity,* Holt, New York, 1965.
Cohen, Sidney: *The Drug Dilemma,* McGraw-Hill, New York, 1969.
———: *The Beyond Within: The LSD Story,* 2d ed., Atheneum, New York, 1967.
De Grazia, Sebastian: *Of Time, Work, and Leisure,* Twentieth Century Fund, New York, 1962.
Dennis, Lawrence, and Joseph F. Kaufman: *The College and the Students,* American Council on Education, Washington, D.C.: 1966.
Fingarette, Herbert: *The Self in Transformation,* Basic Books, New York, 1963.
Fromm, Erich: *The Art of Loving,* Harper, New York, 1956.
———: *Man for Himself,* Rinehart, New York, 1960.
———: *May Man Prevail,* Doubleday, Garden City, N.Y., 1961.
———: *Beyond the Chains of Illusion,* Simon & Schuster, New York, 1962.
Herzberg, Frederick: *Work and the Nature of Man,* World Publishing, Cleveland, 1966.
Jencks, Christopher, and David Riesman: *The Academic Revolution,* Doubleday, New York, 1968.
Jones, Kenneth, et al.: *Drugs and Alcohol,* Harper & Row, New York, 1969.
Lingeman, Richard R.: *Drugs from A to Z: A Dictionary,* McGraw-Hill, New York, 1969.
Maslow, Abraham H.: *New Knowledge in Human Values,* Harper, New York, 1959.
Matson, Floyd W. (ed.): *Being, Becoming, and Behavior,* Braziller, New York, 1967.
May, Rollo (ed.): *Existence,* Basic Books, New York, 1958.
Nowlis, Helen H.: *Drugs on the College Campus,* National Association of Student Personnel Administrators, Detroit, 1967.
Osmond, H., and A. Hoffer: *The Hallucinogens,* Academic, New York, 1967.
Overstreet, Harry A.: *The Mature Mind,* Norton, New York, 1949.
Parsons, Talcott: *Social Structure and Personality,* Free Press, New York, 1964.
Polyani, Michael: *Personal Knowledge,* Harper, New York, 1964.
Rivlin, Harry N. (ed.): *The First Years in College: Preparing Students for a Successful College Career,* Little, Brown, Boston, 1965.
Ruitenbeck, H. M.: *The Individual and the Crowd: A Study of Identity in America,* Mentor, New York, 1964.

Strecker, Edward A., Kenneth Appel, and John W. Appel: *Discovering Ourselves,* Macmillan, New York, 1958.
Tournier, Paul: *The Meaning of Persons,* Harper, New York, 1957.
Volks, Virginia: *On Becoming an Educated Person: The University and the College,* Saunders, Philadelphia, 1964.
Vroom, Victor H.: *Work and Motivation,* Wiley, New York, 1964.
Weinberg, Harry L.: *Levels of Knowing and Existence,* Harper, N.Y., 1959.
Whyte, Lancelot Law: *The Next Development in Man,* Mentor, New York, 1962.
Yablonsky, L.: *The Tunnel Back: Synanon,* Macmillan, New York, 1965.

4. SEX AND MARRIAGE

18.

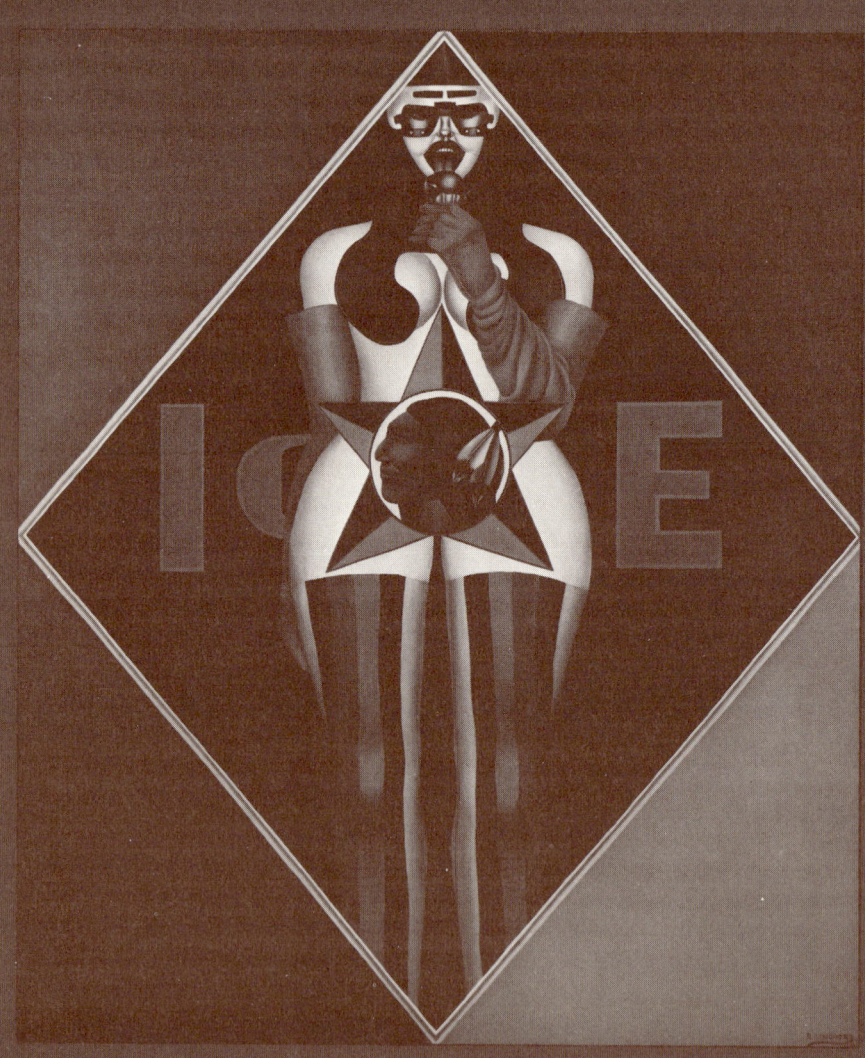

SEX AND SEXUALITY

Sex heads the list of preferred discussion topics among college students. It is a subject of endless fascination. There is enormous curiosity about sex—not confined to college students. In the Western world the wonderment about sex begins in the early years of childhood and runs throughout life. We wonder about ourselves; we wonder about the other sex.

Repression versus Freedom

Because we have grown up in what has been a sexually repressed society, much of our curiosity has a morbid twist. Many people who cannot talk freely about sex are nonetheless fascinated by the thought of it. Further, this fundamental part of our nature fills many with neurotic fears. Far too many people express these fears in various forms of dysfunction. Guilt becomes a large part of the sexual experience. An elaborate system of what is wholesome and what is degenerate is structured by most people.

Fortunately our society appears to be moving away from the repression we have lived with for several centuries. In the process of transition from one set of standards to another, confusion is rampant. Some members of society believe in total freedom and complete libidinous expression of their sexuality. Others continue to maintain the traditional standards of morality. The social controversy, which will become increasingly more vigorous as we move toward greater freedom in sex, is a healthy sign. However, conflict will also rage within individuals. Unless such conflict is resolved, it will have crippling effects upon the persons involved.

While college students contribute a part of the confusion, they would like to feel free of it. If given the opportunity in classes, some college students would discuss the subject endlessly. At the same time, large numbers in any class are unwilling to venture a thought on the subject. Ideas that are expressed may be loaded with misconceptions. Only after a comfortable atmosphere has

Richard Lindner, "Ice," 1966. Oil on canvas. Collection, The Whitney Museum of American Art, New York. Gift of the Friends of the Whitney Museum. Geoffrey Clements, photography.

been established do honest questions begin to appear. These questions often reflect a combination of sophistication and naïveté. Why is this so? In an age when there is probably more literature on sex than ever before, there is still a remarkable amount of confusion. At a time in life when interest in sexual behavior and research is apparently greatest, there is still an astonishing amount of ignorance.

The Difference between Sex and Sexuality

Most of the information available centers around sex, but very little of it considers *sexuality*. Briefly, the distinction between the two is this: Sex refers to our biologic endowment for reproduction. Sexuality, a broader term, refers to all that is involved in our identity as a sexual being.

The biologic and physiologic elements of our being are not difficult to understand. Information common to all people can be gleaned from books on sex and reproduction. We can study the anatomy of sex through charts, diagrams, and pictures. We can even study own own anatomy from life.

But our sexuality is in a different category altogether. Each person has his own unique sexual identity, which has been developing since infancy. An integral part of his response to life, it influences the way in which he sees himself in every relationship.

Since one's sexuality is so much a part of what one is, it has a marked influence upon the physiologic functioning of one's sexual machinery. The frigid woman has problems in her identity as a sexual being. The impotent male's sexuality is distorted. The homosexual cannot manifest his sexuality in the usual way. One's appetite for sexual activity may be strongly influenced by the rejection of his own sexuality. One's unwillingness to participate in a sexual encounter at a particular time is probably due to his concept of himself as a sexual being.

Our sexuality influences everything we do in life. Conversely, what we do in life influences our sexuality. For example, the person who has experienced himself as a failure may be left with a residue of this in his sexual identity. This need not mean that he will therefore be blighted in his sexual activity. But perhaps these experiences of failure may drive him to compensate in the area of sex. The man who fails in business may attempt to establish his masculinity in the realm of sex. The woman who believes she is a failure as a woman may attempt to compensate for this by unchecked sexual exploits.

The Nature of Conflicts about Sex

It is in the area of understanding our sexuality that we are confused. It is in the realm of becoming a new sexual being that conflicts develop, which probably accounts for the combination of sophistication and naïveté which young people manifest about sex and sexuality. In addition, most of us feel the effects of the sexual repression which has existed so long in our society, and efforts to break out of this have led to social and personal distortions about the place of sex in life. Therefore it is extremely difficult for many people to see their values about sex in a realistic and useful perspective.

Basically the conflicts of college students about sex center about three interrelated elements: establishing a set of values about one's sexual conduct which are uniquely one's own; the way one sees oneself as a sexual being, in contrast to one's peer group; and one's assessment of one's worth as a person.

In setting values for oneself, the problem is to sort out the conflicting elements of one's nature—the glandular drives toward sexual gratification versus one's conditioning—the restrictions and taboos inculcated into a person from past experience. Much of the past has been markedly influenced by parental concerns. In the United States, generations of young women have lived with the horror of becoming pregnant out of wedlock. They believe their own worth as people is at stake. If they commit the grievous error of violating social custom, they must face the stigma of social condemnation.

Furthermore, the middle-class attitude about virginity among females has been a source of conflict for young people. Both men and women have been influenced by this. Some young women, bent upon "saving themselves" for their husbands, are confronted with their own desires for sexual fulfillment and the need to respond to the demands of the men they care for. Some young men, conditioned by the value that virginity is a mark of purity, find themselves confused about engaging in a sexual relationship with a women for whom they care.

At the same time these young people have companions who believe quite differently. The idea of sexual freedom for both men and women is becoming more acceptable. Among some young people a less puritanical view is held. They are freer in their view of premarital sex. Even the idea of premarital pregnancy is not always threatening. This view is represented in the comment of a a young woman speaking in a class discussion: "What's really so wrong about having a child outside of marriage? It doesn't mean that the world is coming to an end."

The cross currents of these conflicting thoughts create anxieties for the young person in transition about how to manage his own sexuality. All these factors have worked together to establish the irrational attitudes many people have about sex. Reason and objectivity are often the last things that come into the picture when we think about this area of human experience.

Because it has been such a difficult area to handle, the subject of sex is rarely mentioned between parents and children. If it is, the chances are that it is mentioned in restrictive terms. How often we have heard of sex in terms of "getting in trouble." How often young people have been conditioned to sex through admonitions about what people will think. How often girls have been cautioned about the lustful tendencies of boys. The result, of course, has been that an undue amount of apprehension surrounds a fundamental and powerful part of our nature. When, in the course of a person's growth, "sex rears its ugly head," the new feelings which surround the event are disturbing.

What is one to do with these feelings? Many a young person has wondered about his worth as a human being when the biologic drives toward sex have manifested themselves. How can I, the young person wants to know, discover what is right? To some extent I believe my parents. I certainly love them and want to honor their values. At the same time I believe I should find what is right for me in my own way. But how do I go about it? Do I have sexual intercourse with the first likely person who comes along? If I do, how will I feel about myself? How do other people deal with this problem?

These concerns lead to the long discussions about sex and matters sexual. But for many, even in these discussions, there is little comfort. Some companions attempt to create the impression that they are not only knowledgeable but skilled and experienced as well. What is one to believe about one's own inexperience and lack of knowledge? Should he join the party and create the impression of equal sophistication? Or should he honestly admit that he is a novice with many fears, doubts, and hang-ups? What will his friends think if he looks like a chump?

This is the dilemma for most young people. It is particularly a problem for males who believe that they should be experienced. They frequently judge their worth as men on this basis. Most young men, once they have had sexual intercourse, feel themselves to be remarkably and mystically changed. Never again will they be the same. A new and exciting era has opened up for them. And yet, at the same time, they may also experience a vague sense of uneasiness about what they have experienced. Somehow the experience was not totally fulfilling. Why? Is there something wrong with them? Did they do wrong? Should they have behaved in another way? What about the girl? Suppose she becomes pregnant?

The young woman, for her part, feels equally changed. But for her there is apt to be even more profoundly disturbing residue of feeling. She may feel her physical being has been violated. Her most secret part had been invaded. Unless the event was conducted with the utmost tenderness and concern for her feelings, she may think of her partner as a thief who has stolen something that is irreplaceable. She too will never be the same. How can she think about herself? Is she evil? Has she cheapened herself? Will she be acceptable to her future husband?

Many of the questions raised by both men and women cannot easily be explored in an open discussion. Any sense of shame makes such an exploration difficult. Any feeling of inadequacy in the sexual encounter is examined only with the greatest courage. Too often no examination of feelings is made; they are tolerated until they sink below the level of consciousness. They may be forgotten, but they are not without their influence.

These concerns influence the sense of self. Whatever guilt results from our sexual encounters registers within us and causes us to devalue ourselves. Whatever false values grow from the experience likewise register. The boy who feels, because of a sexual experience, that he is now a man is obviously deluding himself. The girl who believes herself to be dirty is also deceiving herself.

The literature about mental health is heavily laden with sexual overtones. We have erroneously concluded from this that most problems of mental illness are sex-oriented. It would be more appropriate to conclude that these are problems of identity formation. The value we place upon ourselves grows directly out of our experience. As we evaluate this experience, we place a value upon ourselves in the experience. We conclude, through the watchful self, that we have succeeded or failed, that we have been good or bad, that we are mature or childish. These values we carry forward into the future, and unless the conflicts within our sexuality are adequately resolved, we carry them forward into marriage. Our values about ourselves as sexual beings will haunt us until we have them in perspective.

The man and wife who cannot establish a mutually satisfying sexual relationship have not worked out the hang-ups they have about themselves as sexual beings. The woman who thinks her husband is "sex crazy" may not have sex in perspective herself.

The man who is unable to risk marriage may not see himself as capable of being a husband. The woman who remains unmarried may have identity problems vis-à-vis men.

Much can be done during the college years to work out the difficulties we have about sex, although it is a bit late to begin working on them. However, in a society as confused about sex as ours is, people must address themselves to the problems of their own sexuality wherever they can. It is a rare situation where these concerns can be adequately worked out in isolation. The very nature of the sexual encounter indicates that there must be some dialogue between individuals to get things in perspective. Some of the dialogue must be done in groups. Other portions of it must be undertaken between two persons of different sex. A great deal of continuing dialogue is necessary in the intimate relationship.

In any dialogue that is to be meaningful, a two-way communicative process must be at work. Listening is an important part of any dialogue. Unless we listen carefully to what others are saying, little can be gained. We must listen, as the noted psychiatrist Theodore Reik has said, "with the third ear," or we will miss much of what is being said, because many people who cannot put into adequate words what they believe about their own sexuality *do* get it across in the totality of their expression. Their silences sometimes say more than their words.

We must listen to ourselves, as well, if we are to gain insight into the conflict. The difficulty with listening to ourselves when we talk to others is that we are so engrossed in getting our ideas formulated and expressed that we do not really hear what we are saying. It is frequently helpful if others can reflect to us what we have said, if they can let us know how we have come across *to them.*

There is no reason why young people cannot establish groups to discuss their concerns about their sexuality. They may do it on their own or, better still, they may invite respected faculty persons to participate. If persons can enter this experience with the desire to be open and honest with one another, much good can come of the situation. It enables them to *identify* what is bugging them. Then they can begin to search for ways of dealing with it. If they do not know what it is that bothers them, they have little real chance of working themselves out of the bag they are in.

Some Specific Concerns

Volumes could be written about the specific concerns young people have about sex. The issues are raised here with only enough comment to open the subject up for further discussions by readers.

Role Identification

Role identification, while mentioned elsewhere in this book, cannot be overlooked here. One of the marked changes which have taken place on the American scene is that the roles of men and women have become blurred. With the advent of the woman in the labor market, in industry, and in the professions, one of the sharpest lines of demarcation has been erased. Men are no longer exclusively dominant in these areas. Thus a major area of identity satisfaction for men has been invaded. Does this mean that other areas of masculine achievement must be developed? Men with working wives often take over many of the duties which once were the exclusive responsibility of women. Are the men then less masculine for having done so? Women, in turn, have to clarify their own feelings of feminity. If they no longer identify themselves in terms of the roles of housewife and mother, they need to understand the qualities that constitute femaleness. The changes have been widespread. They show themselves in relationships, in conversation, in status, and, since one's experiences influence his sexual performance, in sex. These changes have certainly complicated the problem of understanding one's sexuality.

The paramount value for both male and female is one of personhood. When we attempt to characterize what constitutes a good woman and a good man, we recognize that we are really describing a good person. Let us take the characteristics of sensitivity, gentleness, understanding, intelligence, responsiveness, patience, consideration, self-assertion, capability, courage, and humility. Are any of these specifically masculine or femine? Clearly, they are qualities we would like to see in a person regardless of his sex. They are also characteristics we would like to see in our mates.

The person who is role-bound may discover that he must sacrifice one or more of these characteristics to fulfill the role he structures for himself. By doing so, he negates some of the qualities which make him a person of worth and integrity. For example, a man who believes he must be decisive often dominates his wife to the exclusion of her need for expression.

In a social context where the roles of male and female are carefully spelled out, as they have been in the earlier traditions of American life, men and women have been strongly influenced by economic determinants. Men were traditionally the breadwinners; women were confined to the home. The changes of today demand that both men and women find a sexual identity which is uniquely theirs as individuals. Resilience and adaptability then become important traits.

One's maleness or femaleness has two points of verification: with members of the other sex and with members of his or her own sex. In every relationship something unique is demanded of us. The mature person is capable of making the various necessary responses. The immature person finds himself more bound to a role and may be so intent upon living up to the role he envisions for himself that he misses the vital essence in the relationship. For example, the woman intent on freedom and individuality may become insensitive to her husband's needs.

The conflict inherent in being ourselves but at the same time responding to the needs of our mates demands of us an ongoing sensitivity. It further emphasizes the necessity for a constant dialogue through which we learn what others expect of us. In a committed relationship we grow through this dialogue toward an identity which is mutually satisfying and which develops the essential features of our masculinity or feminity. Maleness and femaleness are in part, then, a matter of responsiveness.

Fears of Being Homosexual

Often the young college student has a fear of being homosexual. Both men and women find themselves attracted to members of their own sex. This is a perfectly natural phenomenon, but it may make them wonder if they are inclined toward homosexuality. Close associations with members of the same sex are a precurser to establishing heterosexual relationships and, in fact, can be thought of as a developmental task.

Without any definite guidelines as to what is uniquely masculine and feminine, young people are often confused about themselves. Styles of clothes, hair, and behavior make this more difficult to ascertain. The confusion, associated with the attachments people sometimes have with members of the same sex, is often frightening.

Probably as our social attitudes toward homosexuality are broadened, the fear of it will be relieved. However, this doesn't help the young person who is concerned about himself in this respect. It may help him to gain some perspective if he can see how others see him. Often he is surprised to find that there is no question in the minds of other people about his sexuality. The others can see quite clearly that there is no problem. The person who does not know this may find himself bringing the self-fulfilling prophecy into being. In spite of all evidence to the contrary, he will act out and thus prove what he believes about himself.

One young man, finding that he had an unusual degree of sensitivity, a characteristic often not thought to be held by men, became concerned that he was too effeminate. In seeking out a person of mutual interest he found another young man. As they became close friends, he found he had a growing interest in being with his friend. All the while he became more and more fearful that he had strong homosexual tendencies. It was not until he learned from a mixed group of other young people of his attractiveness to women *because of this very sensitivity* that his mind was put at ease. Until it was, he endured unnecessary anxiety and stress because of his suspicions about himself.

Another example of this phenomenon is seen in the case of Cynthia.

> After two years at college and two relationships with college men that ended unhappily for her, Cynthia found herself strongly attached to her roommate. One evening walking home from the movies her roommate took her hand. At first Cynthia was surprised but, leaving her hand clasped with her friend's, found that she enjoyed the experience. Though the relationship became closer after this, there were no further physical advances. They continued to walk hand in hand upon occasion but nothing more. However, one day Cynthia overheard some other students discussing her relationship with her roommate. At this point she began to worry about her delight in the physical contact with her friend.
>
> It was not until Cynthia spoke with a member of the counseling staff at the college that her mind was put at ease about what she thought were homosexual tendencies.

Cynthia's major problem had been her fear about herself. The gesture of holding hands had resulted from the shared enjoyment of the film which had been particularly moving. She was not any more homosexual than anyone else.

Menstruation

The menstrual period is surrounded by all sorts of confusing ideas and attitudes for a woman. Her male friends may know the physiologic facts but may not really understand what it means in emotional terms. A man is reluctant to enter the shroud of secrecy which surrounds the whole experience. He treats the subject in the same way he would treat the death of a friend's parent. He stands with hat in hand, abashed, knowing that something is called for from him but feeling incompetent to comply. He mutters some inadequate phrase and lets it go at that. What else can he do? he wonders.

Women themselves may not understand all there is to know

about menstruation. While they may have the physiologic and emotional facts, handling the information in the context of their daily lives is another thing entirely. Attitudes established around this experience can range from embarrassment about it to pride. They may feel differently about it at different times, sometimes using it as a means to get sympathy, sometimes discussing it with another person as an act of intimacy.

Sexual Experience Now or Later?

To engage in sex now or later is a vital question for young people. If the question has not arisen before the college years, externally imposed but internally adopted forces have been at work. The crux of the issue is in the modification of these internalized values which constitute sexual identity. For most young people the increased freedom experienced in early adulthood demands some consideration of the values of the past which they still hold. Conflict may be avoided by adopting a firm position with no intention of changing it. However, this limits the possibilities of growth and in the long run may interfere with the quality of one's response to the circumstances of married life.

The changing roles of men and women are a factor in the issue of premarital sexual activity. The role of the woman appears to be changing more than that of the man. She has experienced some emancipation from traditional standards of sexual behavior and is moving toward further freedom. In many ways this movement is characterized by the breaking down of the double standard of sexual behavior. Women are beginning to recognize that their womanliness is not dependent upon the incorporation of demure chastity in their identity.

This makes possible a much greater range of acceptable behavior than before and an individuality which is freer of the role imposition that has been known in the past. However, the existence of these possibilities does not mean that all individuals are free. Furthermore, many see the need to move toward a greater freedom but are unable to do so without some cost to themselves. The young woman strongly conditioned to the middle-class values of morality may find considerable difficulty in taking an emancipated position.

Since there are several points of view, little can be gained by flatly stating the rightness or wrongness of premarital sexual encounters. Several issues may be explored with profit. Among both men and women some feel that a committed relationship offers a greater possibility of pleasure and satisfaction. Indeed, there may be some persons for whom the expense in terms of guilt and anxiety may negate altogether any satisfaction from more casual sexual activity. Others, however, may be able to move through these feelings rather rapidly, so that they may be able to enjoy a casual relationship quite fully.

The assumption that sex should be engaged in only when there is love often leads to self-deception. Under the duress of opportunity and the excitement of making out, some individuals may feel it is necessary to convince themselves that they are in love. In the belief that this gives them license to follow their inclinations, they then engage in behavior which later precipitates considerable anxiety and confusion. It may also lead one person to use deception to exploit another. Many young people are familiar with the male tendency to declare his love so that he may get what he wants from a girl.

No one wants to be deceived. It is a painful and humiliating experience and has long been a source of distrust among women. For this reason many unmarried women find themselves in an ambivalent position on whether or not to give in to the advances of their more aggressive partners. Out of this has grown the assumption that the woman is responsible for determining how far things will go. Men have readily adopted this notion and have consequently failed to take responsibility when they should have shared it with their partners. The controls built into the woman by this situation are not easily relaxed immediately after the wedding ceremony. Depending upon their intensity, controls may last for some years into marriage.

Among some other women there is a growing attitude that sexual intercourse before marriage is quite acceptable, even if the relationship is only a casual one. These women would prefer that the casual nature of the event be openly recognized between the participating partners. At least, they feel, there is no deception involved. A premium is placed upon honesty of intent and subsequently honesty of enjoyment and satisfaction.

In spite of the apparent increase of liberated attitudes, there are still young women who emotionally have not reached this point. They may be eager to participate in sexual intercourse but unable to accept themselves fully for having done so. Even in the act itself they may feel so much anxiety that they are unable to enjoy what they are experiencing. One result of this may be a sense of frustration and inadequacy. Recognizing their inability to respond, they may draw the conclusion that they or their partners are lacking in some important quality. This produces further anxiety with an increased inhibition toward satisfying function.

The following set of questions indicates the variety and range of feelings that a woman might have: If I engage in sex with this man, what will he assume about me? Does he want me for the satisfaction of his sexual urges alone? What if this relationship doesn't last? Assuming it is not permanent, will present sexual experiences influence the man whom I will eventually marry? Can I keep this person interested in me without sex? Is there something abnormal about me if I don't want sex? If men are free to engage in sexual experiences before marriage, why can't I? Should I engage in sex just for the fun of it? Don't I need experience before marriage?

The man has a different problem. He is driven toward seeking sexual gratification, but at the same time he may still have strong feelings that he would like his wife to be virginal when she comes to him. Since he associates his own masculinity with sexual competence, he may wonder how well he measures up to the sexual partners his girlfriend may have had. If he feels threatened in this area, he may strongly prefer his girlfriend or wife to have had no sexual experience with other men.

The man does not want his beloved to have been the topic of indiscriminate conversation among other men. Because he loves a girl, he wants others to respect her. If they do not respect her, he wonders, how can they respect him? If his girlfriend has been known by several other men, what do they think of him? He feels that his privacy has been invaded.

The concept of the cuckold is an ancient one. It is loaded with emotional content for the offended man. Some elements of this emotion influence feelings of the young man who wonders about his girlfriend's previous sexual experiences. In one sense he feels she has betrayed him. At the same time he must recognize that he has no prior claims on her chastity, but nevertheless he is often uncomfortable when forced to think about the possibilities.

If he must accept his girlfriend's sexual encounters prior to his relationship with her, he wants to believe that each experience was one in which the girl felt she loved the other person. This feeling tells us something. The young man too is concerned about the relationship between love and sex.

This is a complex situation, about which young men and women need to do a lot of talking. Because neither fully understands the feelings and motivations of the other, much identification of these motivations is necessary. There are many more complexities than space permits discussing in this volume. More issues will be raised in a good group discussion than can be identified by one individual. And as groups of persons begin to explore the feelings which surround sex in our society, insights will develop. These insights will not be the same in every group but will differ as much as the insights particular individuals hold for themselves.

But no group can do all that is necessary to explore the issues fully. Therefore it is important that individual couples engage in a mutual examination of their feelings about their own sexuality. An open discussion should be entered into. Sensitivity to oneself and to the other person is essential. Since some persons may not be able to discuss these things readily, it may take time before the topics can be raised. But because the confusion about sexual feelings exists today and will probably exist for another generation at least, conflicts will develop. These can be dealt with only by facing them, recognizing what is involved, and becoming more comfortable as a result of the knowledge gained.

Sex in Perspective

When we find ourselves in a situation in which the motivations toward sexual fulfillment spontaneously generate, it is often extremely difficult to turn these feelings off. Our whole being pushes toward the next step. This is the way we are designed, and out of this much of our greatness grows. The drive toward fulfillment has led to most of the great scientific discoveries and to political achievement. However, in the area of sex we are constrained to hold back when every fiber of our being tells us to go ahead.

Within the context of our social conditioning, whatever we do in the area of sexual expression is fraught with consequences that are limiting. If we move toward affirmation of our sex drives, we must resolve the feelings of guilt which ensue. When we refrain from fulfilling ourselves, we build up much in ourselves that must be unlearned in later years. Restraint of powerful drives is usually the result of equally powerful self-discipline. Once these restraints have been established, it takes an effort to free ourselves from them.

If these restraints were equally established in all persons, we would enter marriage with similar sexual appetites. However, since the restraint of the sex drive is usually established more strongly in the female, there is often an unequal element of enthusiasm for sex between a husband and a wife. This poses a dilemma to which there is no one answer. The premarital years are a time when some degree of exploration should be attempted. A bit of healthy experimentation has rarely hurt anyone as long as precautions are taken that conception does not take place. There is little to be gained by condemning ourselves for this experimentation.

Two questions frequently arise when students discuss sex: First, is sex on a purely physical basis possible? Second, is the idea that sex should be associated with love a natural or enculturated factor?

Since we are symbolizing and value-conscious creatures, it is impossible for sex to be experienced on a purely biologic basis. We cannot divorce ourselves from the meaning-giving proclivities we have. We will always be impelled to give meaning to those events in which we participate, and the meaning we give will always be conditioned by past experience. According to the residual content of our past experience we will be influenced by what happens in the present. Therefore it is impossible for us to experience sex on a purely physical level. We have been too heavily conditioned about the meaning of the sexual encounter for it ever to be free of symbolic significance for us.

The second question is related to the answer to the first. Though there is a natural drive within us toward fusion with another, we have invested this drive with particular value. Since we can care about ourselves only in relation to others, for many of us the only fully satisfying sexual encounter is in a relationship in which we care about the other person. Therefore we cannot fully divest ourselves of the association between sex and love.

The so-called sexual revolution is rapidly having its effect upon young people. If trends of the past few years continue, more and more young people will believe that love and sex do not have to be related for enjoyment of sex. At present probably a large number of people in our society are aware of this, but few have been able to escape the cultural conditioning in which love and sex go hand in hand.

In terms of health and self-actualization what, then, is the part of wisdom? Probably no definite answer can be given. It is for each person to discover for himself. This can come about only through an experimental approach to living. Probably most persons will have to go through some degree of exploitation in their interpersonal relationships before they can achieve a relationship in which there is a mutually supportive search for self. However, the person who attempts to superimpose upon himself some standard of exploratory behavior before he is ready for it is probably motivated by reasons which in themselves are to be questioned.

What Is Normal

What is normal in a sexual encounter? The question of normalcy and degeneracy is another source of confusion among young people. Here again, many young men and women may have some degree of intellectual sophistication. Nevertheless they have had years of conditioning which make it difficult for them to function effectively within the wide range of what is healthy sex play. At this writing, the growing social controversy about nudity, sensuality, and sexual exposure in films and on the stage represents the schizophrenic attitude that our society has about these things. Regardless of the artistic integrity of these dramatic productions, one must recognize that they are a reaction to the sexual repression we have had in our society for many years. How the controversy will be resolved is not yet clear. The chances are that the social confusion is probably reflected in many individuals as well.

Each of us has been conditioned in one way or another to the idea of the "dirty joke." Usually it is a joke which has some sexual overtones or references to bodily processes. The very fact that we refer to these things as dirty says something about our way of viewing an important part of our nature. Some of us have escaped or overcome this kind of conditioning. Some of us, for example, can think about oral-genital sex as wholesome. Usually men are more easily freed from the repressive background than women. There are probably fewer women than men who can imagine themselves engaging in fellatio or cunnilingus without some feelings of revulsion. And yet, with mutually consenting partners, there is little if anything that is "wrong" about these practices.

Those who have overcome their feeling of nastiness about such practices have found them, when mutually satisfying, to be wonderful additions to the sexual relationship they have with their mates. The range of sex play has been broadened. The sensual experience of sex has been increased. The appreciation of their own bodies has gone far beyond the usual genital-genital contacts of sex. Most people who engage in the free use of experimental contact in their sex play have found that their sexual relationship has become more joyous and more satisfying. As long as we continue to classify these practices as degenerate, we will be inhibiting our ability to bring our mates the pleasure we would wish for them, and we will continue to remain in the zone of immature sexual experience and ignorance of what is possible in the sexual encounter.

Simple engagement in unusual sex acts is not by itself the sign of a mature sexual relationship. How we feel about what we do is of equal importance. When one person engages in acts which he feels are degrading for the sake of another, he must be able to handle the emotions which result. If he cannot, a barrier rises between the two people which will be extremely difficult to surmount.

How can this be dealt with? First, a thorough exploration of the feelings one has about the subject of sex should be undertaken in heterosexual groups. This will give the person an opportunity to recognize what he does believe and feel and to compare his attitudes with those of the others. This is part of the process of bringing things into perspective which is so important in the resolution of conflict. There should be no limit on what might be examined by the group. Limitations create either fear or curiosity about the restricted topic, neither of which contributes much to healthy self-actualization if ignored for long.

The second way to deal with the question of what is normal in sexual encounters is for the two people involved in a relationship to discuss it openly. Not that one individual should try to convince another against the latter's wishes or get the best of the other in an argument. The aim should be exploration, a mutually enlightening process of self-discovery. What follows, then, will be the result of growth.

The Sex Act

The sex act itself is another area where young people have doubts. So much can be written about it that one small section of one chapter can offer only a limited glimpse of what is involved. Many other books, however, have dealt with the details of foreplay, coitus, and afterplay. Furthermore, in the same sense that the detailed specifics about painting, written in a book, will be of little help in producing a masterpiece, so the specifics of the art form of love making will not produce great lovers.

What needs to be emphasized is the implications of the fact that sexual intercourse is an involvement with another person. If that involvement exists in the context of a larger relationship, a marriage or other love relationship, a high premium must be placed upon the mutuality of the experience. Although sexual appetites do differ, little is gained if one person is satisfied while the other is left wondering about the value of the whole experience. Worse than that, if one is not satisfied in the sexual experience, he or she is apt to feel exploited. These attitudes must be revealed and handled by the couple.

Conflicts which grow out of sexual involvements are somewhat different from the other conflicts discussed in previous chapters. They, more than the previously discussed conflicts, directly involve two people and the feelings generated between them. When the sexual relationship is one in which there is little more invested than the desire for physical gratification, conflicts are less complex. But when there is a caring relationship, a part of the self moves out toward one's partner. The result is that one is never totally himself again. He has made direct contact with another. He has become involved in a situation which makes demands upon him.

If he is able to meet these demands, he brings satisfaction to himself and his partner. If he is not, the resultant feelings are confused by a sense of failure and frustration. Immediately the complexities increase and questions arise: What does the frustration come from? How was I responsible for the failure? What should I have done that I didn't do? What did I do that I shouldn't have done? These questions must inevitably occur to the reasonably sensitive person.

The next sequence of questions will have to do with the other person. To what extent was the failure and frustration attributable to my partner? What did my partner bring to the situation which made it unsatisfying?

Even these questions may not provide an answer which is really adequate. If the questioning ends here, little of a constructive nature is brought to the relationship. Some progress may be made in assessing the motivations that led each person to the sexual encounter. If, for example, the woman felt that she was "giving" herself to the man and entered into the sexual encounter with this as a motive and the man was not able to give appreciation for the gift, some frustration is bound to ensue. If on the other hand, the man had to "con" the woman into "coming across" and she was able to yield only with reluctance, his satisfaction is apt to be limited also.

These factors need to be examined with the utmost sincerity by both partners in the relationship, and each needs to develop skills of communication with the other to make this possible. It may mean putting aside one's embarrassment to enter into a frank discussion of the feelings involved. When we are able to do this, we not only open new areas for satisfaction in a relationship; we also develop skills which are useful for the future.

When two people are able to discuss their feelings about their sexual involvement, they add immeasurably to their enjoyment of it. They learn to use the sex act as a means of communication for expressing their love. It enables them to become more sensitive to one another, reducing the possibility of misunderstandings, and thus reducing the possibility of confusion and conflict within the relationship and within either partner.

One more problem may be mentioned here. It is not specifically a problem for the college student, but it is one which is rather frequent among young married people. The skills which are developed around discussing sexual attitudes in the premarital years should make it easier to resolve the difficulties which center around the *differing sexual desires* of the partners in a marriage. Marriage counselors state that this issue is the most frequently raised. Because none of us has had the kind of experience necessary to establish some *sense* of what is normal, we wonder about our own sexual performance in marriage.

Since frequency of sexual encounters ranges widely from couple to couple, it seems that normalcy has to be determined by the couple themselves. In the early years of marriage, when some emotional preconditioning must be overcome, it is easy to imagine difficulties arising over this point. Wives may feel that their husbands are overly interested in sex, and at the same time the husband may believe that his wife is frigid.

Once again, it is essential that men and women learn to explore these differences together. When they can lay aside their tendency to blame and together try to improve what exists, they will achieve a great deal for one another.

This may mean learning some of the skills of sex play. It may mean that new dimensions of patience and sensitivity must be developed, that each person must relinquish some of his cherished ideas about himself, that each person must recognize that they are novices, that each must take mutual responsibility for the failures which they experience together. It may mean admitting some of the innermost fears of each.

When we can do this, we take the strides toward full humanness which can come about *only* when the tasks of marriage and life are approached with humility. Too often humility, compassion, and tenderness are absent in human relationships. They are in great demand in any intimate relationship if it is to produce growth in the persons involved.

Conclusion

When we examine the status of sex and sexuality in the Western world, it is clear that too much has been forced below the level of easy discussion. Too many of us are unable to recognize how we feel about our own sexuality. It is even more difficult to admit these feelings to others. Therefore, there is a great deal we do not know about this vigorous and vital part of our lives. We badly need to communicate our attitudes in the area of sex and sexuality, so that they fit into the pattern of life as they should.

There is hope that average individuals can accomplish much of what is necessary for themselves. The seriously crippled person, of course, is excepted. Free discussion will not take the place of psychotherapy, but it *can* assist in growth.

A wide-ranging program which enlists the interest and energy of all young people is essential. Since sex is such an important element in the relationship between two persons in marriage, it is essential for the health of the two persons in the marriage that they learn to understand one another as sexual beings. It is essential to the health of the children who are born of that marriage that the sexual problems of the parents be resolved. Unless they are, the very sources of difficulty for the parents will be passed on to the children.

19.

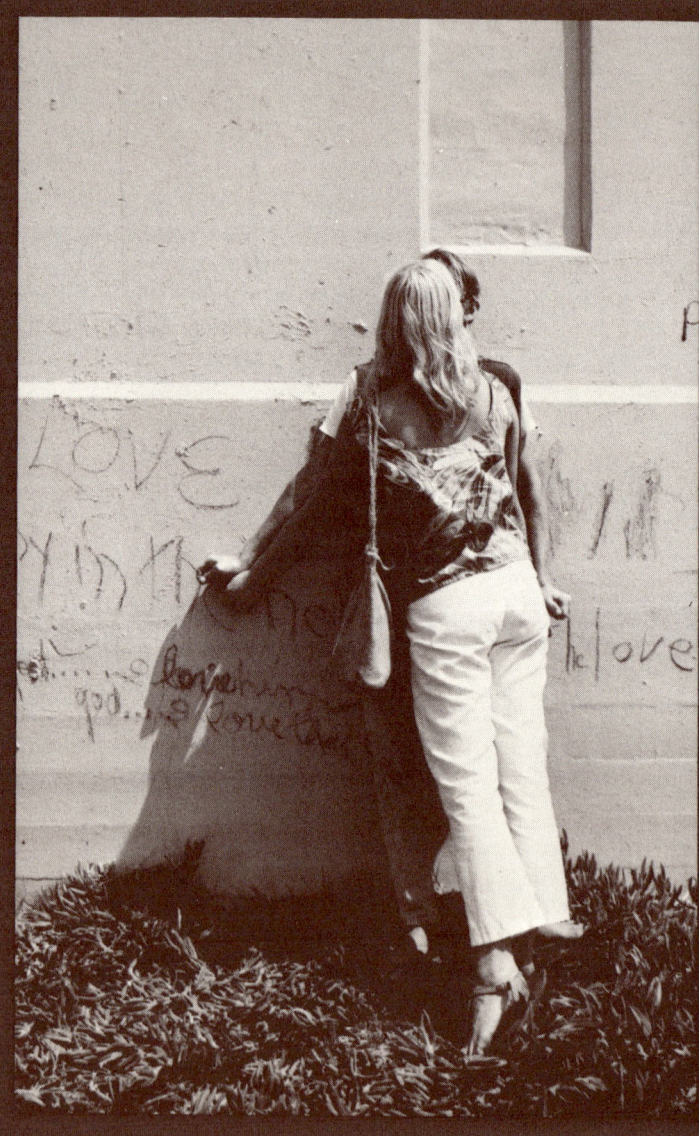

DATING: EXPLORATION OR EXPLOITATION?

If our actions were motivated solely by the emergence of our own inner being, we would be free from many of the pressures we feel. Almost any area of growth is subject to several outside and extraneous forces that frequently make it impossible for us to be ourselves and difficult for us to determine what our real selves are. These forces can be categorized conveniently as the biologic, the social, and the personal. Our interaction with them constitutes our experience.

Each of these forces has a profound influence upon the quality of our response to the dating situation, and each has a certain compelling power which must be taken into account as we assess our lives during the college years. If we ignore these forces, there are always consequences in the development of self.

Biologic Forces

The biologic forces are rather well known and often easily recognized by their influence upon us. Usually they impel us toward some form of sexual gratification. Not all people have an equally strong drive toward sexual satisfaction. It is difficult to say whether this is because of enculturation or because of a hereditary endowment. It is probably safe to say that both experience and heredity play a part. The drive varies also at different times in one person's life.

Since there is no question that the drive toward sexual satisfaction varies among individuals, it is reasonable to assume that it differs between some men and some women. For many young women, a date can be an enormous success even if it has very few sexual overtones. This would likewise be the case for some young men. However, men are more apt to have at least a vague hope that some overt physical encounter will result from the dating situation.

Magnum Photos, Inc.

If there is some physical encounter between the couple, even if it is so mild as hand holding or a good-night kiss, the man is more apt to be biologically aroused than the woman. If the encounter reaches preliminary sex play in the form of petting or caressing, it is almost certain that the man will be aroused. His companion will not necessarily be aroused in the same way. This difference, be it biologic or social, is a fact. It will influence the residual feelings and attitudes about the date and about the other person. It certainly will become a factor in determining whether or not a succeeding date will be sought by the young man.

Social Factors

In a dating situation it is extremely difficult to determine which influences are personal and which are social. We are meaning-giving creatures, and since we always give meaning to our experiences as a result of social conditioning, the social and personal become inextricably interwoven in the structure of the self.

The social role cast for the young person by his peer group becomes a dominant factor in the way he sees and conducts himself in the dating situation. Most young people see dating as an important part of the identity they must assume. When they are unable to date, for whatever reason, they feel a need to compensate.

As we have already noted, many devices are employed by young people to make themselves acceptable to themselves if they are not able to date. Some resort to study to fill the void. Others rationalize by saying that dating is not important to them. A not uncommon device is for an individual to become a kind of confidant and "close personal friend" of members of the other sex. Through this, they develop a sense of worth vis-à-vis members of the other sex and do not feel totally ignored by them. In most such cases some self-deception is involved; yet, the long-range results are not altogether bad. Others are just plain miserable, because they feel left out.

The young person who suffers through the early years of young adulthood without being able to date often develops character traits which stand him in good stead later in his life. On the other hand, there are those who, because of physical attractiveness or some other engaging trait, have been extremely popular but who, having basked in this popularity, develop traits later in life which make them extremely unattractive, whose personalities seem to have a void which they are incapable of identifying or filling.

When the social pressures are so great that one feels he must date or be considered a failure, unnecessary stress is introduced into his life. He uses false values to judge himself. Distorted views of himself are developed and pressures are created with which he has difficulty in coping. Identity becomes progressively more blurred. The inner self does not unfold, and self-actualization does not take place.

Traditionally, women have played the waiting game in the dating situation. Some take this role seriously and literally wait. Most learn the rules of the game at an early age and proceed to develop impressive skills. A father, brought up in a family of brothers, indicated his amazement at seeing the machinations of his two teen-age daughters as they maneuvered to get two particular boys to invite them to a prom. "The poor dumb fellows didn't have a chance," he said. "Though they didn't know it, they were marked men six weeks before the event." The interesting thing is that the other young men who approached these girls for a date to the same prom were rejected so skillfully that they could hardly wait for another chance to date the girls.

This deceit may be a necessary tactic developed from childhood in a world where women must play an apparently more passive role than males. How else can they exert their own wills? But is this the important issue here? If the tricks of the dating game are all that is focused on, little is accomplished. What is important to recognize is that women view the date in a different way than men. They approach the date with a different sense of role identification, and they view men differently than men view women. Unless this is understood and further efforts are made by both men and women to achieve deeper understanding of one another, the game remains merely competitive, for in essence women are in competition with men to achieve a sense of worth for themselves in the dating situation. Unless skills of identifying and examining the differences in their views of dating are developed, the competition is carried over into marriage. The exploitative nature of both men and women will be projected into marriage, which demands a high degree of open cooperation. Most marriages fail simply because the two principals are unable to break through the exploitative nature of their relationship to one another.

Men in the dating situation also have an image they are attempting to uphold. The social pressure to be a dominant, decisive type often forces men into a role for which they are not personally suited. To the extent that a young man incorporates the belief that he should be such a person, he succeeds or fails in the dating situation solely on the basis of whether or not he is able to create this image. Since failure as a man is anathema to the young male, he will often go to ridiculous lengths to establish his dominance. Frequently the image is created only in a context where the man exploits the woman.

Men engaged in the task of preparing themselves primarily for a vocation approach dating in a more dilettante manner than women and are inclined to resist the efforts of their female friends to become more serious. As one male college student said, "I can't afford to get serious. I have too many years of hard work ahead of me before I can consider marriage." Many young men look on the efforts of women as a trap to be wary of. But because they are motivated toward dating (even if for different reasons), they cannot easily resist the siren call of the female.

Women resent the attitude of male college students who appear to them to be insincere. The mutual distrust necessitates that a concentrated effort be made to open the subject to cooperative consideration. For many, the skills of effective communication have not yet been developed at this time in their lives. As a result, they use role playing designed to protect themselves from being clearly seen by the person they are dating. In other words, these men and women obscure themselves from one another.

There is much in the dating relationship which lies below the level of conscious recognition. Unless both persons are able to go into the deeper levels of motivation and help each other reveal what is at work, their relationship remains clouded in frustrations which they cannot understand. In each case externally imposed role expectations hamper personal growth. Each person remains at the adolescent level of using the other for reasons which are not worth the effort. To become free from enculturated values about male and female roles during the dating years is consistent with Maslow's goal of freeing oneself from enculturation as one of the components of self-actualization.

Expectations

Generally speaking, young women have a much clearer image of what they expect in a man than men have in regard to women. This picture tends to change during the four years of college life. The woman tends to identify much sooner than the man what she wants in a mate and can enumerate these expectations long before the time for marriage arrives. The man tends to give little thought to the kind of woman he wants for a wife. For him, the college girl is a playmate, and he tends to see himself, or would like to see himself, cast in the role of a playboy. He would like to be cool, sophisticated, indifferent when necessary, and completely in charge of his emotions in whatever situation he finds himself.

There is no mystery about these differences. Society encourages young women to concern themselves with these expectations. It stands to reason that if women are searching for potential husbands, they have to know what they are looking for. Usually this knowledge does not come overnight or as a result of one session of "thinking things out." More often, it is the result of a long, slow process of growth in which attitudes are developed in the girl's home as a result of watching her parents function. The process continues through the high school years, when many influences are felt. Later, the careful observation of many men and their way of relating to women has its effect. The mass media and the male images which are projected are evaluated. Discussions with friends center about this important issue of what a girl wants in a mate.

Males, on the other hand, usually find themselves concerned with other things. Boys begin quite early to realize that their mothers may not be thought of in certain terms. While it is accepted in most homes that a girl may flirt with her father, the boy learns early that he may not do likewise with his mother. His father is a jealous guardian of the relationship between a boy and his mother. The result is that a mother, the first female figure in a boy's life, soon becomes one whose primary purpose is to take care of him. She feeds him, comforts him, picks up after him. He cannot approach her as a woman. Often, he is at the same time dominated by her in a way that is not consistent with what he later believes his role to be.

Since he does not have to woo her, a boy often becomes indifferent to what kind of person his mother is. He usually finds that she will love him regardless of what he is. This is the nature of a mother's love. It does not have to be won; it is there for the asking. Since he does not have to woo her, a boy is free to do things which are of interest to himself. He does not need to develop the skills of responding to women in a loving way. He has found that they will love him regardless of what he is. If this appears to carry the idea too far, it can at least be said that his only problem is to conform to her wish that he "behave himself."

From this stage of development he moves into the realm of boyhood with a freedom from the other sex that a girl does not have. If she is to get attention and love from her father, she must learn how to play up to him. Through this she learns skills which she carries over into the realm of playing up to other males about whom she cares or from whom she wants attention. Not only are these valuable skills, but they also require some thought and some experimentation. In the process, the girl soon learns to value particular characteristics in a man. It rapidly becomes a part of her nature to use her wiles to "catch a man" and becomes a major influence in her life. This ongoing task, in fact, becomes a part of what she is, permeating her thoughts not only about what she is but also about how she can become what she feels she must become. It is no mystery, then, that she begins to observe men with an evaluative eye long before a boy even begins to think about the need to do so about girls.

When asked what they expect in a woman, many young men will rate rather high her ability to make him feel important. By this they mean that she is willing to defer to him in decision making, that she accords him the status of dominance in their relationship. He usually does not feel that he should have to work for this. He believes that this is his right simply because he is a male. He has to *learn* that there is more involved in a male-female relationship than existed between himself and his mother.

The opportunity to learn the skills involved in being an effective man is not readily found in our society. Society demands that he learn how to be a boy among boys, and later how to compete successfully with other men. It is only at a relatively late stage in his life that he realizes that a woman is something other than a gratifier of his needs. In fact, he may not learn this until he is already married.

Because he is not primarily concerned with what a woman is and what is necessary to woo her (except in superficial ways), he has no clear picture of the kind of woman he would like to marry. For him, being in love with a particular girl usually just "happens." He is often surprised to find himself loving a particular girl. He may even resent feeling pulled toward her and away from what he believes is his major purpose in college. He cannot devote his full energy to the problems of successful academic competition. He finds that he has mixed feelings about the girl he loves. At the same time that he loves and desires her, he resents what she is doing to him. But because there is some degree of status in our society to being attached to a member of the other sex, he goes along with the situation.

Many times his conflicting feelings lie below the level of conscious cognition. He is surprised at the external manifestations of his inner confusion. He often finds himself openly hostile to his beloved. He becomes involved in arguments with her which he cannot explain. He is usually unable to identify the nature of his feelings or communicate them to his girlfriend.

On the girl's part there is equal confusion. It is difficult for her to understand why this man who professes to love her can be so aggressive toward her. She wonders why he appears to be insensitive to her needs. It is difficult for her to comprehend the conflicting emotions he has. As she looks at her feelings, they seem quite simple: She loves the man. She wants to share his life. She looks forward to marriage and making a home with him. How, she wonders, is it possible for him at one moment to give every evidence that he cares for her and in the next to indicate that he thinks that she is using him? How is it possible for him even to believe that she is interested in anything but what is best for them both (defined by her as a continuing relationship which will lead toward marriage)?

Though the young woman has ideas of what she wants in a man and though she has given much thought to what kind of husband he will make and even what kind of father he will be, she still is not equipped to identify the specific issues that upset them. She may even be unwilling or unable to attempt to explore these issues. The prospect may be too frightening for them both to face. The usual alternatives are to suffer through an unproductive relationship, to break the relationship off, or to adopt subterfuges to enable the relationship to continue. None of these alternatives is a creative one. None leads to satisfaction or to growth. The first and the last may actually be destructive of the need to actualize.

Personal Factors

The distinction between the above-mentioned social factors and those which we call personal is in some ways arbitrary. The personal factors too are universal in that they stem from basic needs inherent in every human being. However, they bear the stamp of unique personalities.

All people share the need to discover their own personal meaning in life, to find out what and who they are, but the drive toward knowledge of self is manifested in different ways by different individuals. In some, severe anxiety may be associated with self-discovery. One of Freud's greatest contributions is the discovery that the great cause of much of our psychological illness is the fear of knowledge of oneself—of one's emotions, impulses, memories, capacities, potentialities, and destiny. When this kind of fear becomes dominant in our lives, it becomes one of our greatest blocks to self-actualization.

Often we fear any knowledge that would tend to cause us to despise ourselves. If we are led into circumstances which make us think of ourselves as weak, destructive, inhuman, or otherwise reprehensible, we tend to behave in ways which will obscure this knowledge. Hence the young man who finds himself in a situation which will result in the realization that he is being unmanly (by whatever standards of manliness he has set for himself) will do everything he can to distort the circumstances so that he does not have to view himself in this unfavorable light. He will not only blind himself to the truth; he may also fail to recognize that what is really distorted are the expectations he has for himself. And he refuses to submit these aspects of the existential situation to critical evaluation.

In the dating situation, when unrealistic expectations are held, the tendency to obscure the innumerable opportunities for gaining self-knowledge is strong, for the simple reason that in order to develop such insight it is necessary to expose oneself to the critical examination of one's partner. Hence one is led not only to blind oneself to the truth but also to so manipulate one's partner that he is rendered helpless to assist in the task of self-discovery.

The statement "To be completely honest with oneself is the very best effort a human being can make" is attributed to Freud. In many life situations, to be completely honest with oneself often demands that we expose elements of the self which we do not wish others to see. A young woman, believing intelligence to be unfeminine, will often hide her intelligence from her date. At the same time she hides from herself the fact that she is obscuring her intelligence. She not only robs herself of one of her best tools for self-actualization but projects a deceptive image to her date. In the long run her intelligence will be revealed in one way or another. When it is, her boyfriend will feel deceived. He may even feel threatened by her intelligence, and perhaps doubly threatened because he cannot easily identify what is threatening him, since it is masked. Rather than work together with the young woman in question to acknowledge her superior intelligence openly and use it for their mutual benefit, he may cooperate with her in obscuring it. Neither, then, will understand what is at work. Each exploits the other to protect images which are not worth protecting and which will produce nothing of value in the relationship.

Those couples who are able to mutually explore the dynamics of their own makeup are ahead of the game. They have begun to develop the skills of self-discovery and mutual self-revelation that will serve them well in future interpersonal relationships.

When young people, in the course of the dating years, are not able to discover their own meaning in life, they become frustrated and frightened. The problem is all the more vexing because it cannot be identified. The result is an intensified sense of confusion, followed by an anxiety which makes the college years rather unstable.

To avoid this anxiety, people tend to lock themselves into patterns of response which are not always productive but serve merely to allay the anxiety by obscuring the source. As we have seen in Chapter 15, young people are able to fit into their peer group only through the severest kind of conformity. By doing so, they create the illusion of having no problem. For a time this illusion works, but in the long run it is merely a temporary soporific. Perhaps the worst part of any personal problem is that one feels intensely that he is alone, that no one else has ever had such a problem, and that no others can really help him. His feeling of being cut off from his fellowman is probably the motivation for the remarkable peer-group conformity which manifests itself throughout adolescence and into young adulthood.

The desperate need for a soul mate in such circumstances is apparent. Being cut off from most people is not too bad if we can have at least one person whom we know we can count on to share our woes. We reach out toward this person with tentacles which draw him toward us in an enveloping and often destructive symbiosis. Often our need for affiliation with another is so great that we not only surrender all our claims to freedom and autonomy but also expect the other person to do the same. This is true exploitation, a use of the other person for one's own ends. Whether or not it is mutual makes little difference. In fact, when another person cooperates in the exploitative relationship, the results are insidious and enormously difficult to detect. This renders each one of the couple helpless to extricate himself from the limitations which put him there in the first place. It is the antithesis of self-actualization.

Another protection against the anxiety of loneliness is to alienate ourselves from our own feelings. If we can somehow convince ourselves that none of our concerns really matter, we do not have to suffer the frustration or the confusion associated with them. Through alienation, anxiety is measurably decreased, too. How can this be done? In the first place, a subtle attitudinal adaptation takes place. We become less and less in touch with the feelings which develop. We deny their existence.

We are then unable to respond in an appropriate manner. When an occasion for being sad arises, we are not able to be sad. We do not allow ourselves to feel any emotion that causes pain. When something embarrassing happens, we do not let ourselves feel the normal feelings of embarrassment, since the feeling does not fit the image we wish to project. The result is a detachment from the realities of life and an inability to relate to others in any way which will evoke in ourselves the feelings we so fear.

To others we do not seem real. Because we do not show the feelings which they expect us to show and which they themselves would feel in similar circumstances, they cannot recognize us and, in turn, cannot relate to us. The effect of this is to cut us off from the very sustenance we need in order to achieve our full humanness. Others, in our presence, feel manipulated by us, because they are caused to have emotions when we do not.

All these personal factors—the need to discover our own meaning in life, the necessity to examine ourselves, the pain of such examination, and the defenses we raise against this pain—strongly mark our conduct in dating situations. We are driven to utilize every situation to resolve antithetical motives. We use the dating situation, we use the persons we date, we distort reality, we confuse issues, and we suffer. During periods when these drives are in strongest conflict, when two people are engaged in a mutual relationship, they are each strongly tempted to exploit one another for their own personal gain.

While exploitation as a steady *modus operandi* is juvenile, it is not altogether deplorable. Exploitation is a stage to be gone through. When we are in it, we should recognize that we are. Recognizing this, we should then attempt to do what is necessary to move beyond it. The following pages are devoted to some alternatives to exploitation.

Exploration

The only acceptable countermeasure to exploitation in dating is exploration. Several important areas can be explored, depending, of course, upon the makeup of the individuals involved. One area to be explored is the range and capacity of feeling one person can generate for another. A second is the background of motivation we bring to the dating situation. A third consists of our hopes, expectations, capacities, potentialities, and abilities. Then there is the entire realm of the other person. What is he or she like? What does he expect from me? How does she respond to me? Finally, we may wish to explore the nature of dating relationships.

This means that one must be willing to live with some degree of adventurousness, shedding a familiar role and not bound by the past. Does this mean that every life style one has developed for himself is to be abandoned? Definitely not. The exploratory process may begin by examining what we are involved in and our basic beliefs. For example, one might well ask what his beliefs are about being a man or a woman. When this is identified, one might explore with another person how these beliefs are lived out in one's life.

Examining Our Beliefs

Generosity

Most of us have been brought up with the belief that it is better to give than to receive. Early in our lives this concept is inculcated by a variety of coercive measures. We are taught to share our playthings. We are expected to take turns. We are often forced, in one way or another, to yield to another person what we believe to be rightfully ours.

The effect of this is to establish feelings of guilt when we do anything which is in any way self-centered. Even though the early stages of a love relationship are selfish and incorporative, many of us assume that it should be otherwise. We feel guilty when we are not selfless and openly giving.

The dating relationship often accentuates some of these complex feelings. We are driven toward dating a particular individual for selfish reasons, but we feel guilty about it. We want to take and we feel we should not take. In the process of exploring the beliefs one has about generosity, many facets of one's personal makeup may be revealed. How much give and take should there be in the relationship? What constitutes giving and what taking? When one gives and the other takes, what are the subsequent feelings for each? What influence will these feelings have upon the relationship and the individuals in it?

If sex is thought of on a give-and-take basis, there is much to be explored. Young women, for example, often feel that they have given something of themselves when they have participated in a sexual act. Usually they expect some measure of giving in return. The trade is made when some symbolic declaration of love is received from the man. How does each person in the relationship view this trade? When one person is unable to give the expected symbols, how does the other one feel? Is the woman willing to engage in sexual intercourse without the declarations of love from the man? If he declares his love but indeed does not feel it, how does he feel? Is the woman able to detect this deceit? Can they discuss what is involved in terms other than accusatory ones? Are they able to work out compromises which are mutually satisfying to them? Or will the compromises result in the feeling of being exploited? Can these things be discussed?

These are but a few of the questions which might be used in the exploratory elements of the dating relationship. When less than this happens, the relationship is relatively superficial. This is not to say that it is meaningless. As already mentioned, often some degree of exploitation is necessary before a more mature arrangement can be established.

Honesty

Obviously, unless people can be honest with themselves and with one another, communication tends to break down. Usually an inability to be honest is apparent to the other person. Some persons' behavior may not be labeled dishonest because of the subtlety with which it is masked, but usually we can spot something unconvincing in the way another person behaves or speaks when we are in a relationship that counts.

It helps little for one person to attack another with an accusation of dishonesty. It is, however, important to spot it in ourselves when it occurs. We should then explore the reasons for it. Often it is helpful to identify what threatens each individual in a relationship.

Because we have been strongly conditioned to the value of honesty, it is difficult to admit that we are not being honest. To do so is tantamount to an admission of failure as a person. When we feel ourselves to be failing, we become defensive, and this often leads to a stalemate in an interpersonal relationship. Dishonesty is often used as a protective mechanism. For example, when we are engaged in a dispute with another person, we may cite supposed authorities to support our side. Frequently this is nothing more than a ploy to gain an advantage over one's debating adversary. In a normal dispute this is so common that it is generally overlooked. In the more intimate relationships of dating it is also frequently used to gain some form of leverage over one's partner. Engaging in such practices develops the skills of competitive dominance rather than the skills of cooperative communication. The subsequent carry-over of this in the personality structure only leads to behavior which must be unlearned in the future. In marriage there is no place for competitive dominance. Cooperative communication is essential. Without it, mutual self-discovery cannot flourish.

Often a girl dates a fellow not because of what he is as a person but because of what he can give her in the form of a good time. The fellow too may be looking for nothing more than a good time. For him, "good time" may mean the thrill of a sexual encounter. It must be underlined here that no pitch against having a good time is being made. The concern is with the ploys to which people resort in order to have the good time. When this necessitates compromising and using another person, questions can be raised about the value of the experience for each person involved.

Faithfulness

One of the basic assumptions of going steady is that the individual members of the couple will date no other person as long as they are involved in the steady relationship. It is probably important to explore the nature of such a relationship. What does it mean to each of the persons involved? Are they interested in going steady out of a desire to tie down the other person? If so, why? Are they interested in the steady relationship because they want to commit themselves to another person? Why? What does each person expect of the other beyond sole dating rights? The answers to these questions may lead to the discovery of invaluable personal information.

Often, however, rather than examine these questions, each member of the relationship prefers to keep the motivations hidden from himself and from the other. To discover why he is engaged in a relationship may lead to the recognition of some aspect of himself that he does not want to recognize. He may feel threatened by the possibility of revealing a weakness to the other person—perhaps revealing that he is involved in the relationship for selfish reasons alone. Again, he thinks of himself as a failure. Who wants to admit this to another person?

However, if we were able to admit these "weaknesses" readily, we would be much better equipped to maintain perspective about ourselves and our shortcomings. We would find that the open recognition of these personality factors was not nearly so bad as we thought it would be. We would be better able in the future to examine other, more important aspects of our makeup. We would be better prepared to work out a creative and mutually satisfying relationship. Furthermore, we would be able to recognize that there is no great fault in selfishness if we are willing to examine it and recognize it for what it is. The very fact of being willing to enter into such an examination with another person would be evidence of an ability to give to one another in a most significant way. The highest evidence of faith in another person is to trust him with knowledge about oneself. By doing so, we say more strongly than we ever could with words that we care a great deal about the other. The rewards of this kind of relationship are manifold. Chief among them is the feeling that we are engaged in something that is important to us. In short, the rewards lie in the fact that we are moving toward the achievement of full personhood, and we are able to know it.

Kindness

Kindness is another of the values with which we are imbued. From childhood on we have been encouraged to be kind and loving. When we are this way, we feel we are successes as persons. When we are not, we feel that we have failed in another important area of our being. The sense of failure for many is acute. When we find it impossible to be as kind as we believe we should be, the subsequent feeling of guilt can become crippling.

On the other side of the coin are the expectations we have for our partner. Often we believe that the partner should be kind beyond the bounds of reason. When he or she cannot live up to our expectations, we are hurt. Feeling hurt, we often attempt to retaliate. Unless the feelings can be opened up to mutual examination, the relationship breaks down. Accusations are made, suffering is endured, and respect is lost. When respect is gone, there is little that can make up for its loss.

We can readily see how the situation might be saved if each person were able to tell the other how he feels when kindness is not reciprocated or when it has been absent. Unfortunately, many times we cannot identify what is missing. We expect kindness to the extent that we cannot believe it is not present. The problem then is that our retaliative efforts focus on areas irrelevant to the basic issues involved. For example, when we share private information about ourselves with another person and we learn later that that person uses the information against us, we are shocked and hurt. The hurt becomes the focus of our attention. We are not able to examine why the other person may have done what he did.

We have little desire to enter into a dialogue with the person who has caused the hurt. We are unwilling to run the risk that we may be hurt further. We believe we have been betrayed. Our major interest is to wall ourselves off from the other person and make ourselves impervious to his bruising tactics.

Not only does communication break down, but we cannot discover the cause. Often what happens is that two individuals withdraw from one another until the hurt subsides. They may not speak to each other; they may not even see each other. When the hurt subsides, they may once again move toward each other, in a tentative and hesitant fashion. But distrust is evident in every move that is made. They hesitate to explore the area in which the hurt took place. Efforts are made by both persons to cover over what has happened. They attempt to act as though nothing had happened. In their mutual desire to be kind and to compensate for the bruising period, they ignore the situation and therefore learn little that is useful to them in the future. About all that is learned is that this is an area that should not be entered again. Each learns little about the other. Neither learns much about himself. What is more, the results of this experience, left unexplored, are usually carried into future situations and contribute to a cumulative process.

Making an exploratory effort in this area might be the most productive thing that either person ever did. Often, at the outset, no clear goal can be seen. Neither person is aware of what specific direction they ought to take. However, if they are able to move into the forbidden zone of feelings, enormous insight is developed. Beyond this, they have the feeling that they are involved with an individual who is willing to travel a rough road with them. They do not feel alone in their hurt. Through this mutual exploration, both grow in knowledge and in faith as well. They have added one more experience of success as a couple to the set of feelings they have about one another.

The Quality of Heterosexual Relationships

A different pattern of dating appears to have been established than existed a generation ago. A much higher incidence of coupling off for protracted periods is one difference. Does this reflect a greater maturity? Are people now ready for this pairing off sooner than before?

As one young man said, "I guess I go with one girl because it's easier that way." He seemed to believe that it was just too much work to remain unattached. It would have meant that he had to exist in the competitive dating market and run the risks of being rejected by every girl he asked to date. When he had an agreement to go steady, this risk was eliminated. For many young couples the agreement is little more than the simple recognition that they will not date anyone else while they are committed to one another.

Presumably this arrangement leads to greater personal intimacy and greater depth of feeling in the relationship. However, there is little evidence that greater personal intimacy does exist. What appears to be operative is a symbolic manifestation of intimacy. The steady dating in itself tends to create an illusion of intimacy. But there is reason to believe that this is a soporific more than anything else. Steady dating, rather than producing increased intensity of relationship, simply eases the tension and anxiety of *not* going steady.

No doubt there is a higher incidence of physical intimacy in such relationships. But this, in itself, is also a matter of symbolism rather than reality. One almost wonders if the disillusionment with marriage is an outgrowth of the long years preceding marriage in which steady dating occurs. The continuing relationship creates something of an illusion of marriage. At the same time, the steady relationship is one in which rather superficial interpersonal dynamics exist.

If, in fact, young people do go steady to avoid the anxiety of *not* doing so, there is reason for serious doubts about the maturity of the relationship. It appears to have a compulsive element. Whenever individuals are compelled to behave in a particular way, questions may be raised about the motivations and about the quality of this behavior as a response to life. In effect, the compulsive individual is not free to become himself. He is not able to resist the enculturating influences of his social environment.

Is there an ideal dating relationship? When this question arose in a discussion among college students about the subject of dating, one young man replied, "I doubt if ideal is a relevant word. It seems to me that a good relationship is one that works." A relationship that "works" is one in which each member can work toward achieving self-actualization. The student characterized such a relationship as one which lasted for some time. Furthermore, he believed that the two individuals should feel committed to one another and within this commitment should attempt to work toward mutual understanding. The relationship should also have a high degree of honesty in it. As each person attempted to be fully aware of the other person's feelings and attitudes, they should also be willing to accept comments about themselves from one another.

While this could be agreed with in principle, it should be recognized that in any human relationship each individual has personal vested interests that he is attempting to protect. For example, a young woman who expects her steady companion to respect her may insist upon this at all times. If she happens to be more skilled at articulating her thoughts and feelings than her mate and it is difficult for her to restrain her use of this skill when the two disagree, frustration felt by her friend might cause him to respond without the respect she feels she is due. Then, marshaling her dialectical skill, she could make a good case for the fact that he was clearly not giving her the respect she believed he should. How could he win? What are the working tasks of such a relationship?

It would be important for each of these young people to be able to identify the sources of the difference. Once this was done, and it could only be accomplished if each of them was able to admit, even if only tentatively, what his and her motivations were, the next step would be to explore the means by which each of them was attempting to communicate with the other. As we have seen in an earlier chapter, communication goes far beyond merely telling another person what you think. It implies listening with a sensitive ear and mind to what the other person is saying with his words, his body, his behavior, and any other expressive medium at his command.

Often to listen only to the words is not enough. Words may be deceptive. The working relationship is one in which one thoroughly sensitizes himself to the other person's self. This goes far beyond the vapid situation which operates only as a security blanket. Such sensitivity requires courage, willingness to change, determination to see things through to a mutually satisfying conclusion. There can be nothing one-sided about a working relationship. If there is, it soon ceases to work as a mutually developmental affiliation. When one person develops at the expense of the other, the quality of the relationship may be questioned.

It is unreasonable to assume that immature individuals can operate in a mature manner. Many people, married for years, still do not have an effective working relationship. But those involved in a relationship which does not work well should not assume that the relationship should be abandoned. Most of us have to do things less than well before we can learn to do them well. Recognizing that we are being immature helps us move toward maturity.

Since most college students are preparing for marriage, there should be times when they are evaluating the nature of their relationships. When they can have the help of another person in the process of evaluation, they are fortunate. Often the other can bring them some objectivity. But when they are in a competitive struggle for dominance with another person, objectivity flies out the window.

Newfound Freedom

The newfound freedom most college students experience when they first leave home is both a blessing and a source of confusion. The young woman who has heretofore been under the supervision of her parents must now exercise controls over herself, free from the coercion of their presence. She can no longer avoid responsibility by deferring to her parents' wishes. If she refuses an offer of sexual pleasure by an ardent young man, it must be totally on her own responsibility. She can no longer plead "getting home on time." Nor can she avoid a weekend party because her parents wouldn't allow it. She is now her own boss and must decide for herself what she will accept and what she will reject.

Though many young men would have others believe that they are sexually experienced by the time they get to college, they may have the same doubts as their coed friends. As long as they were in the moral shadow of their parents, there was some inner excuse for their continued existence in the realm of boyhood. Now, with the freedom from this moral restraint they are faced with the challenge to "prove their manhood." It is now *their* responsibility. Can this responsibility be easily avoided?

The social pressures of peers make this avoidance difficult. Thus, in matters sexual, how free are we in college? Once again, compulsion enters the picture. Instead of parents, peers are now the controlling forces. The direction of the force is different, but the pressure is still there.

What can be expected of a working relationship? First, there could be an open recognition and statement of one's puzzlement. But few young people are willing to admit their naïveté. If it could be admitted, true freedom would be found.

Freedom, then, is not a matter of geography. It is much more a state of mind. The college years offer the opportunity to explore the possibilities of finding this state of being. Those who find it before marriage are fortunate. They have a basis for marriage which is invaluable. Much of the work of marriage will have been accomplished before it has been entered.

What happens in dating relationships either enhances or inhibits the development of the skills important for successful marriages. College relationships are proving grounds for readiness for marriage. When individuals are able to establish open relationships in which communication flows easily and readily, they are well on the path toward readiness. Even precluding the idea of marriage, skills of communication and sensitivity are valuable assets for the healthy life. All one's relationships are richer for it. One's entire life is equally enriched.

20.

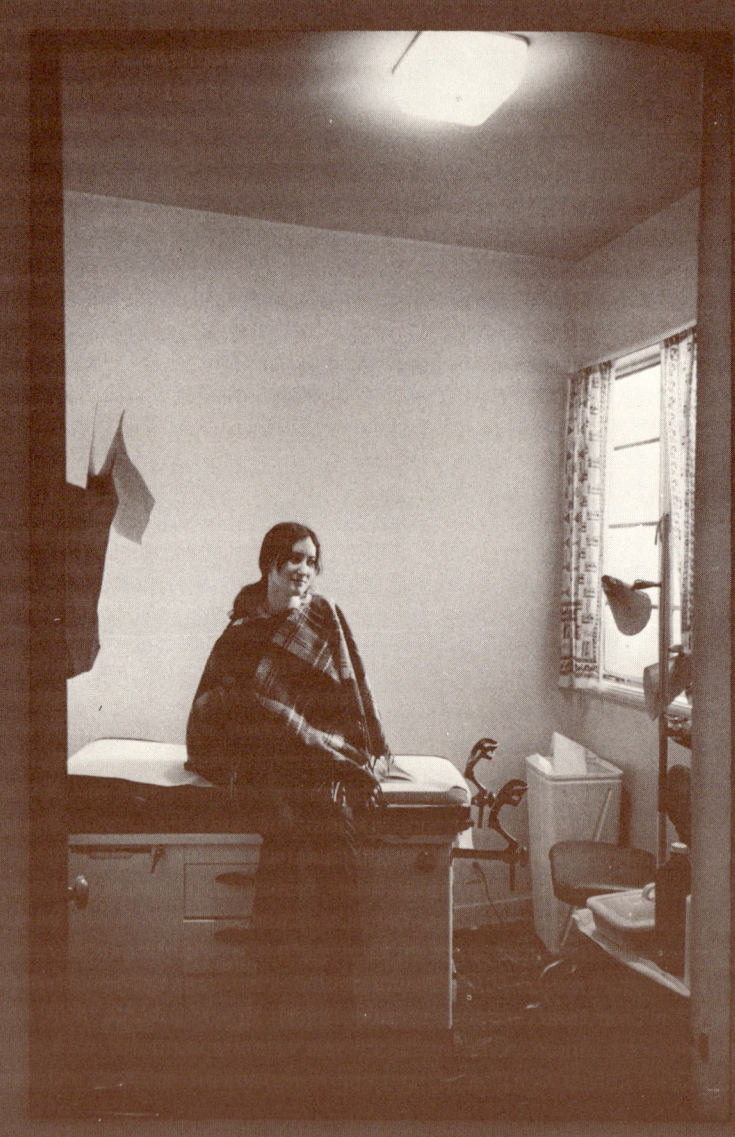

PILLS, PREVENTION, AND PROMISCUITY

Changing Values

We have seen that while the college years bring newfound freedom to many students, the changing values they encounter may urge many of them toward behavior for which they are not ready. The old values are challenged by respected teachers as well as by peer groups. Parental values are often discarded as one would discard last year's coat, but sometimes the student simply dons another garment of values over the old ones, and then, with two layers of values, he attempts to cope with an altogether new life situation. The resultant conflict has already been examined in this volume.

Research about sex on the campus tends to reveal some conflicting findings. On the one hand, it would appear that the sexual relationship among college students is not a casual encounter. Other studies, however, tend to indicate that there is an increasing amount of "one-night stand" activity. What is one to believe?

For the individual dealing with his own sexual problems, it doesn't matter what the surveys show. What is important in terms of health is that he be able to manage the feelings which are generated as a result of his behavior and that he come closer to an understanding of his motivations. Unless he can do this, his life becomes a welter of unexplained and conflicting feelings.

Character of a College Campus

Just as individual persons have personalities which are unique, so do particular college communities. A college marked by the preeminent fact that most of its students are commuting people has characteristics which are different from the college where students live on campus. In commuter colleges, parental controls frequently are in effect and usually influence the motivations of students in regard to sexual activity. Many of these students have a strong tendency to engage in behavior which is antithetical to parental

Dennis Stock, photography. Magnum Photos, Inc.

wishes. The problem of conformity to parental expectation, more often a factor with women than with men, is frequently acute.

For generations parents have been far more concerned with protecting daughters than sons from defamation. The specter of an unwed pregnant daughter looms hauntingly in the minds of middle-class parents, and they tend to place more restrictions on daughters. Curfews are established. Explanations are expected. Dates are watched with apprehension. Probably such families always expect the young woman to introduce to them the young man she is dating.

Reactions to these conditions are bound to follow: Violation of parental codes stands for emancipation. Playing at sex is a sign of adulthood. The person who has had a number of sexual encounters has arrived. But too often the behavior is a reaction *against* other values, rather than a means of self-affirmation.

What's the difference, one might ask, so long as the person is freed from the restrictions and inhibitions which bound him as a child? A valid question, but one which presupposes that such behavior comes without price or penalty. Even though the student may be inclined to go against the values of his parents, their values have been strongly instilled in his own personality in the form of conscience, and unless he can successfully answer his conscience, any behavior which violates these conditioned beliefs will present difficulties.

If the social context of one's campus is such that he is given sufficient emotional support for his changed behavior, he is helped to overcome parental attitudes. The collective experience on the college scene can help him establish a sense of autonomy about his behavior. If the college establishment represents the same values as his parents, the game of getting-away-with-it can be played to the hilt. The situation, in terms of the inner struggles of a young person, is no different than if he were living at home.

Where there is a liberal attitude on the part of the college, students tend to conduct their sexual relationships in a context that is serious rather than casual, especially if the faculty-student relationship is one of mutual trust and esteem. When students feel that it is possible to approach faculty personnel to discuss things of personal student interest, the wise teacher may help students bridge the gap between the more infantile relationships of the student-parent world and the world of mature sexuality toward which they must move to develop into successful adults.

When a mature adult-adult relationship does not exist, students tend to insulate themselves from the influence of wiser heads.

They are forced to find comfort and insight among themselves. While this frequently has constructive outcomes, sometimes the attitude of revolt predominates, the members of a group engaging in behavior which has no other motive than that of negation of the established values.

An Attitude about Sex

A student came into a professor's office concerned about the fact that he did not seem to have any firm ideas about sex. Most of the young people he knew, he said, seemed to know "where they were at." He, on the other hand, found himself moving from position to position according to the strength of the last argument he had heard. His vacillation bothered him. What should he believe?

Together the teacher and the student arrived at the point of view that there really was no one way to think about it. They also came to realize that persons who when young have definite beliefs frequently hold these beliefs either because of their need for security or because they have never really questioned the attitudes that were given them by their parents. Furthermore, they reasoned, if one is really to grow, values must change.

This is not an uncommon experience for young people. It is frequently what they experience just before taking an important step ahead in the self-actualizing process. They are pulled in two different directions at the same time. One leads toward growth, the other toward safety. The process of changing our values is seldom a quick and easy one. As values change, our attitudes about ourselves change. Our estimates about our own worth fluctuate.

Considering the number of influences which promote changed behavior relative to sex, it would be surprising if the set of values one held five years ago remained intact today. The automobile has had a remarkable effect, increasing the opportunities to escape the surveillance of parents or other curious elders. The availability of the motel room for short periods of time also has brought about changes in behavior and frequently in attitude. Motion pictures, literature, and other mass media have introduced many to the mysteries of sexual activity.

What attitude should one take about these things? Are they good or bad? Serious discussion with young people soon reveals that the question of good or bad is not relevant (see Chapter 18). The fact is that changes have taken place. Many of the changes have made it possible for people more easily to rationalize behavior which was once not condoned. The attitude often is, "Others are involved; why not me?"

It is important to see things in the broadest perspective possible. Our point of view in this book is that there are things which must be attempted if we are to develop the autonomous judgment needed for self-actualization. We have already established that sexuality is not an isolated aspect of one's being, that it permeates everything we do and every attitude we have about what we are doing. Whether a young man and woman believe their behavior enhances their sexual image or see themselves engaged in behavior which is damaging to the anticipated image will affect the nature of the relationship and its consequences. In either case they must understand what is happening within themselves. This is illustrated in the following account of a relationship at a small college in upstate New York.

>Marc and Ann had been going together for some months. Each of them felt they cared a great deal about the other. Marc was convinced that this was the real thing. They had talked about marriage but had made no definite plans, for graduation was several years away.
>
>Against Ann's wishes but with her consent, the two young people had begun to be intimate with one another. For both of them it was the first experience with sex that had any meaning. Marc had no doubts about the rightness of what they were doing. He believed it was natural and wholesome for them, since they were in love. While he was troubled by Ann's reservations about their sexual intimacy, he felt good about his role in the relationship. He felt he was playing a man's natural role and felt stronger, more confident, and more sophisticated as a result.
>
>Ann, however, believed that what they were doing was not right. She wanted to give herself to Marc but experienced a great deal of guilt about it. She had been brought up to believe that only a tramp would behave as she was doing. She did not like the sneaky tactics they had to use in order to be intimate with one another. She felt humiliated on the one occasion when they went to a nearby motel for an afternoon of privacy.
>
>Because she was not fulfilling a role expectation she had for herself, she became increasingly uneasy about her relationship with Marc. They had many tearful arguments about what they

were doing. As the weeks passed, Ann showed increasing signs of the tension she was under. It registered on her face, her behavior was less buoyant, she began to do poorly in her academic work.

The quality of Ann's response was obviously influenced negatively. Problems of this sort have been discussed in Chapter 18.

If we proceed with the assumption that people seek personal enhancement which goes beyond the physical in every interpersonal relationship, then that relationship which does not provide it is not a source of self-actualization. When we learn this and then seek to invest something in our relationships, the rewards of the relationship increase. We see ourselves as persons capable of obtaining reward from life. We see others as persons worthy of our regard and our concern. We attempt, then, to develop skills which are mutually satisfying. In the words of Erich Fromm, as he defines love, we have an "active concern for the life and the growth" of one another.

Sex and Symbolism

Any act can become invested with symbolic significance (discussed in Chapter 4). It is in its symbolism that the sexual encounter has its greatest meaning for human beings. For the uninitiated, sexual intercourse is rich with its newness. It is also invested with the belief that one is moving into a more adult world. This in itself has value in that it enables one to see himself in a different light. Problems arise when the act is invested with meaning that is not consistent with the facts.

For example, when one assumes that sexual activity is all that is involved in adult behavior, he is deluding himself. Furthermore, when, after several encounters at one stage of development, no new understanding is reached, there is evidence of retardation. This is a particular problem on the American scene. Too many young people attempt to define their maturity in terms that are not adequate to meet the challenges of mature living but have become behavioral clichés, like smoking, driving, and earning money. Many place sexual activity in a similar category. When these are compared with other signs of maturity like sensitivity, empathy, autonomy, judgment, and creativity, it is obvious that some distortion of emphasis is operating.

When one's sexual encounters are invested with a desire to bring joy and satisfaction to another, he has moved beyond the stage of adolescent fascination with the purely physical elements of sex. He seeks to develop a sensitivity to his partner's moods. He attempts to develop skills which are suited to bringing the greatest pleasure to his partner. He becomes less interested in self-gratification and more interested in pleasing his partner. His greatest pleasure is found in his partner's pleasure.

It is difficult to imagine the development of this kind of skill and sensitivity in a casual relationship. The subtleties of communication require an intimate knowledge of one another that cannot be attained in an encounter of short duration.

A Standard for Evaluation

We need to evaluate the relative worth of the casual and/or promiscuous relationship as against the more enduring one. When we invest something of ourselves in the relationship and are willing to commit ourselves to its larger meaning, we ourselves receive more from it. The sex act itself is enhanced, bringing forth with each encounter a newly found sense of wonder, respect, and joy both in ourselves and in our partner. Sex then is developmental, unfolding some element of our being which we have not known before.

What, then, can we say about the casual encounter? Is it wrong? It *may* be, but the most important thing we can say about it is that it is *limited* in its meaning. It brings limited returns in self-actualization. It may be necessary for the immature person to experience this kind of encounter, with its relative emptiness, before he can go on to something more meaningful. But tragically the limited and exploitative attitudes may remain with those people brought up in a restrictive tradition about sex. They may never reach the levels of appreciation of which they are capable. Many men use sex as an outlet for the frustrations they experience in their work. Women expect that it will relieve them of the crushing boredom of their daily duties as housewives. They feel so bored with the normal pursuits of their lives that they attempt to find satisfaction in the mere physical release that sexual intercourse can bring. When this is the case, sex soon becomes invested with the same monotony as the rest of their lives. A frequently sought alternative to this boredom is the excitement of a new sexual relationship. For some the new relationship not only brings relief but may even be developmental for them as persons. But when others are involved, the mate or children are often hurt. The sense of guilt associated with the surreptitious nature of such relationships often produces problems which cannot easily be handled by the persons involved in them. The worth of the relationship may then be questioned.

Modern Methods of Birth Control

The preceding discussion has concerned itself primarily with the attitudinal aspects of sexual intercourse, with little regard to the possibilities of conception. Presumably, modern methods of birth control have played a considerable part in freeing people from fears which have traditionally exerted controls over their behavior.

The fear of conception has been a controlling factor in the lives of women engaged in sexual intimacies. Because they must go through the rigors of gestation and must face the social disapproval of bearing a child out of wedlock, it is inevitable that they give much deeper consideration to the consequences of sexual intercourse than their male counterparts. The stress and anxiety of seeking some means of aborting the conceptus has been an ordeal which has had no equal in our society. To some extent this stress will undoubtedly be alleviated by changes in abortion laws, discussed later in this chapter, and present-day attitudes about sexual intercourse are strongly influenced by the availability of contraceptive devices. All the same, though few young people fully consider the implications of their acts at the time, the possibility of conception casts a shadow over the thoughts of women engaged in sex acts outside the bounds of marriage.

Men are more concerned with preserving or enhancing their masculine image than with whether the woman becomes pregnant. The remarkable intensity of the male need to bolster his identity through his sexual encounters influences both the male and female attitude toward sex and birth control. Many men have developed a marked sense of irresponsibility. With the woman quite the reverse has developed. How, then, does this influence the feeling about the various methods of birth control?

The kind of research in birth control which has evolved is proof of some of the attitudes that prevail. Most birth control methods render the female incapable of conception. There have been few developments designed to render the male incapable of impregnating his partner. It is quite possible, for example, to develop a pill which would render the male impotent without affecting his ability to function in sexual intercourse. However, most males resist this kind of interference with their peculiarly masculine function. Apparently they would suffer feelings of inadequacy as males if this should occur. The vasectomy, a simple operation, has been rejected out of hand by the vast majority of males. The operation entails a simple slit in the scrotum and then a tying off of the tubules leading from the testes to the penis. The *attitudes* toward this interference with normal function by some males who have had the operation have been such that they have been unable to function sexually. There is no physical reason whatsoever for this to happen. The fact remains that it does.

At present, the responsibility for birth control falls primarily on the shoulders of the woman. On the surface there appears to be no great problem here: the sole criterion is "Does it work?" However, more is involved.

Just as the popularity of a contraceptive designed for men depends upon its effect on a man's feeling about his identity, so it does for the woman. Devices which work may not become popular if the woman must act counter to her idea of acceptable female behavior. The majority of women, as well as men, have come to accept that the responsibility for contraception lies with the woman. Nevertheless a device like the diaphragm (discussed below) remains unpopular with some women. Most claim discomfort about having to take the sexual initiative by inserting the diaphragm, because it implies that a sexual encounter is expected. Since aggressiveness is still not a part of the woman's role concept, this makes her reluctant to use the diaphragm. Some women would rather interrupt the natural foreplay sequence than apply the device ahead of time, as should be done. This, of course, leaves something to be desired in the enjoyment of the sexual act.

The Condom

At the present time the most commonly used means of birth control is the condom. Often called a "rubber," it is a balloonlike sac of fine latex rubber. This sac is placed over the penis and, when it remains intact, usually provides a reasonably effective barrier between the sperm cell and the ovum.

One of the greatest hazards in the use of the condom has been nearly overcome through modern manufacturing techniques. At one time the danger of the condom's bursting was quite real. Since the advent of new materials and more effective production methods, this danger has been reduced substantially.

But another hazard lies in the fact that withdrawal should occur immediately after ejaculation. Since some couples prefer to remain locked in a loving embrace for some time after ejaculation has taken place, immediate withdrawal presents some problems in the enjoyment of the sex act. Furthermore, it is frequently felt by most males and some females that the condom, however fine, results in some deadening of sensation, and many couples report that psychologically there is some sense of separation when the condom is used. The condom is more popular in the casual relationship and, when used carefully, acts to prevent the spread of venereal disease.

The Diaphragm

This is another mechanical device which acts as a barrier between sperm and ovum. Basically, it is a rubber dome designed to fit over the cervix, the narrow neck of the uterus which protrudes into the vagina. Usually the diaphragm is used in combination with a spermicidal agent which is placed inside it before it is inserted into the vagina before intercourse. It is neither as easily purchased nor as easily applied as the condom.

The diaphragm requires an initial fitting by a physician so that a device of the proper size is used. Once this fitting is accomplished and the proper size is determined, it can be purchased in most drugstores. The same device can be used many times and remains reasonably effective until the material of which it is made begins to deteriorate. Usually a properly cared for diaphragm will last about two years.

The cream or jelly which is used in conjunction with the diaphragm lines the rim and the cup of the diaphragm and thus prevents sperm cells from entering the uterus, even if some sperm should successfully pass over the edge, or rim, of the diaphragm itself.

The objection to the diaphragm is that it too creates a sense of separation between the partners engaged in intercourse. Furthermore, there is some effect on sensation for the male, not so much a sense of limited sensation as of the presence of a foreign object. This results both from the diaphragm with its rigid rim and from the vaginal cream used in conjunction with it. If this cream escapes from the cup and coats the lining of the vagina, it provides an excess of lubrication and therefore interferes with the full enjoyment of the act.

Other objections to the use of the diaphragm are usually overcome with use and experience. Some women object to the fact that they must insert their own fingers into the vagina in positioning the diaphragm. Instructions by a physician tend to alleviate other objections. For example, it is usually recommended that the diaphragm be inserted some time before intercourse takes place, so that the procedures which lead up to intercourse are not interrupted. Some couples object to the calculated feeling this imparts to the act. The objection of some women—their reluctance to behave like the aggressor in the encounter—was mentioned earlier. Usually, however, couples who have lived with one another for some time learn to detect signs that a sexual encounter is in the offing. While this does not fully eliminate the problem, it can become a part of the scheme of things which most people using the diaphragm learn to live with.

For correct use, most manufacturers of the various vaginal creams and jellies recommend that the diaphragm be left in place for at least eight hours after intercourse has taken place and, when more than one ejaculation occurs, that an additional application of vaginal cream be used. This is done by leaving the diaphragm in place and simply applying the additional cream with the use of a syringelike applicator. This again has the drawback of interfering with the spontaneous nature of the sexual encounter.

Chemical Spermicides

These are usually in the form of agents which foam up when in contact with the moist lining of the vagina. When properly applied, they cover the upper end of the vagina and cervix. When sperm are deposited, the foam acts as a spermicidal agent. Statistically, this barrier to conception is not as effective as the diaphragm. Furthermore, it sometimes acts as an irritant to the vaginal wall. It also acts to increase lubrication, sometimes to such an extent as to interfere with complete satisfaction for the male partner.

Withdrawal

Probably the least effective and most limited method of birth control is that in which the male withdraws prior to ejaculation. Since there is apt to be some seepage of sperm prior to ejaculation, there is no guarantee that conception will be prevented. Furthermore, as a regular means of preventing conception, withdrawal is virtually guaranteed to establish sufficient frustration in both partners so that it may well act as a deterrent to satisfying sexual intercourse. In the context of carrying on sexual activity as a means of mediating mutual satisfaction, the limitations of this means of birth control are self-evident.

It is understandable that in the frustration that surrounds this means of conceptual control there are bound to be occasions wherein the ability to withdraw is well-nigh impossible. Ejaculation then will take place within the vagina, and only chance determines whether conception will take place or not. As a result the entire act becomes one in which the effort to maintain control over oneself transcends any other consideration in the act.

The Rhythm Method

This means of birth control is based upon the idea that the female fertility period is cyclic in nature and that the most fertile period can be determined with some degree of accuracy. It further asumes that a careful plotting of the temperature cycles of the female will show, just prior to the period of ovulation, a slight elevation ($\frac{1}{2}$ to 1 degree) of temperature and that if intercourse is avoided for about eight days after this, conception will not take place.

Although we have much information about the timing involved in conception, nevertheless this means of birth control is still ineffective. Many factors may delay the time of ovulation, even in a woman whose regular menstrual cycle has been established. For example, a woman with a 28-day cycle should ovulate 14 days before the onset of menstruation. This together with the regular temperature taking (usually every morning just after waking) should provide information to guide the couple in determining when sexual intercourse is "safe." However, if there has been some emotional disturbance about the time of ovulation, it may delay ovulation for several days to several weeks. Also, a slight elevation of temperature can be caused by other factors. This immediately throws off the calculations, and there is a good chance of a surprise conception.

The Pill

Birth control pills effect the hormonal content of the female system. In this way the ovaries can be fooled into reacting as if the woman were pregnant, and they will not ovulate. Conception is then not possible.

The usual method is for the Pill to be taken for 20 days beginning the fifth day after the menstrual flow starts. These pills release into the system progesterone and estrogen, hormones that suppress the follicle-stimulating hormone of the pituitary gland.

This prevents the ripening of the egg in the ovary. At the end of the 20-day period the Pill is no longer taken. Within three days the menstrual flow should begin.

When recommended procedures are followed, this means of birth control is extremely effective. However, the Pill must be taken every day. If it is not taken regularly, ovulation may occur and conception could result. The possibility of human error is therefore to be reckoned with.

Many research projects have attempted to investigate the side effects of taking the Pill. At present there is accumulating evidence of an increasing likelihood that small emboli (blood clots) will form in the woman's bloodstream. When these achieve a size that prevents them from passing through the many valves through which our blood must circulate in completing its cyclic flow, the results may range from muscle cramps to blood deprivation in critical areas like the heart. Why this happens in some women and not in others is not understood.

There have been reports which indicate that the incidence of cervical cancer among women using the Pill is on the rise. Again there is no clear understanding of why this happens. Other side effects have been an increased incidence of headaches and a tendency toward emotional depression.

The Intrauterine Contraceptive Device

This means of birth control is a very ancient one. Historically, many peoples have followed the practice of inserting a foreign substance into the uterus to prevent conception. The contemporary practice is to insert a small plastic object into the uterus. It is not known just how this prevents conception. It is assumed that there is no interference with the fertilization process, but, rather, that the foreign object renders it impossible for the fertilized egg to become imbedded in the uterine lining and that therefore the egg decomposes and is passed off with the normal secretions of the vagina. The great advantage of this device is that once inserted, little more than routine checkups is necessary.

A small plastic coil, or loop (known as the IUD, or the loop), is inserted into the uterus by a physician. Attached to it are several plastic strings which protrude from the cervix to make removal easier if this is desired and to provide a simple test to ensure that the device is still in place. There is no interference with the menstrual cycle or with the production of ova, although heavy menstrual bleeding is a common side effect.

The major problem is that in about 15 percent of women the body will automatically reject the device. This usually happens without the woman's knowledge, and the IUD may be passed from her body when least expected. Subsequently, there is no protection against conception. There is no way to determine beforehand whether a woman's body will reject the device. It happens because of the body's natural tendency to expel a foreign substance. Furthermore, with about 2 percent of women conception has taken place even when the contraceptive device has remained in place.

Contraceptives of the Future

Research continues on various means of birth control, among them, the subcutaneous Spansule tablet. This method utilizes the principle that certain chemical compositions are dissolved by the body at a predictable rate. If a tablet designed to release hormones into the system of a woman at a predictable rate is placed under her skin, it can be used to control fertility for several years at a time. Such a tablet would have to be replaced from time to time.

Another method which has possibilities is the "morning-after" pill. This pill would also control hormonal balances and work to interfere with conception. It would be taken by the woman the morning after intercourse has taken place.

Injections given by a physician have been experimented with. These also work on controlling hormonal balances within the female system. At present, experimental evidence shows that these injections are useful for a three-month period. At the end of that time another injection must be administered.

In every one of these procedures some shortcomings are evident. But there is no doubt that within the next decade many more contraceptives will have been developed than are available now. This means that we are approaching a time when the possibility of conception will no longer be a factor in the attitudes we hold about sex.

Unmarried Pregnancy

The wider choice among life styles today becomes apparent when the issues surrounding pregnancies are viewed. Only a few years ago an unmarried woman who found herself pregnant was usually forced into one course of action. There were no real alternatives available. Today that picture has changed. Changing sexual values, legalized abortion, and different attitudes about the entire structure of marriage are but a few of the factors which have a bearing on the problem of unwed motherhood. Let us consider some of the alternatives and the problems attendant in each.

Keeping the Baby

It is often the moral issue that motivates young couples in their decision about whether to keep the baby or not. The stigma of the past is so powerful that the couple—or even the young woman by herself—prefer to face this crucial time alone. What is the stigma really? It is nothing more than the open admission of the indisputable fact that sexual intercourse has taken place outside the marriage structure. The unwillingness of the young people to reveal this openly keeps them from seeking help from parents, friends, or even professional sources. The fear of social rejection may prevent them from considering keeping the baby as one possible alternative. The fear of discovery creates panic and horror.

It is conceivable that some young women might want to keep their children. There are some who suggest that it is more immoral and irresponsible not to. For these women, especially if there will be no father, there are practical circumstances to consider. The future possibility of marriage may be affected. The problems of a future marriage are increased. Financial support may be needed, at least temporarily. Provisions for child care will have to be available if the mother is to work. Last, there is the problem of facing the social prejudices of others.

The following is an excerpt from a magazine article[1] written by a mature unmarried young woman with a financially stable career as a newspaper reporter who became pregnant. She chose to keep her child because "[I] felt that what was inside me was not an embryo or a fetus but the essence of life itself. The spark of human existence was demanding that my body clothe it in tissue that it might be born." She made provisions for her own and the baby's care. Even though all practical accommodations were made and she happily anticipated the new facts of her life, she encountered constant prejudice from those who thought that she should have an abortion. After refusing to have an abortion or to put her child up for adoption, she lost her job. Even after the baby was born, the stigma associated with the situation continued. She wrote:

[1] Jane Harriman, "In Trouble," *The Atlantic*, vol. 225, p. 9, March, 1970.

While the unwed mother has to assume almost complete responsibility for her child, society does not really consider her a responsible adult. To give an example, in order to get life insurance, I was told by the salesman that I had to lie and call myself "divorced." Also, the first diaper service I called asked my husband's name, and then, after I said "unmarried," would not accept me as a customer. When I called a second service, I said, with a catch in my voice, "Widowed." The diapers were delivered that day.

The problems inherent in this choice are many, and all its ramifications must be considered before a decision is made. For some women this may seem to be the best decision. Pregnancy and childbirth can be a most exciting and thrilling experience. But much of the pleasure comes from sharing the experience with the father of the child, friends, and family. When the responsibilities of parenthood are shared and when the mother gets emotional as well as practical support, having a baby is a celebration. When the child is unwanted and represents for the mother rejection, shame, isolation, and loneliness, it takes an unusual woman indeed to face the experience and make a success of her life and the life of her child.

It is often assumed that certain ethnic groups are innately promiscuous because there are so many unwed mothers among them. Contrary to general opinion, behavior and choice more often follow along economic stratification than ethnic or racial lines. There are many reasons for this.

In the poverty culture, having a baby out of wedlock is a common thing. There are many homes without fathers. Although there may be no social stigma attached to this, the lower-class mother may feel guilty because middle-class values have been imprinted upon her to some extent. Many young mothers of the lower economic class keep their babies not only because there is no stigma attached to it but also because there are fewer alternatives available to them. That the home is fatherless only perpetuates the maladjustments, monotony, dreariness, and poverty. A vicious cycle is set in motion. No ethnic or racial group is constitutionally lazy, immoral, irresponsible, or depraved. Such assumptions are unfounded prejudice.

Putting the Baby Up for Adoption

For any number of reasons a young mother-to-be may choose to have her baby but to put it up for adoption. These reasons may vary from personal or religious convictions concerning taking the life of the child to the fear associated with abortion.

Accepting the child into the home is often a repugnant idea to the parents of a pregnant young girl. The pregnancy represents evidence of their own failure. The desperate explanation that parents give to neighbors and friends for the girl's absence from the home is evidence of the depth of their feelings. At the same time feelings about abortion, and the moral codes and prejudices of the community they live in, operate strongly. Both the parents and the unwed mother may be victims of strongly entrenched prejudices.

The idea of terminating a pregnancy may be completely unacceptable to some people. "In what way is it different from murder?" "How could I take the life of another human being?" For some girls, finding the right doctor, particularly in states where abortion is illegal, proves to be a stumbling block. As abortion laws become increasingly liberal, this problem will probably diminish. But there may still be many who will not have the finances to support such a venture. Many women, rather than face the horror of revealing their plight to their parents, suffer in secrecy and in silence, hoping that the whole thing is a bad nightmare, until abortion is no longer a reasonable alternative. Perhaps a young woman will attempt to make her own arrangements with a social agency for unwed mothers and try to keep the information from her parents completely. Her desperation often precludes any rational thinking. The importance of getting some professional and objective advice at a time like this cannot be overemphasized.

Adoption is not a satisfying alternative for all. The emotional trauma of having to give her own child away and the fear of the unknown circumstances in store for her baby must be dealt with by the young mother. This is not an easy decision to make. Black women are confronted with the fact that childless couples who can afford to adopt a child are usually white. Thus, there is less demand for their children than for white babies.

Abortion

The incidence of medical abortion has increased in recent years. Many physicians are convinced that abortion is preferable to an unwanted birth. These feelings persist in the face of some strict laws to the contrary. However, legal abortions are now available in several states of the union. In time more and more states will probably modify their abortion laws so that it will be possible to obtain the services of a competent person to perform the operation.

In cases where abortion must be performed illegally, serious risks are run. There can be little or no assurance that the abortionist is qualified or responsible. Hospital facilities are usually not available. The surreptitious nature of the arrangements, the often sordid conditions in which the operation is performed, and the natural guilt that follows make this an unpleasant experience even under the best of circumstances. Serious injury and even death are not uncommon when the patient is handled by inadequately trained persons. When the surroundings are unclean and when the abortionist is unqualified, sterility, infection, hemorrhage, and a severe threat to life itself may follow.

Many women are fearful of abortion procedures because of the horrible stories that have been told to them. Once again the social stigma attached to pregnancy may keep the unmarried woman and her family from inquiring after safe and legitimate abortions. So long as abortion procedures remain illegal, prices will be exorbitant and prohibitive. This closes the door to many people. The desire for secrecy and the lack of adequate funds sometimes moves young women to make desperate attempts at aborting themselves or to listen to friends who say they know how to take care of the problem "because I have a friend who . . . ." Home remedies, such as the use of knitting needles, hangers, and internally taken drugs, are very dangerous and often unsuccessful.

Under optimal conditions abortion is a simple procedure if done within the first trimester of the pregnancy. The risk to the life of the mother is small. Many methods have been used by qualified gynecologists with success: suction, introduction of a saline solution, and dilation and curettage. When these are performed under sterile conditions and provisions are made for unforeseen emergencies, there is little to be feared. There is indication today that strict abortion laws are rapidly on their way out. Thus, safe abortion techniques may soon be available to many more young women. Fleeing to other countries for legal abortions will become a thing of the past.

What are the moral implications of abortion? Some of them pose serious questions, not only for those immediately involved, but for the society as well. Shall we feel free to take a life? When is it permissible? Some debates have centered around the issue of when life begins for an embryo. Does the life within the mother have no rights? Who should have final decision over the matter? Are there other aspects of abortion that take precedence over the life or death of the embryo?

These questions are not easily answered. There are probably no fixed answers for the society or for the individual. In the future the

The Man-Woman Relationship

It is most unfortunate when an illegitimate pregnancy occurs and precipitates behavior that is unwise for the couple involved. Even if the relationship has been a loving and stable one, marriage may not be the wisest course of action to follow, although it may save face for the families and for the young couple. Such marriages begin with added difficulties and stress. Adjustment to marriage is difficult enough without the added financial and personal responsibilities of a new infant. If the relationship is a strong one, however, the marriage may succeed.

When the relationship is an uncommitted one, it is most often doomed to failure. The circumstances of the stress situation, plus the lack of commitment and love for each other, are almost always impossible hurdles. The pressure to keep the facts of the situation quiet may motivate parents to force their children into a hopeless future of unhappiness. This should be avoided at all costs.

Most parents, however, are more understanding and even more helpful than the children expect them to be. At a time when they are needed most, even though they may be very conservative in their views, they usually come through. Parents may be of great assistance, sometimes through their own experience, and should be included in the decision-making process.

The Role of the College

There is ample reason to believe that the college should carefully consider the introduction of programs of education and counseling that are designed to deal with pregnancy, birth control measures, etc. Some institutions, capitulating to neurotic parents, have attempted to maintain a Victorian position in which they refuse to recognize that there is a problem. Other colleges have moved with the times, and while they recognize the value in a student's taking the responsibility for his or her own behavior, they believe that an enlightened program is necessary. Such programs not only provide the necessary help after the damage is done but prevent problems from arising. Information and materials for birth control are dispensed and medical services are provided.

This, however, is a minimal program. Not only is a factually accurate information program essential, but beyond this there needs to be an opportunity to explore the entire process of establishing one's sexuality, with an open discussion of the feelings and conflicts involved and with members of both sexes included. Competent faculty personnel should be involved in these discussions. Such courses, seminars, or discussion groups should work toward developing a sense of mature awareness of the meaning of sex for people of college age.

Student responsibility is essential here—responsibility to ourselves as well as to others. An honest examination of our attitudes about sex and about our own sexuality is necessary. It is important for male students to be open and direct in communicating with female students about their expectations relative to sex. The reverse is also true. We should not be ignorant about what the other sex feels about itself in the heterosexual encounter or about what we ourselves feel about these matters.

As we have already stressed, our culture has been potent in forcing us to obscure from ourselves what we feel about our own sexuality. It is a rare person who can adequately reveal his or her feelings about the particular parts of the body. It is unusual for a man or woman to be able to admit the secret practices he has engaged in. The very fact that much of our attitudinal belief about our own sexuality has been developed in a frame of reference that is shrouded in mystery and secrecy has led to any number of hang-ups in this area. For many of us, what should be a source of joy and pride is cloaked in shame and ignorance. This is a sad commentary on what exists and strongly indicates what is necessary on the part of the colleges.

Venereal Disease

Though campaigns to remove venereal disease (VD) from the area of secret suffering and ignorance have been conducted for several decades, it is still relegated to the world of underground thoughts by those who experience it. This is perhaps one of the most dangerous aspects of the diseases in this category. The shame which surrounds VD often prevents infected persons from obtaining treatment when it is most likely to help. Postponed treatment enables the diseases to establish a hold upon the victim and sometimes cause organic damage from which there is no recovery to normalcy.

Both the common venereal diseases in the United States (syphilis, caused by a spirochete, and gonorrhea, caused by a gonococcus) are transmitted usually by direct contact with an infected person. Unfortunately most of us have been given the idea that VD can be contracted only under evil and disgusting circumstances. Furthermore, most of the education about VD has been of the scare variety in which students are exposed to the horrifying long-range results of unchecked infection. The result has been that persons who contract venereal disease experience a deep sense of shame and fear. They are unwilling to face the fact that they may have the disease and frequently wait, hoping that the symptoms will disappear. In the case of syphilis, they may often be obliged. The initial symptoms may go away within two weeks of their appearance and not return until some weeks later. Again symptoms will disappear if ignored, to reappear perhaps years later in the form of crippling damage to one or another system of the body.

In the case of gonorrhea the symptoms in males are constant and increasingly painful but in females may go undetected until serious damage has been done to the reproductive system. Furthermore, an infected female may spread the disease to countless other individuals who, themselves, may become a part of the infecting chain.

One way to check the spread of venereal disease is to have the essential facts and to act promptly when exposure has been experienced. Another means of preventing the spread of the disease is to render it subject to easy discussion. It should be recognized that VD *can* be contracted from persons about whom one cares. A love relationship, a "good" family background, social position, money, or prestige are no guarantors against venereal infection. Syphilis and gonorrhea are contagious diseases which may be contracted under conditions which are socially acceptable among one's peers. They cannot be treated with silence.

The essential facts, in addition to those mentioned above, are as follows: For gonorrhea the symptoms are a pus discharge from the urethra and a burning sensation during urination. Sterility may result from an infection allowed to last too long. Self-medication is useless. Protection may be increased by using a condom during intercourse and thorough washing afterward. For syphilis the primary symptom *may* be a chancre at the site of entry of the spirochete to the circulatory system. This may be any place upon the body where there is a break in the skin or mucous membrane which has come in contact with an infected person. The chancre may appear from three to four weeks after exposure. If ignored, it will disappear. Secondary symptoms may appear two to three months later in the form of a rash, a swelling of lymph nodes, mucous patches in the mouth, a sore throat, or joint inflammations. These symptoms may not be noticed and will also disappear. The next time the disease makes its appearance may be 25 years later in the form of heart disease, blindness, or any number of other afflictions.

People need to be aware that whenever they engage in sexual practices with other persons, they may have been exposed to venereal disease. The incidence of venereal disease among homosexuals as well as heterosexuals has risen greatly in recent years. Should questionable symptoms appear, immediate medical treatment is indicated. Little is gained by waiting to be sure the symptoms are real. The healthy response is to act in the direction of eliminating the infection. This is best done under the supervision of a physician. Those who discover that they have venereal disease should promptly communicate with others whom they may have infected. Unless this is done, still others are needlessly exposed to infection, and in a single geographic area the diseases may achieve epidemic proportions.

The New Morality

It is important to recognize that a certain amount of experimentation is necessary in the growing-up process. College students for generations have recognized this but have usually advanced some of the wrong reasons for it. A popular belief held by young men is that a couple ought to have some sexual experience with one another before marriage in order to determine if they are sexually compatible. Under the circumstances in which premarital sexual activity must be carried on in our society, this idea is not entirely accurate. Sexual compatibility cannot be determined in the context of secrecy, nor can it be determined in a hit-or-miss occasional encounter, nor on the basis of a fairly regular experience that is free from the usual demands of a committed relationship.

As a society, we would probably be better off if we freed ourselves from the unnecessary guilt which surrounds premarital sex today. This idea doubtless frightens many parents. It takes some getting used to. It is difficult for a parent of today to condone his daughter's sexual experimentation, but when parents are able to view this in perspective, seeing sex as a part of the total development of an individual, it is easier for them to move toward another point of view. Parents too must realize that the developmental influence of what takes place in earlier years has direct consequences in later years, that sexual inhibitions bred into young people usually carry over into marriage, and that these inhibitions must be overcome if a young couple is to establish a mutually satisfying sexual relationship in marriage.

If this important area of married life is fraught with confusion and guilt, there are unnecessary risks in the relationship. The sexual area of marriage ought to be one wherein two people should be able to approach one another with relatively little difficulty. Instead it is an area in which much anxiety exists and out of which many conflicts grow, an area wherein far more difficulty exists than is necessary or reasonable.

Unless a young person is to be brought up in a closed community in which all members share similar ideas and where similar practices are observed, the time is past when a hard-and-fast line can be established about premarital sexual activity. If the development of a mature autonomy is a goal of life, then parents and college authorities should provide a climate of opinion in which this quality can develop. This does not mean a laissez faire attitude should prevail in regard to sex. It does mean that both adults and youth must engage in an honest dialogue with one another about these matters. They must listen to one another with sympathy and an honest effort to understand.

Furthermore, a new morality must emerge, one based upon an honest confrontation of oneself and one's fellowmen in the entire area of sex. This means that young men should put aside, as soon as they are able to, the desire to exploit their female associates. A new basis for heterosexual relationships should be established, and the sooner the better. Since communication is so important a part of marriage, every effort should be made to communicate one's deepest feelings about sex to one's partner. This communication should be a mutual undertaking. As emphasized earlier, listening with sensitivity and empathy is a must. When these things are done, one giant step toward achieving mature sexuality will have been taken.

With the increased availability of contraceptive devices and with the changing attitudes of college authorities about freedom of choice in the realm of social behavior for college students, we are embarking upon a new era of responsibility for college students. The choices are not being made for the student. He must make them for himself, which is as it should be.

Where will this lead? What will be the outcome of this for future behavior? Are we to become a society in which sexual freedom becomes the norm? Probably not. In situations where this freedom has been granted, sexual encounters tend to be carried on in relationships in which there is an important degree of personal commitment. When this occurs, sex is placed in its proper human perspective. It becomes invested with meanings which are important within the framework of marriage. People tend to use these encounters more as a means of expressing their feelings of concern for one another than as a means of revolt and rebellion against the restraints of parents and society.

Members of the older generation may tend to say, "You don't know how lucky you are." This, of course, has no meaning to the young person. What he experiences is the norm for him. As far as he knows, it has always been this way, and he tends to take it all for granted.

Is there anything wrong with this? In and of itself, probably not. But where opportunities for experimentation exist, it seems tragic to waste them. When life is seen as a series of glorious opportunities for self-development, there is a changed way of meeting the experiences of life which in terms of health is to be encouraged.

21.

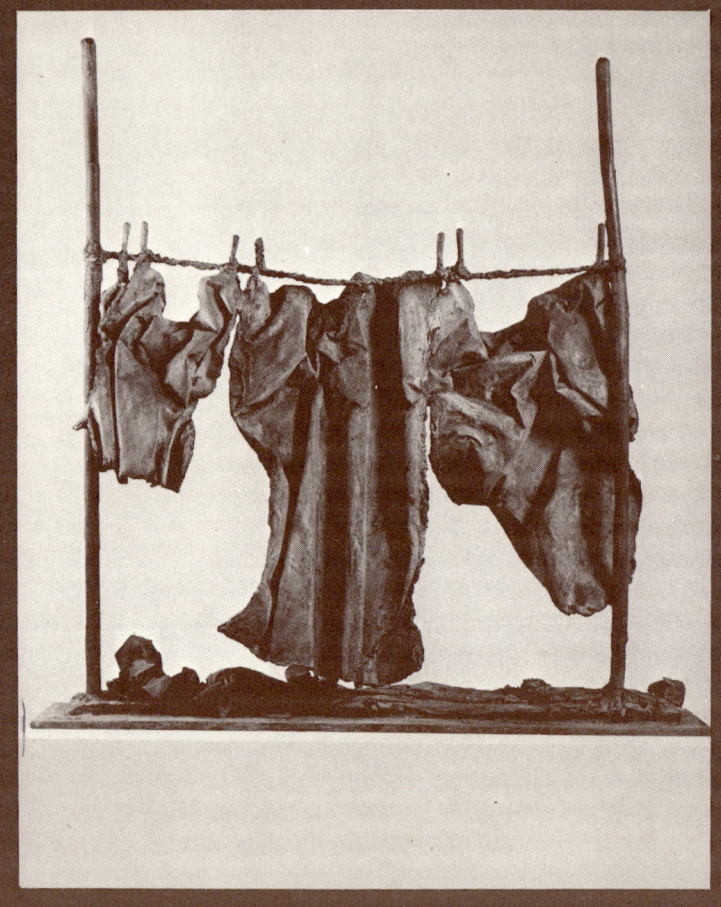

THE INTIMACY OF MARRIAGE

Since a significant part of our experience centers about those periods of time when we are directly and intimately involved in some family situation, it is important to evaluate what happens within the family context. As college students, we have begun the process of separating ourselves from our family of origin and are in the process of finding a mate with whom, presumably, we will spend the rest of our days. At the same time we are also preparing ourselves to fit into the economic structure of society. Sometimes the two efforts run counter to one another.

Attitudes and Expectations

About 90 percent of adults in the United States marry, and the college years are filled with activities having to do with the institution of marriage. Generally speaking, men go to college to prepare themselves for the primary role they believe they will have in marriage. Right or wrong, most males in the United States have the impression, as we have noted, that their major function in life is to be providers for the families that they establish. Many men have this value so stamped upon their personality that they cannot function effectively in any of the other roles they must assume in marriage. They are poorly equipped, by inclination, to be good lovers. They feel totally inadequate as fathers. They frequently chafe at the time necessary to create an effective male image for their children. For many men, home is an escape from the field of combat in their professional or business life. They often return to home depleted and badly in need of the restorative sustenance that only a wife can give. When they find that they must return to the challenges of husbandhood and fatherhood, they are not only dismayed but hostile because of the extra demands placed upon their energy.

While many women on the college scene are oriented toward the search for a husband, they are also preparing themselves for a

Peter Agostini, "The Clothesline," 1960. Bronze. Collection, The Whitney Museum of American Art, New York. Gift of Howard and Jean Lipman. Geoffrey Clements, photography.

career, should the search for a husband prove unfruitful. Young women frequently deny that they are looking for a husband. They believe it puts them in a bad light. The image of the calculating female, coolly surveying the current crop of males for husband material, does not flatter them.

Many young people tend to idealize much of what occurs within the framework of a marriage. In many ways it is well that they do. If they were not able to, there might be a strong tendency to avoid the commitment. Few relationships in our culture are more demanding. The partners must adapt to the differences in what each expects of himself and of the other as well as of the relationship itself. A series of adjustments must be made in order to bridge the considerable gap that usually exists between idealized expectations and the realities of the day-by-day marital experience. These adjustments are part of the developmental work of marriage.

Revolt against the Establishment

The anticipation of marriage is complicated by the new wave of criticism directed at the institution of marriage. At the same time that we are drawn toward wanting to marry because so many other people in our society do, we are inclined to look at marriage skeptically. This is an age of disillusionment for many young people. Many hypocrisies have been exposed through the mass media. We read about, hear about, and see dramatized in films and on TV the shallowness of many marriages.

The wife-swapping antics of which suburbanites have been frequently accused are played up in the news. Extramarital affairs, because of their gamey nature, have been the theme of many contemporary novels. If we used the mass media as a true representation of our marital and sexual mores, we could easily believe that marriage is simply one huge put-on. Associating this with the heavy emphasis on materialistic acquisition and the insensitivity apparent in our lack of concern for human dignity, we might conclude that the American home is doing a poor job of preparing its members to achieve fulfillment. More than ever before, youth have been exposed to critical comments about these shortcomings.

The result not only is disillusioning; it raises doubts in the minds of idealistic young people about the importance of marriage in the classic sense. Young people are drawn toward marriage but at the same time repelled by what it appears to produce. Traditionally, marriage and a family have been one of the major sources from which both young and mature people have drawn their sense of purpose in life. Today there is far less certainty about the value of marriage than ever before.

One result is that attitudes about premarital relationships have changed. One attitude now seems to be, "If marriage is such a sham, why wait for it? Let's get fulfillment while the chance is here."

For many, this is a frightening prospect. Dire predictions about the decline of moral values are made. Many have a sense of living in the midst of decadence and decay. The condition has had its impact upon the young. Some have reacted as though what *appears* to be true is so. They feel that if this is the way it is, they want a piece of the action now. They too have begun to conduct themselves with open disregard for the traditional views on premarital relationships.

Other young people have reacted in a different way. It has been possible for them to recognize that, in spite of the fact that moral transgressions *appear* to be all around, there is something more important at stake. They recognize that marriage still has the potential for facilitating human development. They see it as a relationship more filled with promise than ever before. At the same time they realize that marriage must be based upon a much higher degree of personal honesty than ever before. They believe there must be more behind a marriage than tradition, sex, and economic stability.

These young people are aware that an interpersonal relationship is real and important only to the extent that each member of the relationship is willing to be open in his approach to his mate. For many this means dispensing with the shams and ploys that worked in the past but do not work today. Honesty, rather than manners, realness rather than goodness, are the order of the day. There is almost a desperate hope that this will work.

Mutual Understanding

A class of men of mixed ages ranging from the late teens to the midthirties were asked to separate themselves into several groups The grouping was along age lines, one group ranging from eighteen to twenty-four, the other including those twenty-five and older. As expected, most of the married men in the class were in the older group. They were then asked to discuss and list the essential factors in a satisfying and effective marriage. The single men developed a list of some twelve items ranging all the way from *sex* through *companionship* and *mutual interest* to *similar goals*. The married men came up with one item: *mutual understanding.* The ensuing debate was loud and lusty. In essence the married men thought that the single ones were not being realistic. The single men believed that their older colleagues were too cynical.

As order developed in the discussion, it appeared the older men felt that mutual understanding should be divided into a number of categories. First, marriage should result in progressively more understanding of self. They stated that each individual in the relationship has a definite responsibility to help the other understand himself. In one sense, they were saying that a major task of marriage is to satisfy each person's need to become self-actualized. In the process each will have revealed to him, by his mate, aspects of himself which he had hitherto not known. There should be a progressive unfolding of the potential each has for living an effective and satisfying life.

They believed this cannot be done without conflict. Sometimes, they stated, conflict is essential for one to relinquish old attitudes about himself. Until he is able to do this, the newer insights cannot emerge. This is quite clearly a description of the developmental task.

The married men also underlined the mutuality of the task. They felt it cannot be done in isolation. They had found there was the need for a back-and-forth play between the individuals involved. As the task unfolded, not only did an understanding of oneself grow but also an understanding of the other person. This understanding could be used to aid one another in gaining the insights necessary for development.

The younger men in the group recognized the validity of these concepts. What they did not see clearly was the dynamic nature of the marriage relationship which the older men wished to convey. Understanding another person is getting to know what that person thinks, feels, hopes for, and wants out of life. The younger men assumed that in a few years' time understanding would be achieved and from that time forward things would run smoothly. This can be characterized as static thinking with the consequent failure to recognize that individuals change in the course of a relationship. They continually see themselves differently from the way they did at any previous time in life.

For example, a young woman enters marriage with a preconditioned idea of how a marriage should work. Her ideas result from observations of the relationship between her father and mother. She assumes that she will play a role similar to her mother's role. Frequently, this role is not clearly defined in her own mind. The feeling context of the role cannot be understood. She has been so close to it that she cannot be objective about what happens or why it does.

The role she attempts to play is not one she plans for herself. It is one which *happens* because she is what she is. It is her *self* in operation. Unless some objectivity can be brought to bear upon the situation, she will have great difficulty in seeing herself in a realistic way. It may be that the role she brings to her marriage will work for a time. But unless she is able to shift according to the developing needs of the marriage, both she and her husband will soon outgrow the internalized role.

Factors for Change

To bring about the role changes required by the developing marital needs, a number of subtle factors must come together. The first is an understanding of self. This implies a careful and progressively more objective examination of oneself. It presupposes that the person is also willing to change according to the needs which arise in the marriage.

Another factor is the task of learning what one's mate needs. The young woman, to continue with our example, has brought to the relationship an understanding of the kind of man her father is. Presumably her husband is a different person with different needs. She must learn to respond to him in a manner different from the way her mother responded to her father. The role she must play is different.

Not only must she play a different role, but she must refuse to become locked into just one role. This is where the recognition of the dynamism of marriage is important. A role, once cast, need not be perpetuated forever. If it is, growth has been inhibited. The chances are that the growth of the husband as well as of the wife will be limited.

The refusal to become role-directed is an important skill of marriage. There is a strong temptation to allow ourselves to settle into a role. This appears to be the easier way. It is not the most productive way. Many a marriage has foundered because the two persons were unable to shift roles with the growth of their mates. An illustration of this will be seen later in the chapter.

A fourth factor may be identified as the recognition of what the relationship demands. This is related to the previous task of role spontaneity. Every marriage moves forward at varying paces. At one period of time the pace is leisurely; at another it becomes intense. One or both partners are in active stages of development. Because of this they are excited, perhaps exciting, and frequently irritable. Unless each individual is able to keep pace with these changes by recognizing them as they appear, a void grows between the partners. Further work is then necessary to recover.

When there are other demands upon each person's energies, the developmental work of the marriage is often not accomplished. The demands of their careers, their children, and their involvement in community affairs may be so devitalizing that little energy is left for assessing and dealing with the demands of the marriage.

These factors—understanding ourselves, learning to meet our mate's needs, refusing to become totally role-oriented, and keeping up with the demands of the relationship—require that each person be spontaneous, creative, and flexible. For many of us this is an enormous challenge. Often, even though we are quite young when we first marry, we have learned to protect ourselves by dealing with life in stereotyped ways. We have incorporated rigidities into our personalities which prevent us from being the dynamic persons we need to be.

Living Together

In spite of the fact that we live in a society in which a very high percentage of adults are married, marriage is not for all people. Many young people feel compelled to undertake marriage simply because "it is the thing to do." If it were only the two people who were involved, little real damage would be done. But usually those who marry because it is the thing to do have children for the same reason. Children of a marriage which is not developmental confuse the situation and make it more difficult.

Many young people get married before they are ready to work toward the necessary understanding. To look at themselves objectively is not only impossible; it is threatening, as well. One solution to this problem may be the liberalization of social attitudes toward experimental cohabitation, an alternative discussed in preceding chapters in which we noted that the arrangement provides opportunities for the mutual self-examination that makes for better marriages. As we have seen, two people cannot live together without having to evaluate what they mean to themselves and to each other, and they thus develop skills which will be carried over into later marriage relationships.

If these arrangements could be carried on with the assistance of professionals who could help young couples to leap the hurdles before them, much would be accomplished to establish more effective marriages. Our society has come a long way toward accepting such arrangements. Many parents today are even supporting them. It is to their credit that they are able to do so. By doing this they are standing firm before the critical comments of their peers and also exhibiting a good deal of faith in the importance of better marriages.

The argument against the experimental "marriage" is twofold: (1) that there is a breakdown of the moral values of our society and (2) that what has been good in the past should be good now. The arguments for the other side are that (1) the world is more complex today than it was in the past, (2) the marriages of the past have not produced people capable of standing up under today's stresses, and (3) today, people are expecting more of marriage than ever before. Let us examine each of the second group of arguments.

The Increased Complexity of Today's World

Many more demands are made of individuals today, demands which take people away from the home. Rural life in the United States at one time provided opportunities for home-centered living. The entire family was engaged in the cooperative tasks of mutual survival. Today, with the vast population shift from rural to urban living, more and more people are involved in earning a living away from the home. The endeavors in which we become engaged are usually not the least related to the home. The professional engineer lives in an entirely different world at work than at home. The accountant, the laborer, the factory worker, the secretary—all are occupied in a world totally unrelated to the home. This necessarily diverts energy from the home-centered tasks of making a marriage work. Much more effort is required of people to maintain the channels of communication necessary for a satisfying relationship.

Because the world of vocation is so different from the world of marriage, it offers challenges and opportunities not heretofore available to people. These opportunities create expectations. We feel that we must succeed in our vocation, not just in our marriages. This causes an investment of time and energy in the job which is necessarily taken from the home.

In contemporary life, furthermore, people of both sexes are engaged in the labor market more than ever before, and thus there are increased temptations for extramarital involvements to exist. If the temptation is yielded to, further quantities of energy and time are diverted from maintaining relationships at home.

These three factors, at least, are an indication of the increased complexity of the world in which we live today. They must be recognized and dealt with.

Inadequacy of Past Values under Present Stresses

Because in the past we have been oriented toward values that grew from a more stable world, we have not been able to apply these values to contemporary living. That so many people are growing up poorly equipped to deal with the general problems of life provides reason to reevaluate what we have brought from the past. For example, a value which suggests that the form of a relationship is more important than its dynamics does not work. When we are more concerned with doing the proper thing than with growth and development, we close doors to self-actualization. A value which suggests that a legal contract is more important than a personal commitment leaves us open to a charge of hypocrisy. A value which suggests that family structure is more important than self-realization stunts personal growth.

Living today demands more commitment than ever before. Many young people today are attempting to abandon the economic determinants of their lives. They have said that personal fulfillment is more important than economic success. Some attention should be paid to this goal, however idealistic it may be. The evidence of breakdown among those who have sacrificed themselves to material success is convincing. A better way of life must be found. New values must be established and can come only from experiencing life as we ourselves know it. We need to resist the temptation to borrow the values of others and to develop a do-it-yourself approach to life. When we do, we will be on the road toward self-actualization.

Today's Greater Expectations of Marriage

Young people today enter marriage with high expectations of personal fulfillment. In the past, many had the attitude of once married, always married. Few questions were asked and few things expected. One learned to put up with one's mate. Love may have been a basic reason for getting married, but many marriages soon became an endurance contest.

Heretofore the roles of the husband and the wife were more sharply defined. Each had his tasks and responsibilities. Each has seen these roles acted out in his or her own home by father and mother. The roles had been incorporated through the process of identification. Boys learned to be men by emulating their fathers. Girls learned to be women by acting as their mothers had. Each had a fairly clear idea of what to expect from the other sex in marriage. Today, many people do not want to be defined by these sex roles, but without the limits, they may be unsure of what to expect.

With contemporary emphasis upon self-development and doing your own thing, much more is expected of marriage. Many persons are not willing to accept failure in their marital roles. They believe that there is no point in maintaining a relationship which is so costly in energy. Their frustration tolerance is low when it comes to failure in marriage. People are willing to try again with another mate rather than struggle with a marriage which has few apparent dividends in terms of self-actualization.

What Stands in the Way?

Simply expecting more of marriage does not provide a guarantee that our expectations will be fulfilled. What primarily stands in the way of creative and spontaneous action in a marriage is lack of readiness.

Youthful marriages have a higher percentage of divorce than others. This has been said so often today that it has become trite, but it needs to be examined. Some of those who have failed undoubtedly were not ready for the relationship. The young man who goes from high school directly into marriage is taking on responsibilities which are awesome in the context of contemporary living. He has attempted to bypass some of the very important developmental tasks which must be performed between the ages of seventeen and twenty-two. The young woman has leaped from a period of relative dependency into a role of total responsibility. It would be miraculous if the marriage did succeed.

Without some degree of maturity it is extremely difficult for young people even to anticipate what is involved in marriage. We cannot assess our readiness if we are not ready, but we often operate on the basis of need rather than on the basis of readiness. We believe we need our beloved so badly that this obscures all else. In a society which places so much emphasis upon marriage for love, we have little opportunity to be objective in selecting our mates. As we have seen in earlier chapters, love has its phases, stages, and varying degrees. When we are so concerned with our own needs, it is extremely difficult to think of love in any terms except fulfilling those needs. There is a tendency to be blind to a partner's needs.

The importance of being aware of our mate's needs in marriage cannot be overstated. Unless we can develop a sensitivity to these needs, it becomes impossible to accomplish one of the central tasks of marriage, *mutual self-fulfillment*. When we fail at this, all the expectations of marriage are dashed, and there seems to be no reason for the existence of the marriage. It doesn't matter if there are children or not. When we feel that we are being defeated in self-actualization, we cannot respond at any level with the quality that is demanded by the situation. Our health is poor. We must reorganize values. This may mean returning to a prior level of maturity, or it may mean withdrawing from the stressful circumstances of the present.

Readiness for marriage is not a matter of age. There are young married people who succeed. Somehow in the course of their growing up they have been helped to view life with objectivity without sacrificing warmth and spontaneity, so that qualitatively high responses are made.

How Do We Become Ready?

Exploring the following questions before marriage will bring us closer to readiness: What is each of us looking for? Does the man expect his wife to be a mother to him? Does the woman expect her husband to be a father to her? Do we expect our marriage to function as the marriage of our parents functioned? Do we expect that the same roles of man and woman we saw enacted between our parents will be enacted in our own marriage? Do we expect our mate to conform to some preconceived image we hold for him or her? We do not decide whether or not to marry solely on the basis of discussions of these questions, but we establish a *modus operandi* for dealing with these matters as they arise in the course of the marriage.

There is no way of telling what specific questions will arise in a particular marriage. The areas of uncertainty cover a wide range. Much depends upon the background of each of the partners. The questions deal with such matters as the style and frequency of sex, the management of the home, the raising of the children, money matters, the way people speak to each other, friends, and outside duties. Often the questions center about the status of each of the partners vis-à-vis one another. Emotions are directly involved; the sense of self is directly affected by the outcome of the discussions.

There is no blueprint for discussing such questions. A guidline is that each individual in the marriage is concerned about his own self-actualization. He or she may feel that this is being inhibited by the behavior or attitudes of his mate. How do the partners determine just where to draw the line between respect for each one's own rights and accepting the other person's position? This probably cannot be established consistently, either in format or in content. What happens and how it happens frequently change from day to day or even from moment to moment.

Because both content and process change so frequently, it is essential that married couples be alert to the changes. Since changes take place both in oneself and in one's mate, the relationship itself changes. Unless couples are aware of the changes, often subtle, they may find themselves involved in disputes which are irrelevant, fighting battles which need not be fought.

> Jan and Bob had been married for two years. In the first year Jan had some difficult problems of adjustment to Bob's sexual advances. She had been extremely inhibited in the realm of male-female relationships until she met Bob. He had been the only man she had dated. In fact, until he came along, she had often been openly hostile to boys and men.
>
> After they were married, Bob was much chagrined to find that Jan was unable to relax and enjoy sex. Furthermore, at times she actively resisted his approaches. In time, however, Jan was able to free herself from some of her fears about Bob's "invasion of her privacy." She no longer talked about being "violated." She had not yet reached the point of being able to enjoy their sexual relations with any degree of enthusiasm, but she had changed.
>
> Even though Bob had been understanding and gentle with Jan about her reticence, some feelings of animosity grew between them. Jan felt that Bob was interested only in her body. Bob felt that Jan did not care enough about him. He believed she did not trust him and for this reason was unable to give herself to him fully. Self-confidence was undermined in each of them. Bob felt himself to be a poor lover. Jan believed that she was not normal. They both found themselves less and less able to enter the sexual encounter in a relaxed manner.
>
> In spite of the progress that Jan had made in the first year and a half of marriage, she and Bob continued to function, at the attitudinal level, in the context of what had taken place in the early months of their marriage. Each of them continued to assume that the other still held the same attitudes they had

many months ago. Consequently it became difficult for them to discuss their relationship rationally. They found that they became increasingly confused and continued to defend points of view which they no longer held.

In this case, both people had changed, and the relationship had changed. Yet, neither was aware of the fact that changes had taken place. Although they probably *felt* that they were different people than they had been, because they did not *know* this on an intellectual level, they were discussing issues which were now obsolete.

How is this related to readiness for marriage? If Jan and Bob had been alerted to the fact that people do change, they could more readily have seen these changes as they developed and have dealt with them appropriately.

The Work of Marriage

The work of marriage is basically the revealing, developing, and meshing of the identities of two people.

Initially, as we have seen, it centers around reconciling the differences between expectations and reality. Although the job is not completed when these first differences are resolved, the work of marriage is not necessarily onerous. Frequently it may be engaged in with humor, enthusiasm, and comfort. Although at times there may be a sense of threat and subsequent feelings of fear and insecurity, it is an ongoing process which must be performed anew each day as the years unfold.

How is the work accomplished? For want of a better term, we will use the word *communication* for what takes place. Communication is of two kinds: One is the internal communication one has with oneself, a dialogue between various elements of one's personality. The other is the external dialogue between two or more individuals; it influences and is influenced by the inner dialogue.

There have been various ways of identifying the different elements of our personality involved in the inner dialogue. We may use the Freudian categories of id, ego, and superego, or we may use the concepts of primitive and evolved selves, or the concept of man as a value structure. According to each of these theories different selves are at work within us. The primitive drives we hold (or the id) are satisfied with nothing less than gratification. The evolved self (the superego) has learned to censor the primitive self. These two selves often stand for opposing values. They see things quite differently. The ego is that part of us which attempts to resolve the differences.

In the case of Jan and Bob, we can imagine these two selves at work in Bob. On the one hand, he has the drive to satisfy his sexual urges. On the other hand, the evolved self has concern for his wife's feelings and wishes. In effect a conflict exists, and the inner dialogue is centered about resolving it. For Bob this meant defining for himself a position relative to Jan which was acceptable to him. Could he see himself as a person, as a man, as a husband, in a light which made it possible for him to live comfortably with himself and with his wife? What resulted in the inner dialogue markedly influenced what transpired between Bob and Jan. Until the inner dialogue was complete, the communications between the two would continue to reflect the internal struggle each was having with himself.

Communication skills depend upon the degree of sensitivity to what the other person is attempting to say, upon the insight each person has into himself or herself, and upon the means used to indicate to one another what they are feeling. Verbal communication, because it often (not always) proceeds from the conscious mind of the individual, may be extremely deceptive. For people who do not easily or adequately communicate on the verbal level, the body level of symbolization is a more direct means of expression. This is not necessarily a matter of intelligence but rather the result of the identity-forming experience.

Communication is a two-way process, the back-and-forthness of a dynamic relationship. It is the expressing of oneself and attending to the feedback from the other person. It is the sensitive listening to another individual and then reacting to this in a creative and spontaneous manner. It is the essence of the mutual self-realization process in which two people engage.

The work of marriage can be facilitated if each person is able to make a distinction between what he thinks and what he feels. We are concerned that another person understand how we *feel*. At the same time we want the other to know what we *think*. The problem often is that we do not know the difference ourselves. Too many times we say what we feel as though it were what we thought, and vice versa. The result is confusion instead of communication.

People sometimes assume that because they preface what they say with the words "I feel," they are expressing feelings. This is not so. The following dialogue illustrates the confusion between expressing thoughts and expressing feelings:

"What is it that bothers you?"
"I feel that you are not being fair to me."

"You are not expressing a feeling. You are giving me your opinion."

"But I feel it nevertheless."

"What is it you feel about my not being fair? How does that make you feel?"

"I feel angry."

"Now you are telling me about a feeling."

This confusion is common among many of us. We are not used to telling others about our feelings, and we *feel* uncomfortable when we are asked to do so. We *believe* that feelings are best expressed in other ways than words. But many an expression of feeling in nonverbal terms is threatening to other people, because it is more likely to be misinterpreted, whereas in words it is possible to express feeling accurately enough so that the other person does not react to the nonverbal and uncontrolled cues. If we are able to tell another person of the feelings his attitudes or behavior evoke in us, he will be better able to understand us and also the dynamics of the relationship, and he will understand better how he is seen by others, as well.

In effect we are saying to someone, "I trust you enough to be able to tell you that I am hurt [angry, frightened, etc.] by your behavior." In one sense this is an appeal, a request that the other person help us to deal with the feelings we are experiencing. It is intimacy of the highest order. Because it is a complete exposure of oneself to another, a mutual sharing in the process of self-actualization.

The transition from expectation to reality in marriage is heavily laced with emotion, fraught with interpersonal conflict, and demanding of time and energy. It is erroneous to expect that marriage will always be a haven in which one can let down one's hair without making an effort to respond to one's mate. Although the home is frequently referred to as a place of refuge where one can be oneself, it is not always so. Marriage becomes intimate according to the degree that we work for it. The need for the work of marriage through effective communication is ever present.

Different Backgrounds

Mildred grew up in a home where her father was the typical self-made man. Mildred's father had left school at the end of the eighth grade to work in a local shoe-manufacturing business. Within twenty years he had become the president of the firm, which had merged with those of some of his competitors, and he was recognized as a leader in the industry. He was also a leader in the community, active in local politics, on the school board, and in his church. In his home he was known to be fair, decisive, and "in charge."

Mildred's mother was a pleasant and intelligent woman, who deferred to her husband's wishes, fed him the right lines at social occasions, and played to his strength and dominance. She had found that the way to get along with him was to make her wishes known and then trust his judgment about honoring them. If her wishes were reasonable, he usually went along with them.

Mildred learned very early that the way to get along with her father was to emulate her mother. She believed her father was a wonderful man and often said to her friends that she could never marry anyone who was not a strong man. As she entered young adulthood, her internal radar was set to find such a man.

Tod came from a very different home. His father was extremely timid. In the usual terms of society he was singularly unsuccessful as a businessman. To his son, he seemed even less successful as a man. Tod's mother was domineering, officious, and castrating of the males in her life.

As Tod grew, he became increasingly resentful of his mother's treatment and of his father's submissiveness. He vowed to himself that when he had his own home he would never be like his father. He did everything he could to create an image of masculinity for himself. He became an outstanding athlete and was offered athletic scholarships by three large universities. He happened to choose the same school that Mildred did.

For two years Mildred and Tod knew of each other only indirectly. Tod became a campus hero because of his athletic skills, his good looks, and his easygoing social manner. Mildred was popular because she had the knack of making every fellow who dated her feel important and manly. She was gracious and friendly though lacking in self-assertion. Tod, while a popular hail-fellow-well-met type, was not really a decision maker. He excelled in sports, but he was not a leader. Although he gave the appearance of being a "take-charge guy," he had none of the inner strength to be one.

To Tod, Mildred looked like the kind of girl he wanted for a wife. When they dated, she made him feel manly, decisive, and in charge. Because he was not this kind of person, he needed the illusion Mildred was able to create. To Mildred, because of his popularity, athletic prowess, and outstanding physique, Tod symbolically represented the kind of man she thought she wanted for a husband.

They married.

Within one year they appeared in a marriage counselor's office, confused, angry, and hurt. Each felt the other had let him down. Tod was unable to be the kind of man Mildred needed. Mildred was unable to provide the direction which Tod could not give. In effect each of them was an extremely dependent person, and neither of them could give the kind of support the other needed.

After hearing both sides of the story, the marriage counselor proceeded to have Mildred and Tod examine the relationship of their parents. As they did so, they became more fully aware of the impact of their parents' relationships on their own identities. They were able to see how they had brought these identities into their marriage and from that point on had some basis from which to proceed in their mutual exploration of their own relationship with one another.

Here we have a perfect illustration of the reality gap. The expectations which both Mildred and Tod had for one another and for themselves were a long way from the realities of their personalities. The image each developed had grown from his and her own personal background. Clearly there were many areas of communication which they had to open up. Neither of them was able to see the other realistically. Neither of them was able to see himself or herself objectively. They believed the illusions they projected. For each of them this image had worked for most of their prior life, but in the dynamics of a new setting and a new relationship these identities did not work. Change was essential.

The changes that were demanded created extreme anxiety. It was frightening for each of them to leave an old self and to take on a new one. For Tod it was impossible to admit the fears he had. For Mildred these fears were such a new experience that she had little understanding of what they meant.

Were these two young people ready for marriage? On the surface it would appear they were not, and probably the same can be said for most couples anticipating marriage. But Tod and Mildred were faced with a special problem. Because the identities each had developed had worked so well while they were single, each was deceived by them. This made it well-nigh impossible for them to spot the problem until after they were married.

The intimacy of marriage highlighted the unpreparedness of

each. As they drew closer to each other, each saw the responsibility that the other demanded. When neither could live up to this responsibility, they were miserable. Because each had had a successful life prior to the marriage, they each assumed that the other was to blame for the misery and should be the one to change.

The marriage counselor helped them develop some of the skills of communication they badly needed. They were then able to function more effectively, and the work of marriage was underway.

Premarital Counseling

Few people would deny the importance of medical examinations before marriage. Many, however, give little thought to the importance of premarital counseling, even though this may be far more important in upgrading the quality of their response to one another. Somehow, our society has done little to alert us to the importance of our interpersonal relationships. We scarcely recognize that these relationships have almost everything to do with how we think, feel, and react, much less that they are vital in the formation and the modification of our identities, since few of us are able to think in terms of the dynamic concepts necessary to understand human nature at work.

A few hours of premarital counseling might have made all the difference in the world to Tod and Mildred. They could have explored some of the potential hazards they would face in living together. Specific answers would not have been found, but this is not the purpose of such counseling. More often than not it serves to alert people to what problems may arise and to help people start communicating effectively if they have not yet done so.

Premarital counseling further establishes a point to which the couple can return when they later have difficulties. When married couples find that they have hit an impasse beyond which they cannot move, only a few alternatives are open to them. One is to simply accept the fact that in a particular area no progress can be made. But this leaves them with nothing constructive to do with their feelings. Another alternative is to withdraw from one another until the intense sense of hurt subsides. This response undermines each one's confidence in the other and makes it more difficult to establish the openness necessary for satisfactory communication. In either case the intimacy of marriage is destroyed. The spiritual uplift to be derived from sharing in the growth of another person is lacking.

Premarital counseling is not the sole answer to the problems of marriage. It does not guarantee that henceforth the marriage is going to proceed without a hitch. It does, however, minimize the initial hazards of a challenging relationship. It gets the partners off on the right foot and provides some insight into the mysteries they propose to explore together.

The Perfect Marriage

There is probably no dream more unrealistic than the one of a perfect marriage. As our research techniques for marriage sharpen, it becomes more and more apparent that there is no such thing. Because marriage is an integral part of the growing experience of the two individuals involved, there are bound to be bumps along the road. Most couples experience periods in which arguments are frequent, hope is dashed, and one or the other partner seriously contemplates splitting.

It would be an interesting experience for a young couple approaching marriage to interview five older couples whose marriages they consider to be good. If frankness could prevail, the stories unfolded would certainly explode the myth of the perfect marriage. If the couple could imagine themselves as having similar experiences, they would have a more realistic view about marriage.

Few of us can imagine ourselves as having the problems that most other people have experienced or realize that we are capable of failure in our love relationships. Then, when we experience disappointment, we find it extremely difficult to believe that we can survive the occasion. Margaret Mead, the outstanding anthropologist, in a talk before an audience of young parents, once remarked that the Western marriage is unique in the world in that it is carried on in extreme privacy, isolated from other marriages in its day-by-day functioning. In some other parts of the world the family structure is large enough so that people of all ages live together on an intimate basis. Children see the various stages of development from infancy to adulthood; married couples can observe other married persons whose relationship is open for all to see. When difficulty arises, there are many present who can be supportive and who can help relieve the tensions which commonly generate in marriage.

While the American home has other advantages, each young couples must determine for themselves just what success is. They must decide what standards of belief and behavior they are going to affirm, what frustration they are willing to tolerate, and how they will deal with it. It is one thing to read about what *should* exist in marriage; it is another to see what *does* exist. The discrepancy sometimes leads to panic. When a young bride experiences, for example, a physical expression of her husband's anger, she may feel that the marriage is ended. Because she has been struck and because she assumes that this is a sure sign of disrespect, she believes that she should not tolerate such behavior. On the other hand, when the young husband learns that his wife has been involved in some extracurricular flirtation, he readily jumps to the conclusion that his trust has been "violated." He may think that this is sufficient ground for a campaign of retaliation in kind.

Successful marriage is a day-by-day achievement. It rests upon the willingness of both partners to work together to make things go. It demands a degree of honesty for which we are not entirely prepared in the families from which we come. It necessitates an honest assessment of our own motivations and a willingness to change when necessary, however difficult this may be for most of us.

Erich Heckel, "Two People," 1909. Woodcut. Collection, The Museum of Modern Art, New York. Gift of the Abby Aldrich Rockefeller Fund.

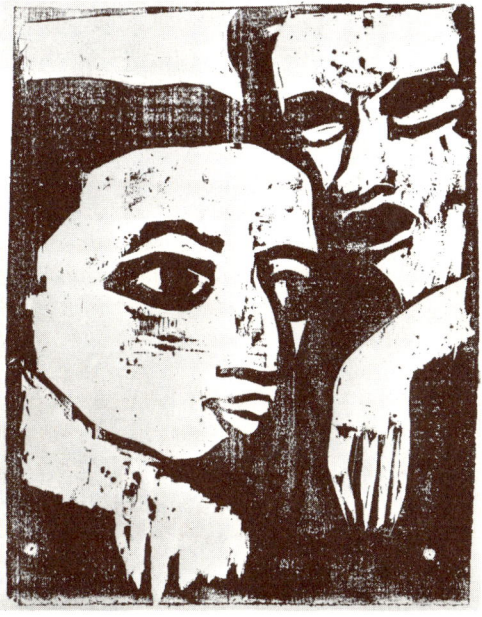

A Man and a Woman

In the successful marriage a man is able to make his wife feel glad she is a woman. Conversely, the woman makes her husband glad that he is a man. Each confirms the identity of the other and enhances the other's sexuality. Each makes it possible for the other to function with confidence and in the knowledge that he is important to his mate.

When a man is confident of himself, he does not need to strive to prove his manhood to himself and his wife. He does not need to compete with her in sexuality. When a woman is confident of herself, she does not have to continually affirm her femininity by going to exaggerated lengths in dress, makeup, or behavior. She projects a confident sense of her sexuality in every aspect of her being and she functions well.

When either one or both of the marriage partners is not confident of his own sexuality, he may blame his mate and function in a manner that is confused and confusing. Both may know they are supposed to act like a member of their own sex, but if they do not know what role to play in order to manifest this image, they are confused and anxious, and they do not project themselves clearly to others. Therefore others cannot respond to them as they wish them to.

There are times in a marriage, particularly in the early years, when mates reject the image the partner presents. What the partner is saying about himself or herself is not consistent with their idea of what he or she should be. An important opportunity for communication is presented at this point. If the mates do not take the challenge, they are failing in an essential task of marriage.

How do we go about making our mates feel glad about their own sexuality? Again there is no blueprint. It is essential to accept the other person *as they are,* without reservation, without a desire to make them over into our image of what we would have them be. Psychologists make a distinction between loving and being *in* love. They believe that being in love presupposes a particular image. They go so far as to say that one may even create the image he is in love with and respond to that.

Being in love with an image leads to distortion. We have seen this distortion in the case of Mildred and Tod. Each of them had an idealized image of the person they wanted to marry. They assumed that the person they married fitted this image. When, in reality, their mates did not act as expected, both Mildred and Tod were disillusioned. As they continued to respond to the idealized image, they frustrated one another. Each attempted to change to fit the role the other expected, but their efforts were doomed to failure, because they could not understand what it was the other person wanted. Tod believed that Mildred did not understand him. Mildred thought that Tod was deceiving her. Because of this they were not able to effectively communicate the experiences they were having. Each of them was playing to an audience that didn't exist. Neither of them received the feedback he expected.

The threat inherent in having to relinquish the ideal image of the lover and one's beliefs about himself is too much for many people. It means entering a world that is strange and unfamiliar, encountering experiences of which we have little understanding gained from the past. It is an adventure in daring to try new things and to reap rewards where they have not been known to exist. This is the realm where the greatest growth may take place. If it is accomplished, we have taken the steps necessary to make our mates feel glad they are what they are.

22.

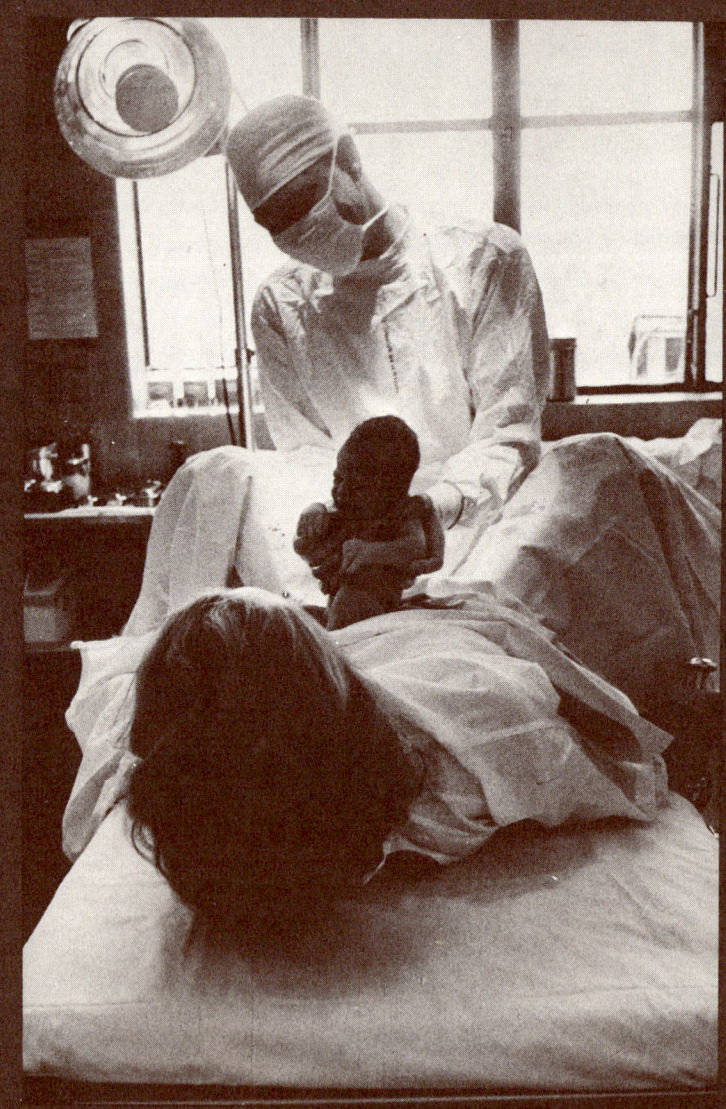

THE MIRACLE OF BIRTH

This chapter is concerned primarily with philosophic issues centering around the miracle of childbirth. As with any other philosophic area of thought, we are influenced partly by the knowledge we have of the subject, partly by the experience and behavior of others, and partly by our own experience. From this amalgam we develop a personal perspective and make our choice.

This chapter will deal with the phenomenon of childbirth as a factor in the dynamics of marriage. No effort will be made to go into the biologic or anatomic details of childbirth. For the reader who is interested in such information, some suggested readings are listed at the end of this part.

In discussing the following concerns about childbirth, an effort has been made to examine some popular viewpoints and to clarify various positions.

1. Are children necessary for a fulfilling marriage?
2. For what reasons do we have children?
3. What are the realities of having children?
4. The prenatal experience.
5. Sex during pregnancy.
6. The experience in the hospital.
7. What is the value of "natural childbirth"?
8. The value of rooming-in.
9. How important is nursing one's infant?

Each couple must evaluate these issues for themselves, choosing a position or arriving at a compromise with which they are comfortable.

In all cases it should be recognized that the influences of past experiences, self concepts, and role expectations will exert pressures in the decision-making process for both husband and wife. Nothing short of a true and intimate exploration will do. Both need to search deeply into themselves to find out how they really feel

Eve Arnold, photography. Magnum Photos, Inc.

about the issue. These feelings should be revealed, no matter how difficult it may be to discuss them or how ashamed one might feel about having a particular reaction. Because the problem intimately involves the two persons, the more they understand about themselves and each other, the greater the chance for a satisfying childbirth experience.

This dialogue is not the time for deception or false bravado, or to feign feelings for the sake of peace. If a woman feels, for example, that breast feeding is disgusting but goes along with it because she knows her husband would like her to, it is likely that she will grow to resent both the child and her husband, whom she silently blames for making her do this. She will have *created* rather than *solved* a problem.

There may be other controversial problems not mentioned here that the couple will need to examine. Each situation is unique. Before any decisions are arrived at, it would be advisable to gather all the information pertinent to the problem. Then each must add whatever personal information he or she can to the body of information, such as fears, apprehensions, limitations. Once a couple have prepared themselves with this foundation, they will be more likely to come to a decision suitable to both of them.

Are Children Necessary?

The decision about whether or not to have children is perhaps one of the most important decisions of marriage. On it may rest the entire direction of the future of the married couple. If they have children, the lives of the couple will at various times be almost totally dominated by the needs of the children. When children are young, great amounts of time and energy must be devoted to their care and feeding. When the children are adolescent, critical strains will develop between parent and child. When the time for higher education arrives, financial strains are often placed upon the resources of the family. There is almost no time when children do not make tremendous demands on their parents.

At the same time having children can bring great rewards. When parents can keep things in perspective, they can enjoy watching a life develop and grow from childhood into adulthood. As they see the individuality develop, they can also take pleasure in the differences between their several children. A child offers parents the satisfaction of knowing another human being in an intimacy that is equaled in no other relationship.

Sometimes, however, people have the distorted view that the

only purpose they have in existing is devotion to their children. Their entire lives center about providing for them. Their only satisfaction comes from seeing their children grow from infancy into independent adulthood. Often the need to play the parent role is so important that it is extremely difficult for mothers and fathers to divest themselves of this role. They find it a great hardship to let their children go. When they do, they often feel that their entire purpose in life is gone, that their lives are over, and that the years ahead will be devoid of satisfaction and meaning.

In spite of the tremendous significance that people place upon children, they often want them without understanding why. Procreation appears to be a basic drive of life. Therefore, people often become parents without giving much thought to what it will be like and what it will mean to their marriage.

In much the same way that our social structure pushes us toward marriage, it also pushes us toward having children. This is so strong a social drive that many people feel themselves to be failures if they do not have children. They feel that something is wrong with them and that their lives have been blighted when they are denied the opportunity to have children.

In the name of health, this idea should be challenged. There is no question that children are a great source of satisfaction and that no other life situation can quite match the challenges of this experience. However, it is difficult to maintain the position that children are a *sine qua non* of the full life. Given all the compensatory capacities of human beings, it is highly unlikely that persons cannot live a full life without having children. No doubt the nature of that life will be different. But the range of possibilities in which self-actualization can occur is broader than parenthood alone. That the vast majority of other people have this experience is not sufficient reason to assume that *all* married couples must have it.

Some people may find self-actualization more readily outside parenthood. Health should not be thought to depend upon particular experiences of life. It may flourish under a great variety of experiences. Single persons find health. Married persons can likewise be healthy. It is the quality of the response that an individual makes to *whatever circumstances* arise which determines and demonstrates his health.

Reasons for Having Children

There seem to be three basic reasons why people have children: ego gratification, definition of our own personhood, and role fulfillment. None of these reasons is mutually exclusive of the other two. Each has its own special area of focus, with some overlapping.

Ego Gratification

Ego gratification is akin to the reason men have given for climbing mountains—because they are there. The possibility of having a child is there. It is part of our nature—we are reproductive creatures. The sex drive impels us toward another person, first, to eliminate the barrier of separateness we feel and, second, to reproduce ourselves in the process of fusing with another. It attempts to satisfy our drive toward immortality.

Because the possibility of reproduction is there, many of us feel that it presents some sort of challenge. If we do not take up the challenge, we assume that we are avoiding it. To many this is anathema. It is not consistent with our need to do what we think we must. Our sense of ego is not satisfied.

When the opportunity to do that which is possible is ignored, some persons feel that they have not fulfilled a divinely established commandment. The biblical injunction to "be fruitful and multiply" is an outgrowth of a profoundly intense drive, and it has had a powerful influence upon all Western people.

Definition of Our Own Personhood

The need to define our own personhood by having children is derived from the assumption that we are not persons unless we have fulfilled the inner commandment to have children. Social sanction to parenthood is so strong that many young adults look upon parenthood, before the fact, as a matter of having arrived. Many adults will assume that the most important thing they can say about themselves is that they have children.

Role Fulfillment

Role fulfillment is a strong motivation in many of us who feel bound by a particular social role. The role of parenthood is learned in our childhood. Our identity as men or women is carved out in particular terms. Unless we can fit into the mold that has been structured, we have feelings of guilt and inadequacy.

What Is Real?

There is nothing wrong with any of these motivations toward parenthood. However, they are not complete, and they are inadequate for achieving what we hope for from them. The ego will not be adequately fulfilled only by having children. In an important sense, ego fulfillment may even be limited by parenthood. The same may be said for each of the other motivations. Many parents are so bound by fulfilling the role of the serving parent that they never become persons in their own right. When parents become so involved in the lives of their children that they ignore their own needs and depend upon their children for fulfillment, the children find it extremely difficult to break away from their parents. One of the tasks of parenthood is to work oneself out of business. If ego satisfaction and the development of a sense of personhood depends upon having children in our lives, we never develop beyond the role of parent.

It would be healthier for both parents and children if, before having children, people were able to realize what it will mean to them. The subsequent disillusionment will be lessened, stress would be avoided, and a more mature relationship between parent and child could be achieved. A woman would not find the cute, cuddly baby changing into a demanding monster who gives her few moments to herself. A man would not discover, too late, that all male children were not born to become athletic heroes.

A greater degree of realism in planning for children would lessen the frustrations attendant upon their development into independent beings. A greater amount of freedom would be accorded children to develop their own potential, with less tendency to cast them into restricting and inhibiting molds. The health of individuals and the health of families would be greatly improved if children were seen in proper perspective before they arrived on the scene.

The increase in the number of cases of the battered-child syndrome, where parents have brutally beaten and murdered their own children, indicates that many people are not ready for the responsibility of parenthood. Such cases have become so numerous that now it is required in many states that doctors report suspected cases to police authorities. The irony of this is that once again society deals with the problem *after* it occurs. How can we produce a future stock of mature and responsible parents?

Some of the answer must be found in the values held by society. In a materialistic culture which at the same time glorifies individuality and conformity, the inherent conflict will be reflected in the families of that society. What little we know about comparative child-rearing styles will inevitably be judged by the standards of our own culture. For example, Bruno Bettelheim,[1] in his study of

---

[1] Bruno Bettelheim, *Children of the Dream*, Macmillan, New York, 1969.

children raised in kibbutzim in Israel, points out that the children, brought up in cooperative nurseries and tended by parent surrogates, become remarkably adjusted and cooperating people. However, creativity, initiative, and individuality are found to be limited. Since we value these qualities, the loss of them raises questions about the parent-child relationships in that situation.

The extremely limited experience of the communal family structure which has developed in the United States in recent years yields little valid information upon which to base conclusions.[2] In these circumstances the children are allowed to relate to various members of the larger family structure and live for varying lengths of time with another set of parents. About all that is known at present is that when these children become teen-agers they are determined to leave the commune and return to the type of society from which their parents fled.

What kinds of parents the children raised in these circumstances will become remains to be seen. To suppose that the child-rearing practices of some of the island cultures can be adopted in our society with unquestioned benefit is illusory to say the least. Too many other factors influence the development of the individual to lay all credit and blame at the feet of parents.

The Prenatal Experience

Once a young couple have placed their desire for children in proper perspective, they are better prepared to enter the period of time between conception and birth. The birth of a child has the potential for being one of the most significant experiences in marriage. It seems obvious that a husband and wife should share the experience of childbirth together. Yet, this is not always so.

Often one of the early developmental tasks of marriage is for people to learn to share the individuality of their experience with one another. It is possible for two people to live a lifetime together without ever knowing how the other person experiences something which they have gone through together. Two people hearing the same lecture in class experience it differently. A meal with friends is experienced differently by each person there. The role they have vis-à-vis one another certainly is experienced in totally different ways. The importance of communication, as we have seen in the previous chapter, is that it serves as a means for two people pro-

---

[2] Sara Davidson, "Open Land," *Harper's Magazine,* vol. 240, p. 91, June, 1970.

gressively to understand how each of them feels, thinks, and reacts to the events of their life together. In marriage, not only do two individuals experience things differently, but men and women view life differently. When these two sets of differences are shared, their life together becomes more rewarding. Each person develops a stronger appreciation of the other and can, through effective communication, develop a heightened sensitivity to the other.

The mutual sharing of the prenatal experience is not easily accomplished. For one thing, the exigencies of the workaday world usually make it difficult for a husband to go along when his wife visits the obstetrician. Presumably, consultations with an obstetrician begin sometime shortly after the wife has missed her second menstrual period. Visits to the doctor continue throughout the nine-month gestation period. Unless an expectant mother can communicate to her husband all that transpires, he may begin to feel left out.

Even though this feeling is unrealistic, if it exists, it is an influence on the quality of the husband's response. He may internalize his left-outness with a shrug of the shoulders, or he may complain about it. In either case it is something to which young persons should be alert. If complaints arise, the wife would do well to listen with sympathetic alertness to what her husband says, even though she may feel that she is the one who really has the problems. For his part, the husband will profit if he attends carefully to what his wife tells him about her side of the experience. Each will be served well if these feelings are shared sympathetically with one another.

Husbands may play one of several stereotyped roles when their wives become pregnant. One is the usual sentimentalized role we often see portrayed in American motion pictures. Upon learning of his wife's pregnancy, usually at some time when he has been blissfully or brutally unaware of what has transpired, the husband turns into a simpleton whose only thought is that his wife should sit down. Presumably this is meant to convey the idea that from this point on he will be willing, eager, and able to respond to her every whim until she delivers a lusty baby boy.

Another role in which the husband is often cast is that of the unsympathetic brute who upon learning of his wife's pregnancy immediately finds himself a mistress. At this point the viewer is supposed to recognize that the husband feels abused, denied, and hostile. The beast then seeks comfort in the arms of another woman. There is no question where the sympathies lie among those who view such a drama. Among Americans, the sacred institution of motherhood is violated at one's peril.

With these roles before him, *and having some of the inclinations portrayed in each of them,* the young husband often finds it difficult to project himself and his feelings uniquely. He may need help in identifying all the feelings he has. When he is given such help, he will probably respond with gratitude to his helper.

The wife, for her part, is filled with a mixture of awe, fear, excitement, and curious anticipation. Her pregnancy is usually more on her mind than she is willing to let on to others. She is incredulous that it can all happen to her without others being aware of it. She wants to tell everyone about what is going on inside her. At the same time she feels silly for wanting to spend so much time talking about it.

Both husband and wife are caught in a complex of confused feelings which they cannot fully identify. They assume that they should feel love for the unborn infant. Yet this love exists largely in fantasy for them. With this knowledge, a mild sense of guilt develops. There is thus a great need for communication.

To illustrate the different ways a situation can be handled, here are two conversations between two different couples after the wife has made a visit to her obstetrician.

> *Wife:* I went to the doctor today.
> *Husband:* Well, what did he say?
> *Wife:* Everything is fine. It was just routine.
> *Husband:* Are you all right?
> *Wife:* Yes.

Another couple, who are used to sharing their uncomfortable feelings, might have this dialogue:

> *Wife:* I went to the doctor today.
> *Husband:* Well, what did he say?
> *Wife:* Everything is fine. It was just a routine examination. But the doctor had to examine me internally, and I hate it. It's so embarrassing.
> *Husband:* Tell me about it. What don't you like about it?
> *Wife:* For one thing, the position you have to get into is so awkward! Your feet are up in those stirrups, and I just feel so uncomfortable! Here I am, going to be a mother, and I'm acting like a child myself about a silly thing like this. You'd think I'd be more mature about it.
> *Husband:* I guess that is an uncomfortable experience. I think I have some funny feelings about it, too. Maybe we should talk about it.

By itself, none of the factors mentioned is of great significance. Each will probably be transcended by the excitement that both prospective parents feel. But more can be added to the life of the young couple if they attend more fully to the feelings they have and to the importance of communicating them to one another. When this is done, an added dimension of appreciation and insight enters their lives and is stockpiled against the future. It becomes a building block for a sounder and more satisfying relationship, giving each partner a greater feeling that he or she can be understood by the mate. It helps in alleviating the sense of aloneness that all people have unless they feel that they are understood by others. If the sense of aloneness persists in marriage, one of the most important elements in marriage is missing: understanding companionship.

A number of hospitals and obstetricians have undertaken group discussions with their prenatal patients. Under the leadership of a psychologist, in conjunction with the attending obstetricians, many of the feelings experienced by couples who are expecting can be identified and examined. Discussing the attitudinal elements of the progressing pregnancy in the group provides a basis for further exploration of these feelings by the couples on their own. Those who have participated in such meetings report that they are a very satisfying and illuminating practice.

But not all of what is needed can be done by the professionals. Much must be accomplished by the couple concerned. As time progresses, feelings will change. Once the newness of the experience wears off, other feelings will manifest themselves. Somewhere along the line, doubts about one's ability to care for the child adequately will arise. Feelings of annoyance will inevitably develop. Pregnancy imposes limitations upon any couple. Life cannot go on exactly as it has before. Coupled with the sense of annoyance, doubts about one's own worth arise. Can we, the young couple wonders, be adequate parents if we are annoyed at the very process of becoming parents? These feelings are all grist for the communication mill.

Most young couples will have an opportunity to meet together with a public health nurse or some other professional who will instruct them in the care of the newborn infant. Husbands will have an opportunity to ask questions about their role. Wives will be reassured through such instruction. This is an important service and should be sought. But it does not take the place of the aforementioned group discussions or personal discussions in which feelings are examined.

Some hospitals offer an opportunity for the expectant parents to review the procedures through which the mother will go when her time for delivery arrives. They may be shown a film on childbirth. They may visit the labor room, the delivery room, and the nursery in which the newborn infant will be kept. Questions are encouraged and answered.

Sex during Pregnancy

The obstetrician will state the limit of sexual activity for the expectant mother. In most cases few or no restrictions will be placed upon her. Masters and Johnson, from a survey of a little over one hundred pregnant women, concluded that many of the former prohibitions regarding sex during pregnancy were not founded on objective and individualized study. They made the following four recommendations:[3]

> 1. For the overwhelming majority of women, there is no reason whatever to refrain from sex during the first three months of pregnancy.
> 2. For the overwhelming majority of women, there is no reason whatever to refrain from sexual activity during the second three months of pregnancy.
> 3. Late in the final three months as delivery day approaches the problems become more complex.
> Some physicians warn against intercourse toward the end of pregnancy for fear of infection. Dr. Masters and Mrs. Johnson regard this as a "residual of the pre-antibiotic days." There is no more risk of vaginal or cervical infection late in pregnancy than at any other time, they state; and if infection should occur, it can be as readily and effectively controlled as at any other time.
> More relevant is the fact that in some women toward the end of pregnancy the baby's head engages in the cervix, and the cervix descends into the main axis of the vagina. *After* this descent occurs, vigorous coital thrusting may cause the glans of the penis to strike the infant-laden cervix. A little "spotting" or bleeding may result. In this case, Dr. Masters and Mrs. Johnson conclude, coition should be given up. But they point out that in many women, especially those who have had babies before, the baby's head does not engage and the cervix does not descend until labor actually begins. There seems little reason to prohibit intercourse for these women merely because the head has descended into the cervix in some *other* women.
> 4. After the baby is born, three factors may properly delay resumption of sexual intercourse. The wife may not feel like it. The surgical incision made to ease the birth of the baby—the episi-

---

[3] Ruth Brecher and Edward Brecher, *An Analysis of Human Sexual Response*, Signet, New American Library, New York, 1966, pp. 94–95.

otomy—may not have healed fully. And there may still be some uterine or vaginal bleeding or spotting. All three of these conditions, Dr. Masters and Mrs. Johnson report, usually (though not always) end after the third post partum week.

The Masters and Johnson research on human sexual response revealed a great deal of variability among women in their desire for sexual contact during pregnancy. An important finding was that while almost three-quarters of the women surveyed had been advised by their obstetricians against having intercourse for periods ranging from one to three months before delivery and for the same period after delivery, less than one-third of the women who had been so advised stated they agreed with, understood, or honored the prohibition. Many of these women were concerned about the effect of the prohibition on their husbands. Therefore they voluntarily entered into sexual relations against the direction of their physicians.

That so many of the subjects of the Masters and Johnson research violated the precautionary restrictions without ill effects leads us to believe that a more highly individualized approach should be taken. Furthermore, whatever restrictions are suggested, *both* the husband and wife should be carefully instructed about the reasons for the prohibition. This should alleviate the tendency toward arguing about interpretations of the restriction and avoid stress that might even jeopardize the marriage.

The Hospital Experience

A high percentage of American babies are born in hospitals under conditions common to the experience of most of the couples. There is good reason to believe that the experience leaves much to be desired in terms of the health of the family.

When the expectant couple arrive at the hospital, they are excited and perhaps confused. The wife is registered at the admitting office and taken away in a wheelchair, while the husband is asked to wait in the waiting room. He is informed that the doctor will notify him "as things develop." As he stands in the hallway, feeling useless, and perhaps guilty, he waves feebly as his wife is wheeled away. The nurse may brighten the atmosphere with some sally such as "Don't worry—we've never lost a father yet." Much heartened, he turns to the opaque stares of fellow waiting-room occupants and settles down to the blank perusal of limp and battered periodicals.

The Father: Waiting or Watching?

Compared to what he could experience were he able to be present at the delivery *if he so desired,* the waiting-room experience is for some a trying ordeal. It is not that he cannot stand the anxiety, the sense of guilt should something go wrong (a possibility constantly present in his imagination), the frustration of his uselessness, or the sometimes endless waiting. It is not that he does not realize that his wife's ordeal is far more demanding physically. The real trouble is that within the framework of marriage *as a sharing institution* he is unable to share the experience with her. He wants to be his wife's protector; he may strongly desire to be with her in the hours of labor and may want to be a part of the mystery (to him) of birth. Because of hospital policy he cannot.

This policy, some hospital authorities say, is well founded. Husbands are an added burden in the delivery room. When emergencies arise, they say, greater anguish must be endured by the husband than he undergoes in the waiting room. Fainting husbands would interfere with the delivery-room routine.

These reasons may be valid. But adequate preparation would reduce the possibility of the fainting father. The experience of being present at the birth of a child can be more than rewarding. It can be one of the most wonderful experiences of a man's life. One young husband stated it neatly: "I was so filled with awe and wonder at the astonishing sight of seeing my child born that words are not adequate to describe the feelings I had. I gained a never-to-be-forgotten respect for my wife. Even now, I look at women who have children with a sense of astonishment. I reflect in wonder at the fact that every one who ever lived was born through the same amazing process."

Some hospitals have developed programs of preparation so that husbands can be present at the birth of their children if they so desire, and they find the practice highly satisfying to all concerned. The choice is left entirely to the couple. Both husbands and wives have reported that the experience meant a great deal to them. Wives say that their sense of pride was increased, that the presence of their husbands comforted them, and that they, in turn, gained a new respect for their husbands because the husbands wanted to be present. Such respect is durable. It stands in good stead at times when the going is rough, as it sometimes is in marriage.

The argument on the other side is equally vigorous. Men who do not wish to be present say that they cannot stand the sight of their wives suffering through labor. Others state that they do not wish to see their wives going through the bovine animalism of childbirth. For them, it detracts from the romance of marriage. They want no part of it. Individual preferences should be respected when they have been given careful and thoughtful evaluation.

The Mother's Experience

Some women have noted that the first intense emotional impact of childbirth occurs at the moment when they are separated from their husbands in the hospital lobby. The wife has the sudden awareness and often fear that she is alone in this endeavor. Realistically, of course, she will not be alone. She will have the support of the hospital staff and her obstetrician. Nevertheless, a familiar, loving face by her side or someone's encouraging hand to hold would probably alleviate her fears.

At this time the expectant mother is usually in her first stage of labor, which is the longest. She is taken to the labor room and prepared, or "prepped," for delivery. The pubic hair is shaved and an enema will be administered to ensure as sterile a delivery as is possible. Thereupon, the waiting for the vigorous and more frequent labor pains begins.

Labor experiences vary greatly in duration as well as in the amount of pain among individuals. The average duration is approximately 16 hours for a first child. The experience is so different among individual women that some claim to have experienced no discomfort at all while others describe extreme pain.

The most difficult stage of labor is the second stage, when the head of the fetus moves through the birth canal and into the world. Some women have heard numerous accounts of what it will be like, many of them contradictory. No doubt this is an anxious time if they have had no preparation for it. Many women imagine, since they have heard so many different stories, that some of the women to whom they have spoken have not told them the truth so as not to alarm them. Others assume that most of what they have heard is probably an exaggeration of the weaker members of the sex and therefore expect no pain or discomfort at all.

The pain of childbirth is an interesting phenomenon. Even among those who report that it is the most intense pain they have ever felt, the memory of the pain is short-lived. The psychological elements of the labor experience have not received enough attention in spite of the fact that this aspect is of great concern to the expectant mother. The whole subject is still in a sea of emotional confusion. Most women just don't know what to make of the situation until they have been through it themselves.

Dr. Grantly Dick-Read, the author of *Childbirth without Fear*[4] and probably still one of the most widely read authorities on the subject, believes that the pain of labor is greatly intensified by fear. That a hospital is so often associated with pain, that we are a pleasure-oriented society and have increasingly rejected the idea of painful hard work, and the conditioning influence of years of hearing how painful childbirth is, precipitate fear. All these preconditioning elements work to increase the tension which in childbirth leads to pain.

Some truisms about the labor experience are that it is almost always a lot of hard work; that the less fear and tension the mother feels, the more likely she will be able to allow the muscle elasticity to operate without inhibition; that having emotional support at the more difficult time unquestionably helps; and that the more information she has about the procedure and what is to be expected, the less likely the fear of the unknown will create havoc with her emotional state.

The Case for Educated Childbirth

In recent years so-called natural childbirth has evoked much controversy. Its advocates speak of it as a foolproof, painproof method of having a baby. They exalt it as an essential experience in learning to love one's child fully. The skeptics rail against it as a Spartan cult in which pain is glorified and unnecessarily endured. They regard many of the claims of the natural-childbirth advocates as so much hokum. The layman is curious, confused, or apathetic. Usually the expectant mother will yield to whatever method her obstetrician follows and leaves the decision up to him.

Probably natural childbirth ought to be called and thought of as *educated childbirth*. In educated childbirth the expectant mother is trained to the work she must undertake when her baby is born. She is taught how to do what she *can* do to make her labor easier. She is taught how to cooperate with her physician. Her husband is included in the educational experience, and his help may play an important part in the birth process.

The general principles of educated childbirth include exercises and practices which may be followed before the terminal stages of pregnancy are reached. Techniques that tone up muscles and

---

[4] Grantly Dick-Read, *Childbirth without Fear*, Harper, New York, 1953.

teach the woman to gain control over certain areas of her body will enable her to relax when it is necessary and to contract at other times. Breathing skills may be experimented with. She and her husband can take a course so that both learn what the hospital experience is going to be like. He will learn, along with her, what the exercises do to help and which ones should be used in the various stages of delivery. During delivery he may help her to time contractions and breathing and allay any fears that may beset her.

There are many variations on this approach, with different emphases. The Lamaze method of childbirth preparation is based on the theory that it is impossible for two areas of intense concentration to operate in the brain at the same time. Therefore, the concentration exerted on breathing detracts from the impulses going to the pain center of the brain. Lamaze too supports the idea that fear is a large factor in producing pain. When expectant mothers are informed of what to expect and when their confidence in their ability to meet the experience is supported, there is less tension (always associated with fear) and therefore less pain (often associated with tension).

Most physicians, regardless of their orientation to natural childbirth, avoid using sedation and anesthesia until it is necessary, because drugs present risks to the unborn infant. Sedation may slow down labor and increase the time of stress for the infant. Some drugs have toxic effects upon the infant. The infant's respiration rate or circulation rate may be depressed if the drug reaches him through the placenta. Although tremendous strides made in the administration of anesthesia have minimized these risks, the real difference between the traditional methods of childbirth and the natural-childbirth method is in the preparation and education of the mother. A common misunderstanding is that in the natural-childbirth method no anesthesia is allowed, when actually, except in cases of emergency, the decision to use anesthesia rests largely with the woman. If she feels that she can no longer go on without some sedation, she may ask for it, and her physician will then prescribe it.

The aftereffects of going through labor without sedation are usually satisfying. The feelings of confidence generated are a valuable asset in self-evaluation. However, the mother who expects to go through labor without sedation and then finds herself in need of it feels disillusioned for having "given in" and may experience a sense of failure. This possibility should be dealt with in the prenatal training course. It should be fully understood that the object of natural childbirth is not to see how much pain one can bear.

356   SEX AND MARRIAGE

The physician should make it quite clear that if the patient becomes too uncomfortable, there is nothing wrong with asking for some drug relief.

Rooming-in

Another standard practice in hospitals is that of keeping the newborn infant in a nursery separate from his mother. The infant is then brought to his mother on a schedule which increases efficiency of operation for the hospital staff and administrator. This practice has its limitations in that mothers feel a sense of deprivation if they cannot have their baby when they feel the need to hold and caress it. This contact is important to both the mother and the child. It develops a bond of closeness between the two which is nourishing for each. Many physicians believe that an infant has as much need for fondling as he has for food. The mother often worries about whether the busy nurses can give her baby the necessary attention. The argument for the other side is that mothers need rest after the work of bringing the child into the world. Furthermore, it is argued, in the years ahead the mothers will have countless opportunities to be physically close to their children.

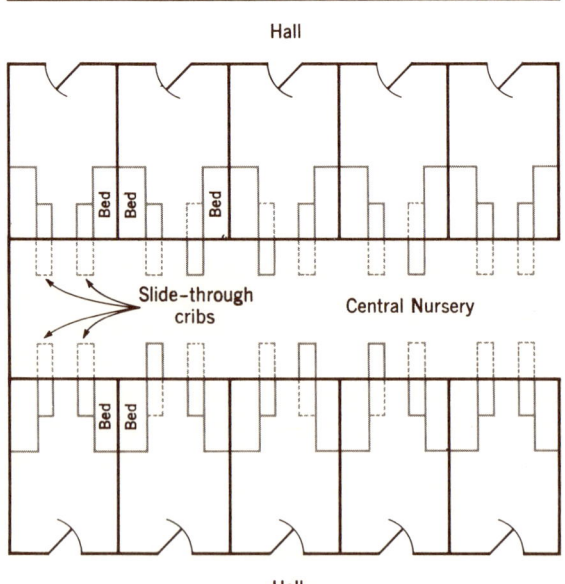

An alternative arrangement to the separate living quarters for mothers and infants is the practice of *rooming-in*. The physical setup is shown in the diagram on page 356. This arrangement allows the hospital staff to care for the infant while making the infant accessible to the mother when she wishes to hold it. All she has to do is pull out the drawerlike infant's bed, lift her baby to her, and hold him close. When she wants to rest or feels that the baby should be alone, she may place him back in the crib beside her bed.

Some hospitals have been built so that rooming-in is possible. It has been found that once the rooming-in arrangement has been made possible, it is just as efficient as the nursery system.

Nursing the Infant

To breast-feed one's baby or not is another area of controversy. Psychiatrists have promoted the idea that when this is not done, an important experience is omitted affecting the relationship between mother and child. The arguments on both sides tend toward exaggeration. On the one hand, we are led to believe that artificial, or bottle, feeding, being based on modern, scientific calculations, is actually superior to the "old-fashioned method." On the other hand, we are told that the mother who fails to nurse her baby condemns it to appalling hazards, to sundry diseases, to an ugly lower jaw, and even to a faulty background in filial piety. A hard-and-fast line on either position has its limitations. Some young mothers, for a variety of reasons, may not be able to breast-feed their babies. They may even prefer not to, and any emotional upset about this may make it impossible to do so.

There may be physical reasons why it is inadvisable for the mother to nurse her child. If this is the case, what about the potential psychological "damage" to the child? Perhaps the best approach is to use common sense in conjunction with scientific knowledge and consideration of the mother's personal emotional disposition. If it is possible to breast-feed and if the mother is inclined to do so, it probably should be done. If inclination is there but the physical factors do not make it entirely possible to breast-feed, some supplementation with bottled formula may be used to advantage.

The advantages of breast feeding are many:

1. Human milk provides natural immunization to certain diseases for the infant in the first stages of life.

2. Breast milk is normally clean.
3. Stomach and intestinal disturbances are rare in breast-fed babies.
4. There is more food value per ounce in human milk than it is usually possible to introduce into a formula.
5. Breast feeding hastens involution of the uterus (the recovery of the uterus after childbirth).
6. Breast feeding is usually more convenient for the mother.
7. Breast feeding is more economical.

The merits of artificial feeding are likewise several:

1. Mothers who follow the instructions of the doctor rarely meet difficulty in feeding their babies artificially.
2. The formula is constant in composition and quality. It can be revised according to the need of the infant.
3. The mother does not have to be present at every feeding. This has obvious advantages, especially if the mother is employed.
4. Artificial feeding is less tiring to the mother, so that she regains her strength more rapidly.

Breast feeding has other values besides those listed above. Both mother and child gain from the close physical contact, even if the child is nursed for only a short time. In this time, the baby's need for close body contact with his mother will have been fulfilled. The mother will not feel that she has deprived her child, and she may then be ready to give her attention to her child in another way.

The decision to nurse one's infant should be discussed by both parents. Many fathers have strong feelings about breast feeding but are reluctant to discuss them. The father may feel that he must abdicate any feeling in the matter, because it is the mother who is directly involved and the decision should be hers. He may recognize that it is good for the baby, and if the mother has no objections, he may feel he should not interfere. He may be quite ashamed of his feelings, but it is essential that they have a place in the decision-making process.

It is not uncommon for the father to have some feelings of jealousy at this time. Many men feel separated for the first time from the closest person in their lives and may resent the intruding stranger. Or he may feel excluded from the closeness of the two most important people in his life each time feeding occurs. He may want more opportunity for himself to hold and feed the infant. He may not like the restrictions placed upon the couple's freedom. He may even wonder about the effect that nursing may have on his wife's shapely figure.

It cannot be emphasized enough that the concerns of both the mother and the father need to be aired. Some of the aforementioned attitudes may sound a bit bizarre to some, and yet to others all of them may have some familiarity and truth. Nevertheless, there is no need to decry whatever feelings *do* exist. Decisions that are going to affect both mother and father should be arrived at mutually. The emotional implications that will influence decisions must be put in balance with as much reliable factual information as is available. Some excellent sources of information can be found at the end of this part.

Conclusion

One of the great strides in increasing life expectancy at birth results from the dedicated work of men in medical science. Their efforts to reduce the incidence of infant and maternal death during childbirth has added years to the average life expectancy. This has been largely the result of cutting down on the chance of infection and of reducing the complications of normal birth.

However, in the process several other factors have been overlooked. One is the personal feelings of expectant mothers and fathers. Medical humanism has been sadly lacking. Both mothers and fathers have been asked to surrender their autonomy completely to the obstetrician, who has made all the decisions. Hospitals have caused a fragmentation of families when babies are born. Husbands are separated from their wives. Mothers are separated from other children in the family. Newborn infants are separated from their mothers. Hospital routine has superseded individual personal needs.

Every one of these criticisms can be answered with logic and reason, but together they amount to the creation of conditions which leave much to be desired. While there is a sloppy sentimentality about the cliché of "togetherness," at the same time the total experience of childbirth can become a tremendously significant element in the lives of the young couple if it is shared fully by each of them or an extremely lonely and frightening experience if they are separated. The fully shared experience has been made possible by hospitals that have established practices in which husbands and wives may share the experience together and in which the mother and the newborn infant are together from the moment of birth until they leave the hospital; by obstetricians who see to it that husbands are fully informed; and by doctors who function without the excessive paternalism that robs the young couple of autonomy.

The concept of family-centered obstetric care offers much in the way of restoring medical humanism. It takes into consideration factors other than just those of biologic sterility, recognizing that health is as much a product of what people experience as it is a result of protection against disease-producing organisms and that the nonspecific elements of emotional stress are as devastating as physical factors alone.

Young people should know that there may be alternative ways of experiencing the birth of a child. When a choice is available, the expectant parents should select the hospital which will allow the kind of experience they think they want.

Although the experience of childbirth has the potential for being a devisive influence, it can be one that brings the husband and wife closer in harmony and growth.

SUGGESTED READINGS FOR PART 4

Atkinson, Ronald F.: *Sexual Morality,* Harcourt, Brace & World, New York, 1966.
Bach, George R., and Peter Wyden: *The Intimate Enemy: How to Fight Fair in Love and Marriage,* Morrow, New York, 1969.
Bell, N. W., and E. F. Vogel: *A Modern Introduction to the Family,* Glencoe Press, New York, 1960.
Bonaparte, Marie.: *Female Sexuality,* Grove, New York, 1965.
Bowman, Henry A.: *Marriage for Moderns,* 6th ed., McGraw-Hill, New York, 1970.
Brecher, Ruth, and Edward Brecher: *An Analysis of Human Sexual Response,* Signet, New American Library, New York, 1966.
Chase, Herman B.: *The Universal Fact,* Dell, New York, 1965.
Committee on the College Student, Group for the Advancement of Psychiatry: *Sex and the College Student,* Atheneum, New York, 1966.
Crawley, Lawrence Q., et al.: *Reproduction, Sex, and Preparation for Marriage,* Prentice-Hall, Englewood Cliffs, N.J., 1964.
De Beauvoir, Simone: *The Second Sex,* Knopf, New York, 1953.
De Rougemont, Denis: *Love Declared: Essays on the Myths of Love,* Beacon Press, Boston, 1963.

Dick-Read, Grantly: *Childbirth without Fear,* 2d ed., Harper & Row, New York, 1959.
Duvall, Evelyn M.: *Love and the Facts of Life,* Association Press, New York, 1963.
———: *Why Wait Till Marriage?,* Association Press, New York, 1968.
Eichenlaub, J. E.: *The Marriage Art,* Dell, New York, 1961.
Ellis, Albert: *The American Sexual Tragedy,* Lyle Stuart, New York, 1962.
———: *If This Be Sexual Heresy,* Lyle Stuart, New York, 1963.
Ellis, Havelock: *On Life and Sex,* Signet, New York, 1962.
Farber, Seymour M., and Roger H. L. Wilson: *Teen-age Marriage and Divorce,* Diablo, Berkeley, Calif., 1967.
——— et al. (eds.): *Man and Civilization: The Family's Search for Survival,* McGraw-Hill, New York, 1964.
Ford, C. S., and F. A. Beach: *Patterns of Sexual Behavior,* Harper, New York, 1961.
Fried, Edrita: *On Love and Sexuality,* Grove, New York, 1960.
Friedan, Betty: *The Feminine Mystique,* Norton, New York, 1965.
Goodrich, D. W., and Boomer, D. S.: "Experimental Assessment of Modes of Conflict Resolution," *Family Process,* vol. 2, pp. 15–24, 1963.
Guttmacher, Alan F.: *Pregnancy and Birth,* Signet, New York, 1962.
Havemann, Ernest: *Birth Control,* Time-Life, New York, 1967.
Hettlinger, Richard F.: *Living with Sex: The Student's Dilemma,* Seabury, 1966.
Jackson, Don D.: *Human Communication,* Science and Behavior Books, Palo Alto, Calif., 1968.
Johnson, Warren R.: *Human Sex and Education,* Lea & Febiger, Philadelphia, 1963.
Karmel, Marjorie: *Painless Childbirth,* Dolphin, New York, 1965.
Krich, Aron (ed.): *Facts of Love and Marriage for Young People,* Dell, New York, 1962.
Laing, R. D., and Esterson, A.: *Sanity, Madness and the Family,* Basic Books, New York, 1964.
Marmor, Judd: "The Marriage Relationship," in Salo Rosenbaum and Ian Alger (eds.), *Psychoanalytical Perspectives,* Basic Books, New York, 1959.
May, Rollo: *Love and Will,* Norton, New York, 1969.
McKinney, Fred: *Psychology of Personal Adjustment,* Wiley, New York, 1959.
Mead, Margaret: *Sex and Temperament,* Mentor, New York, 1962.
———: "Marriage in Two Steps," *Redbook,* vol. 127, July, 1966, p. 48.
Reiss, Ira L.: *Premarital Sexual Standards in America,* Free Press, New York, 1960.
———: *The Social Context of Premarital Permissiveness,* Holt, New York, 1967.

Schienfeld, Amram: *Your Heredity and Environment,* Lippincott, Philadelphia, 1965.

Stone, Hannah M., and Abraham Stone: *A Marriage Manual,* Simon & Schuster, New York, 1952.

Understanding Conception and Contraception, Ortho Pharmaceutical Corp., Raritan, N.J., 1967.

Womble, Dale L.: *Foundations of Marriage and Family Relations,* Macmillan, New York, 1966.

5.

CONCLUSION

23.

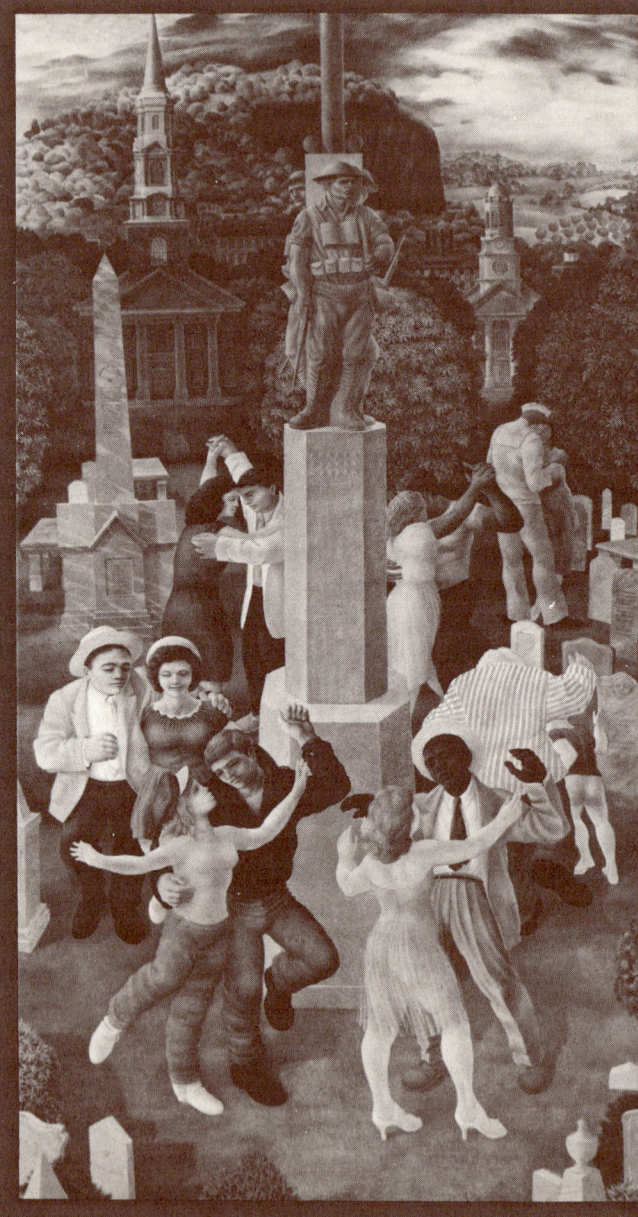

ARE AMERICANS HEALTHY?

Dr. Lawrence Hinkle, Jr., director of the Human Ecology Study Program of the Cornell Medical Center, has stated an important principle about the study of man, his health, and his environment.[1] He says, "For modern man, the aspects of the environment that are perhaps the most important are not the physical but the 'social' and 'interpersonal' features." He further suggests that as far as health is concerned, there is a mutual relationship between men and their environment.

Our actions influence others who then, in turn, respond and interact with us. We have all seen, for example, how our behavior has caused our parents to react to us and then how we in turn respond to what they have done. Conversation is a perfect example of this mutual interaction.

What we are not so aware of is that what we do also has an influence upon the less personal aspects of our environment. Changes are wrought from which we either benefit or lose. The educated person is not ignorant of the extent to which our industrial inclinations have polluted our environment, nor is he unaware of the influence that this pollution has had upon us. Increasing amounts of research show us that atmospheric pollution, for example, is a factor in the rapid increase of emphysema among our population. Some evidence indicates that atmospheric pollution is more dangerous to man than smoking.

The tendency of modern man has been to concern himself more with the obvious elements of his environment and to ignore the less obvious. Though it is odd that the person with whom we are conversing should be more obvious than the air we breathe, we have made it this way. We have taken the air for granted. Because the person demands more of us on the intellectual level, he is more obvious.

This is part of the problem of modern man. He is willing to utilize his time and energy only where the results of his effort are

---

[1] Lawrence Hinkle, Jr., *Health, Human Ecology, and the Hungarian Revolution*, lecture given before first Regional Medical and Science Reporting Workshop, Tarrytown, N.Y., April, 1958.

Wynn Chamberlain, "Celebration," 1954–1955. Egg tempera on composition board. Collection, The Whitney Museum of American Art, New York. Gift of the Pastorale Fund. Geoffrey Clements, photography.

more readily seen. Very few people can image that as individuals they are able to influence what happens to the air they breathe. Yet, it is *individuals* who set policies in industry, who allow pollution to be spewed forth into the air, who drive their cars when they could more profitably walk, who befoul our rivers, our sidewalks, our beaches, and our parks, and who ignore the rights of others so that all are endangered as a result. If health is to be seen in the quality of our response, can these individuals be considered healthy?

The impact of a polluted environment is becoming more obvious every day. The mass media have brought before us all the evidence of its influence upon the physical elements of our being. Lungs, skin, and eyes are markedly influenced by air pollution. Circulation difficulties and heart attacks are related to labored breathing during times when the atmosphere is particularly foul. In every large city the death rate jumps whenever a temperature inversion traps pollutants and inhabitants together for a day or two. When the environment is polluted with noise for significant lengths of time, people become deaf, first temporarily, then, if the noise level continues, permanently.

These are a few of the obvious changes which result from environmental pollution. There are others, however, which are perhaps even more damaging to individuals and to society. We see ourselves always in relation to the environment in which we live. Our sense of self is in part made up of the perspective we have of ourselves and our ability to cope with our environment. In many urban areas today millions of people see themselves totally unequipped to deal with the enormous hazards to existence.

In the midst of affluence all of us are poverty-stricken in certain areas of our lives. Too many of us are stricken by poverty in every area of life. When we give up hope that we ourselves can change things and when we see many around us with an equal sense of hopelessness, we tend to transform our feeling of despair into behavior. We litter as a matter of course, we surrender responsibility as a part of a life style, we tend to grasp what we can and let the devil take the hindmost. The cyclic effect of this is obvious.

In part health is the result of having our basic needs met. We have already seen that the cycle of deficiency-need satisfaction enables us to move forward to the satisfaction of growth needs. When our environment itself prohibits the fulfillment of deficiency needs, individuals feel threatened. It is when this sense of threat permeates the entire context in which we live that many of us experience despair. Deprivation and despair are linked, and wherever our environment creates a sense of overwhelming poverty from which there is no escape, despair is the inevitable result.

The effort to escape through diversions of a materialistic nature or through drugs, alcohol, or other sedation does not eliminate the sense of despair which people feel about the world in which they live. The pace at which many live creates the impression that they are desperately trying to run away from things which bother them. This works as long as the effort continues, but in the long run it is depleting and nondevelopmental.

It is fortunate that we have awakened to the hazards of our polluted environment. The situation cannot be corrected by governmental agencies alone, nor can industry, by itself, do the job. It is necessary for the millions of our population to realize the subtle but powerful influence of a polluted environment upon us and our style of life. When we begin to evaluate this, we will more readily respond to, and cope with, its demands.

Social Surrender

At present, far too many individuals have made what can be called a social surrender. *They have given up their autonomy in the face of the collective proposition*—the "You can't fight City Hall" syndrome. Since we believe this to be so, we do not bother. Only when we are supported by large numbers of fellowmen are we willing to face up to the establishment. Only when we have a union, an organized group, or an emotionally aroused mob to back us are we willing to take up the challenge to change what bothers us. The tactic works. Collective bargaining will probably be the predominant factor in change in the immediate future. But in the process of using this tactic, we have abandoned one of the basic precepts upon which our nation was founded: the idea that each *individual* has rights, each *individual* should be heard, each *individual* has a stake in the collective whole. Unless each individual asserts these rights and *assumes the responsibilities* attendant upon these rights, we are doomed to being manipulated by the politician, the ad man, and the influence peddler.

In abandoning the principle of self-determination, we have lost a significant element of our humanity, the very thing which makes us unique. We have lost a sense of selfhood.

Why have we done this? If we can address ourselves to this question, we move toward discovery of what it is to be a human being in a collective society. No doubt fear is involved. Somehow, in the early years of our lives we have been conditioned to the fear of being different. We have a vague vision of freedom, but we have been kept from exercising what freedom exists in our early years. We have allowed ourselves to be coerced into being like everyone else. As we have moved closer to our neighbors, we have learned that they will not tolerate our individuality. As we have moved from the rural to the urban environment, we have had to consider the other fellow more than ever before. To avoid treading on his toes and suffering the consequences, we have surrendered a bit of ourselves. We have also convinced ourselves that this is no great sacrifice. In fact, because it is for the "common welfare," this surrender has been valued.

The other side of the coin is that when others have exerted their independence, we have retaliated in such a manner that others learn the same lesson we have learned. The consequence is both comic and tragic. We are now at the point where it is only the person who does not "give a damn" about the rights of others who asserts himself. When he does step on toes, our *inhibitions against asserting ourselves* have prevented us from using our influence to curb the violator. How many of us, for example, would be willing to risk the retaliatory insults we would receive if we asked another person to pick up the cigarette wrapper he has casually tossed on the sidewalk? Unless we are aroused to sufficient anger by what another person has done, we will not act. When we act only out of anger, reason is often lacking in our response.

Since anger has also been downgraded in our society, we often feel guilty following an outburst of justifiable wrath. The only alternative many of us have found is to dissociate ourselves from the collective scene. If we can turn off our feelings of anger about the wrongdoing of another person, we are not called upon to act. We have effectively accomplished two things: We have insulated ourselves against the influence of others, and we have voided ourselves of responsibility to act. The combined effort appears to have protected us from frustration.

Why so much concern about frustration? What is so important about remaining frustration-free? The answer probably lies in the fact that other areas of our lives are so heavily laden with frustration that we cannot tolerate any more than is absolutely unavoidable. If our lives are frustration-filled, can we be healthy people?

Fighting Expertise

This is the age of the expert. Specialization, which has become the order of the day, serves two purposes: First, it enables an individual to pursue an area of knowledge which is of value and renders him fit to serve. At the same time it removes the expert from the zone of criticism by laymen, that vast amorphous group to which we all belong. The expert is then safe in his ivory tower, and his only struggles are with his fellow experts. The layman is unknowing in the expert's field and feels inadequate in dealing with the expert's manipulations.

Few of us are "universal men," and yet never has there been greater need for the universal man, a person who appreciates the place of all things, who has his own life in perspective with the lives of others, and who interacts with creativity, efficiency, and maturity with the totality of his environment. The universal man is able to appreciate the place of the specialist but does not surrender his own autonomy. He does not let the expert dominate his life but rather is willing to listen with understanding to what the expert has to say, and then exerts his own judgment in implementing whatever suggestions are made about his own life.

The so-called expert impinges upon our lives at every point. He is represented in each of the professions of law, medicine, education, and religion. He is preeminent in the marketplace. Science has created countless experts who dominate our lives. The effect has been that we have lost confidence in our own ability to manage our lives. Hence we cannot make the decisions which are necessary to live with satisfaction. We are unable to respond with a sense of *self-directed responsibility*. Lacking confidence, we cannot respond appropriately and therefore suffer diminished health.

Finding the Middle Way

What is the answer to this dilemma of modern man? Do we decide all things by ourselves or attempt to take all the advice we get? Do we resort to the coin-flipping method of dealing with life? How can we manage to affirm our own judgment or utilize the expert according to what the situation requires?

To some extent the answer is a willingness to experiment in order to find the middle way and then to assess the value of our efforts. As we accumulate experience, we may hope for wisdom. Wisdom, however, does not always follow experience. Rather it grows out of an evaluation of what we have done in the largest perspective we can place it in. Wisdom also presupposes that the individual will use his educational resources to review for himself all the information that is available at the time. He need not take one expert's opinion. He can search out recent findings for himself and make an educated decision.

We may not like the fact that so much of living must be on an experimental basis. In an age when the expert has had a great influence upon our lives and to maintain sanity the only alternative lies in being experimental, the expert and his assumptions direct our thought and often our behavior.

David Riesman[2] makes the distinction between three basic personality types—the tradition-directed person, the inner-directed person, and the other-directed person. The other-directed person is bound to the values of his contemporaries. These others become the dominant source of direction for him, setting values for him and providing the standards by which he judges himself. They inflict penalties for being different from themselves.

The inner-directed person exerts a greater degree of autonomy. He finds his direction within himself and is less concerned about what others think. He lives his life with a greater degree of freedom than either the tradition-directed or the other-directed person.

Riesman suggests that other-directedness characterizes Americans to a high degree. We are, he says, more uncertain of our values than other peoples. Hence, presumably, we are less willing to assert ourselves as independent of our contemporaries.

The concept of inner-directedness, while not the same thing as Maslow's concept of self-actualization, is a worthwhile point of departure for the achievement of health. Linked together with the idea of self-actualization, this concept gives us some idea of what is necessary in the confusion of our times. It gives us some direction for finding the middle way in the struggle to achieve a sense of selfhood in the age of the expert.

The Consumer Society

In a society where much of the well-being of people depends upon the gross national product, a tremendous amount of importance is placed upon the consumption of goods. This, in itself, is not an evil. The problem is that the emphasis on consumer purchasing tends to cause people to value themselves according to their ability to become a part of the acquisitive scramble. People then become the means to acquire the *things* of life, and the essence of life is lost.

Acquisitiveness and the submission to the expert work hand in hand. The public can be sold on the idea that they need a hairpiece, a facial cream, a gold toothpick, a purple shoelace, almost

---

[2] David Riesman et al., *The Lonely Crowd*, Yale, New Haven, Conn., 1963, pp. 9–19.

anything! The sale of these items is virtually assured when they are recommended by physicians, dentists, or public figures in the theater or sports world. This is well known by the advertising experts. Drug quackery has become one of the most profitable fraudulent practices ever to be perpetrated upon the American public. This condition can exist only in a society where the people have come to believe that others know what is best for them.

This consumer orientation has been a particular problem of most people who are currently of the older generation. Young people who have been brought up in the affluence of the post-World War II era may have a different view of life. It is too early now to make a definitive statement, but if the youth movement of the late 1960s is a reflection of a truly different view of the meaning of life, we are in for a change. If it is only a passing phase and the old economic determinants of life are once again accepted by contemporary youth as they begin to assume responsibility for their own well-being, then similar problems to those we face today will prevail. People will once again either be caught in the traps of the consumer society or have to resist these snares with great determination.

The task is not an easy one. One must have the courage of his convictions to resist the bombardments of a materialistic society. Unless one can find friends with an equal set of values about living, one is continually faced with the problem of keeping up with the Joneses. The status given to the highly paid ad man, for

J. Paul Kirouac, photography.

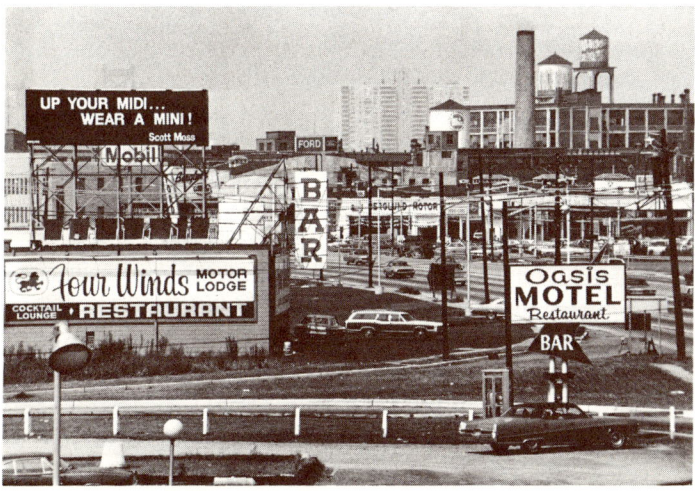

example, is altogether different from that accorded to the shoe clerk. The two persons have an entirely different standard of living. In terms of clothes, recreational pursuits, luxuries, education, life styles, and so forth, the ad man can offer much more in the materialistic sense than the shoe clerk. However, in terms of values which are more humanistic, there may be little difference in what each can offer to his children or contribute to society. However, the personal sense of deprivation is apt to be much greater in the family of the shoe clerk.

The sense of deprivation may so permeate the family experience that every member of the family may feel that disaster is imminent. This cannot help but mark the attitudes of each member of the family. This type of experiential conditioning undoubtedly has its influence in the way people view their lives and their own worth.

Many persons of the older generation have been influenced by this kind of experience. This probably accounts for the heavy emphasis upon economic materialism. The person who has been so influenced cannot help but distort the events of his life. The quality of his response is bound to be affected and his health therefore limited by his view of life.

Social Commitment

In our effort to protect ourselves, we have withdrawn from commitment to anything other than our own interests. Only a few people will become involved in community endeavors to serve its citizens. The vast remainder ride along attending, with varying degrees of success, to their own lives. In a community of 15,000 no more than about 500 are willing to become really involved with the life of the community in any service capacity. These are the people who do the volunteer work in hospitals, health agencies, churches, synagogues, and other service organizations.

Some of these people are compulsively driven to serve, while many more find that expanding their horizons through service is personally rewarding. But since so few people in the United States are involved at all in service to others, one wonders how much of the malaise of the day would disappear if more people would give themselves to endeavors which were larger than they. Some persons are fortunate in that what they do for a living provides opportunities for service to others. Compare the opportunities to serve others which are associated with medicine and with assembly-line work, or think of the difference between teaching and selling.

Our intention here is not to downgrade any of the manufacturing or marketing occupations but merely to point out that certain types of work usually offer more opportunities to get the feeling of service to others. Since this feeling has much to do with one's sense of worth, it is an important consideration in the choice of vocation. It is also true that many professional people in our consumer society have a far lower sense of worth than others whose work involves the manufacture or marketing of goods.

Many of us are discouraged from engaging in work involving service to others because we think that little can be done by one individual. However, every volunteer organization was started by one individual. United Cerebral Palsy, Synanon, the American Cancer Society, the Congress of Racial Equality (CORE), the Muscular Dystrophy Association—all were started by one individual who saw a need and moved to fill it. Many of these organizations have an interesting history. Often they have opened up whole new careers for the founders. An example of the kind of thing that can happen is to be seen in the founding of a chapter of the United Cerebral Palsy Association in one of the wealthy counties of the East. It was started by a school nurse. She became interested in the work when she discovered that several children in her community were not receiving an education because of their handicap. Within five years she had a project involving services to sixty children and thirty-five adults with a professional staff of twenty operating on a budget of over a quarter of a million dollars a year underway. In the process this woman grew tremendously as a person. Her interests in life broadened. Her hopes for the future grew. Her personal sense of satisfaction and worth became stronger with each passing year.

There is no lack of important tasks to be performed in our society. Obvious areas have already been noted—the improvement of race relations, the upgrading of living conditions for the poverty-stricken, the need for population control, the establishment of programs to fight pollution. There are many other jobs that need doing, as well. One of the functions of volunteer organizations is to identify and call to the attention of governmental agencies those jobs that cannot be done well by volunteer organizations.

If we judge health by the quality of one's response to life, we must see life in its largest perspective. When individuals are able to live effectively within the sphere of their family and profession and community, they achieve something important for themselves. But there is more to life than this. The area of service to others must get equal attention if one is to be considered fully healthy.

Full humanness means that each of us identifies more fully with our fellowman and is able to transcend himself and his own miniscule problems. The self expands and becomes more inclusive of other human beings. The sense of self also grows, and with it the sense of satisfaction and confidence in one's ability to live life fully.

The search for a larger endeavor itself is a mind-expanding effort. The very fact that many young people today are interested in psychedelic drugs for their supposed mind-expanding qualities is an indication that the limited life that many of us live is not satisfying enough. Nothing expands one's mind more than a creative effort to become involved with other people. This involvement, when it goes beyond the mundane concern with today's weather, is rewarding.

There are programs which need doing which have not yet been identified. Every community has problems which are crying to be solved. The imaginative person who undertakes such a project will do something not only for his community *but for himself as well.* This principle has been used in hospitals for the rehabilitation of the mentally ill. When patients assume varying degrees of responsibilities for one another in the rehabilitative process, they are able to leave the hospital sooner and with a higher degree of competence for living.

Some of the more effective programs for rehabilitation of drug addicts have used similar methods. Daytop Village, an extremely successful institution for the rehabilitation of drug addicts, involves addicts in a mutual program of self-help. Working together in groups, the residents of Daytop Village help one another to identify what it is that has caused them to become addicted. They have a much higher rate of cure of addiction than any other methods so far utilized. One of the major problems with the rehabilitation of addicts is the high rate of recidivism. According to the director of Daytop[3] the number of recidivists has been three out ninety-nine. This remarkable record emphasizes that when persons become involved with others in a mutual effort at improvement, all are helped.

The principle is not a new one. Many fraternal organizations and societies have been founded on the idea of involvement with others. The early Christian church was an organization of persons concerned about one another. Out of this organization grew the concept of the "beloved commmunity." It worked because it took

---

[3] Dr. Daniel Casriel, address before Westchester Mental Health Association, White Plains, N.Y., 1969.

people out of themselves, got them interested in a larger aim, expanded horizons, and enabled people to put their energies into something other than their own small world.

Beating the Institutions

A serious problem faced by many people today is that their lives have become institutionalized. They have found an identity by being part of an institutionalized segment of society, an economic class, educational group, religious group, or racial group. They have become role-bound in the larger projection of themselves as well as in the microcosm of the family.

To a point this is important and serves us well. When we have found an identity in something larger than ourselves, we grow to fit that identity. However, for many of us the institutionalization of identity is limiting rather than expanding. It prevents us from finding and being ourselves.

Often we leave it to the institution to accomplish what we want for ourselves. Even if we do not want what the institution decides, we go along with it "for the greater good." For example, many teachers find themselves in conflict over salary issues. They believe they should be paid more money than they now receive for what they contribute to society. To obtain salaries commensurate with their desires, large numbers of teachers have resorted to the institution of the union. Although an individual teacher may not feel that he wants to engage in a strike, if one is called, he goes along with it for the greater good. Even when not a union member, he may be unwilling to cross a picket line and is therefore controlled by the institution.

College students are influenced by institutionalization. Many young people want to attend name institutions for the status value. Others are overly concerned about getting into fraternities or sororities. Those who are successful sometimes develop a false sense of value about their institutional affiliation. Many who fail to get into the status organizations feel themselves to be of less value than those who succeed. If this is the primary basis for feeling oneself to be a success or a failure as a person, then, clearly, distorted values are at work.

Distortions of this kind influence most of us to a large extent, sometimes causing us to lose our sense of our own worth. Even when a teachers' union, for example, is successful in obtaining a raise, the teacher may feel that he himself has done little to fight for that raise, and doubts may arise within him about his worth as a person. Usually these doubts are rationalized without too much difficulty, but when the need for such rationalization becomes a predominant factor in life, some lack of self-respect develops.

When an institution stands for us, we have no sense of standing for ourselves. Our identity is amorphous. It has no real substance for us. Hence, the quality of our response is limited, distorted, or inappropriate.

Health and Technology

In contrast with the foregoing problems of institutionalization, social surrender, consumeritis, and expert-orientedness—all signs of diminished health and autonomy—another phenomenon of modern living creates the opposite illusion. Our technology has eliminated many of the problems which plagued man a few centuries ago. The development of vaccines, the increase in knowledge about preventing infection, the protection of food supplies, and improved medical practice have created the illusion that we are healthier people.

As noted in an early chapter, because infection and communicable disease were major killers a hundred years ago, we assumed that any person who avoided these was healthy. He may have been, but the reason for his health was not necessarily that he remained disease-free. More likely his health was in his ability to respond to life in such a manner that he did not contract disease and infection. This is a fine point but an important one. A person may remain disease-free because he has not been exposed to disease, and he therefore gives the appearance of being healthy. However, as soon as he is exposed to the conditions which, combined with nonspecific factors, produce a disease, he succumbs. He is not able to respond appropriately to these circumstances of his life and thus collapses in the face of them. Other persons may be exposed to disease agents time and time again without ever contracting the disease. These are the healthier people. They have the constitutional makeup, the adaptive machinery, the view of life which enables them to cope successfully with the disease-producing circumstances. They have been able to develop and conserve the potential resources which most people have for fighting disease and infection.

The mere fact that the death rate for tuberculosis is lower now than ever before is no evidence in itself that we are healthier people. Our technology has protected us from tuberculosis. That death due to pneumonia is rare today does not mean that we are healthier. Medical technology has virtually eliminated this cause of death. That very few people contract polio today does not mean that we are healthier, for, again, medical technology has saved us. Food poisoning is a rare cause of death today. Is this a sign that we are healthier? Hardly. Food-protection practices have kept this hazard to a minimum.

With the remarkable increase in protection we have gained over the past one hundred years through the efforts of medical science, the burden of proof about our health is directly upon each one of us as individuals. In every age some individuals have measured up to the challenge of being able to cope effectively with the circumstances of their lives. Today too many people, while not succumbing to infection and disease because they have been immunized against them, nevertheless show many other signs of inability to cope with life and its problems.

The extremely high incidence of mental illness is indicative of the fact that many people are bent upon destroying themselves. Other signs of this are seen in the high and increasing rate of alcoholism, addiction, crime, suicide, and homocide. Despair as a forerunner of much disease, coupled with the disease rates of today, indicates that many persons have given up. They see no future for themselves. They do not want to go on living and move toward death in one way or another.

If we become complacent about our health simply because life expectancy has increased, we delude ourselves in equating quantity with quality. An increase of empty years adds little to life. The person, retired at sixty-five, who has fifteen more years to live has little to look forward to if he loses his raison d'être along with his job. Technology has protected his life, but it has not promoted his health.

A Reason for Being

In 1969 a dying man was interviewed on a TV program about the meaning of his life. As he looked back over the years, he found to his dismay that his life had amounted to very little. He had been a "good" man, clean, honest, and diligent. He had saved money against the time when he would be able to retire and do all the things he had dreamed about. But, tragically, before that time came, his life seemed so pointless to him that he saw no reason for living. He became one of those whose sense of despair totally replaces a sense of hope.

The expression of pain on his face spoke to the TV viewer of the agony the dying man felt as he realized the emptiness of his life. As one listened, one thought that probably a causative element of the cancer he was suffering from was the fact that his life had been so meaningless. One did not need commentary to the effect that a will to live had been lost in the process of nonliving as one heard him comment reflectively, "All those weekends that I only cleaned my apartment."

Healthy persons are marked by an enthusiasm for life. They transmit this enthusiasm to others around them. They have a reason for being. They approach all of life with the expectancy that it will provide them with the food that is necessary for men to become fully human. The biblical statement that "man does not live by bread alone" is profoundly apropos. All things in life are of value at least equal to that of the physical necessities for sustaining the biologic processes of life. Without a balance of these elements, without a variety of living experience, an involvement with other people, and a commitment to ideals, man does not survive *as man*. The dying man on the television program had concerned himself only with earning a living and doing what others expected of him. He did not live for himself; he did not do what was necessary to actualize his potential.

The meaning of our life in an affluent society will be found less in economic survival than in the range of our experiences. It will be found in the quality of the way we spend our time, in the degree to which we discover what our inner selves can do.

It may be that this potential will best be utilized in the marketplace. Other people may use it better in research. Some will find satisfaction in teaching, medicine, accounting. Few will find their talents fully developed in their vocational endeavors. If we attempt to, we do ourselves the great disservice of limiting ourselves to one area of experience, which brings only limited rewards.

A Concern for Human Values

The most serious indictment of us as a people is that we have confused our goals and our means of achieving them. Our desire to upgrade our standard of living has caused us to put aside some basic human values. That we have not only ignored the rights of a large segment of our population but also exploited minority groups is a national tragedy. The combined sense of oppression and outrage has resulted in the crippling of countless persons. It has made communication between minority groups and the larger middle-class society extremely difficult. It has built threats and destructive defenses against these threats into the beliefs and life styles of people on both sides of the controversy, making it impossible for us to understand one another.

We have seen that communication is essential in the resolution of conflict and that the stress of conflict often causes people to seek means of eliminating or escaping the stress rather than move toward the changes necessary to resolve the conflict. In the United States today there are a wide variety of techniques for avoiding any effort to change such as the use of clichés like "Blacks are shiftless and lazy, and will never amount of anything" or "I worked hard. Why can't they?"

When we hang on to slogans like these, we create for ourselves a frame of reference in which realistic thinking is impossible and try to combat monsters which do not exist. Much energy is thus diverted to unproductive channels. What is worse, antagonistic feelings are created in persons who hold a different point of view. Each side feels its integrity is at stake, and neither is willing to budge. Consider, for example, the effect of "You can never trust a white man" on both the person who believes it and the one about whom it is said. It is impossible for either to conduct himself so that he is understood by the other.

The intensity of the debate over our use of armed power in international affairs is closely related to the issues concerning human values. The diversion of manpower and money into this effort clearly detracts from our ability to upgrade living conditions for that segment of our population that has not had an opportunity to develop its personal resources for living with satisfaction and dignity.

The exploitative aspects of our society need thorough examination before we can consider that we are a healthy people. This requires dispelling the ignorance we have about what others believe and the way they live. The mass media are vital in shedding light upon the conditions of life among the various groups of our population. But more important is for each individual to take it upon himself to find out for himself. Each of us must open our minds to the basic ideas of others. The Black Panthers, Students for a Democratic Society, and other radical antiestablishment groups have an important message for us. Conservative groups are also saying important things. We need not capitulate to either side, but we should examine what they are basically saying about the American way and about themselves. To close ourselves off from criticism of what we believe in can lead us only to disaster.

Social change may be correlated with personal growth, which as we have seen in this book, is essential for health and well-being. When we interfere with it, we downgrade the quality of our response. The existential circumstances of life in the United States demand change. The status quo no longer works, and change has a national priority of the highest order.

Are Americans Healthy?

This question can be answered in any way and have a measure of truth in it. Much depends upon the standards we use to determine health. We have seen that great advances have been made against the traditional factors which have impaired and endangered life. This has given many more people the opportunity to experiment with their lives. More people are living longer and are therefore carried into the age where reward for living fully has been found. The majority of us have been freed from grinding poverty. This has placed us in a favored category in the animal kingdom. We can spend considerably less of our energy gathering food and staving off starvation and can put this energy to satisfying endeavors in the development of talents which would otherwise lie dormant.

These are all gains. They are the benefits of living in an enterprising society. The critical tendencies of the times often make it difficult for us to appreciate these advantages. The contemporary inclination to knock many of the freedoms which grow out of these advances is possible only because we *are free* to do so. It is a curious fact of man's nature that he apparently is never satisfied, but must turn much of his energy to negating what he has.

What should be more carefully examined is that so many of us are so negative. If, as we have seen in earlier chapters, our lives are stress-filled because of our expectations, some care should be given to evaluating these expectations. When they are such that we cannot appreciate the opportunities which lie before us, we should recognize that we are negating ourselves. This is hardly a sign of health.

The great frontier before every individual is internal. He may commit himself to endeavors which others can see and which produce material signs of his efforts, but unless the inner frontiers are pushed back, the external efforts are of little worth in health. If, in the process of making our mark on the world, we cannot discover our own inner essence, our mark will be of little value to us.

To balance out the inner discoveries with the external endeavors is the trick of life. Self-actualization shows itself in action, but action does not necessarily produce self-actualization. Good works alone are not the sole criterion of the satisfying life. The development of an inner sense of well-being is equally essential. The college years are ones in which young persons are setting direction for themselves. If this direction is toward goals which are primarily oriented toward good works, an important reevaluation is essential.

The hippie movement has produced some weird and destructive things, but it has also brought to the attention of the thoughtful observer some values which have been too long honored only *in absentia*. Embodied in the one word *love*, these values underline the importance of human relationships. The cry of hypocrisy has been raised by the hippie. He believes that we have been far too hypocritical in our dealings with one another. We have, on the one hand, said that we place a high value on individuals. At the same time we have too often ignored the influence upon human lives of our economic endeavors. We have not only ignored the value of other people but of ourselves as well. In the process of accumulating things we have sold ourselves short, because we have not allowed ourselves to develop other qualities along with those of our acquisitive nature. Out of this our sense of emptiness has grown.

But a choice always lies before us. Our lives need not remain empty. We have seen in the earlier chapters that there is a drive within us which propels us toward the realization of the potential we have. Given our nature and the developmental way stations along the path from primitive, undeveloped humanity to the full flowering of our humanness, our choices will enable us to remain at any of these way stations, or they will allow us to move forward toward the undefined goal. As we approximate this goal, it becomes more clearly defined. Both frustration and glory lie in the fact that it is never fully known. We must be content with striving toward it.

The goal we set for ourselves, the path we follow, and the means we use in traversing that path all constitute our health. Because we have control over each of these features of our journey, our health lies quite directly in our own hands. One of the characteristics of contemporary man is that he seems to have forgotten this. He has lost confidence in his ability to manage his life. He has surrendered to the fears and frustrations of modern living.

This is tragic when it occurs in an individual life, but it does not have to be so. When one sharpens his sensitivity to what is happening within and around him, he takes a giant stride toward liberation. A second stride is taken when he can evaluate what is happening in his life. The final stride toward full and rich living is his use of this sensitivity and critical thinking to adapt creatively to what lies before him. He is then moving toward the achievement of what he is, and he reaches toward the future. He becomes a man in the fullest sense.

INDEX

Abortion, 310
Academic pressure, 226–231
   and the future, 226–228
   the nature of, 222–223
   and past conditioning, 225–226
Adaptation:
   creative, 119–131
   and goals, 128–129
   and guilt, 130–131
Addiction, 233–250
   and social factors, 235–236
Adoption, 309
Alarm reaction, 101
Alcohol, 240–242
Alcoholism, 240–242
Allport, Gordon, 57, 156
Amphetamines, 242
Analyzing, conflict resolution, 185
Anxiety:
   reduction of, 228
   sources of, 143
Attitudes:
   importance of, 8–9
   about marriage, 319–337
   about sex, 264–267, 297–299
Autonomy, 33, 96
Axline, Virginia, 24–25

Baldwin, James, 134, 151–152
Barbiturates, 240
Becoming, 48–51

Being, 83–84
   reason for, 377
   unity of, 88
Bettleheim, Bruno, 58
Birth, 341–360
Birth control, 301–317
   rhythm method, 305
   withdrawal, 304
Braceland, Francis, 65
Breast feeding, 357–359

Cannon, Walter, 42
Casriel, Dr. Daniel, 374
Categorizing, conflict resolution, 184
Childbirth, 341–360
   educated, 354–356
   father's role, 352
   Lamaze method, 355
   mother's experience, 353–356
   natural, 354
Children:
   in marriage, 342–344
   reasons for having, 343–344
Cohabitation, 324–325
Cohen, Sidney, 124
Commitment, social, 372–375
Communication in marriage, 331–332
Commuter college, 199–201
Competition, 221–231
Conception, prevention of, 295–317

Condom, the, 302
Confidence, sources of, 144
Conflict:
   and age levels, 171–172
   and health, 173–176
   and identity, 191–207
   interpersonal, 159–161
   intrapersonal, 161
   origin of, 178–179
   resolution of, 171–187
   and sex, 257–260
   signs of, 179–182
   sources of, 176–177
   types of, 159–161
Conformity, 209–219
   meaning of, 210
   why, 214–215
Consciousness and values, 149
Consumer society, 370
Contraception, 301–317
Cooperation and conformity, 218
Counseling, premarital, 335
Creative person, 122–123
Creativity:
   and identity, 201–205
   meaning of, 119–121
   predisposing factors, 125–128
   and response, 97–98
Cultural conditioning, 93–94, 156–157
Culture and suggestion, 156–157
Cunnilingus, 269

Dating:
   biologic motivation, 275
   expectations for, 278–281
   exploration, 284
   faithfulness, 287
   freedom, 292

Dating:
   generosity, 285
   honesty, 286
   kindness, 288
   personal factors, 281–284
   social motivation, 276–278
Davis, Ossie, 120
Death, causes of, 11
Demand principle, 144
Dependency, drug, 233–250
Depression, 65–66
Developmental task:
   and experience, 164–170
   and frustration, 162–163
   and identity, 169–170
Diaphragm, 303
Disease:
   causitive factors, 110–114
   some concepts of, 104–110
   and emotions, 110–114
   the germ theory, 104–105
   people in search of, 103
   the psychogenic theory, 108
   the psychosomatic theory, 107
   the resistance theory, 106
   the stress theory, 105
   the symbolic theory, 109
   venereal, 313
Disease-prone, 103–104
Dropping out, 9–10
Drug dependency, 233–250
Drug problem, 233–250
Drug use:
   risks of, 246–248
   motivation for, 236–238
Drugs in perspective, 236
Dubos, Rene, 105, 106

Ecology, 365–381
Emotions:
   deceptive nature of, 53

Emotions:
   and disease, 110–114
   negative and positive, 54
   purpose of, 55
Enculturation, 33
Engel, George, 111
Environment, control of, 17–19
Exhaustion, stage of, 101
Existential moment, 73–74
Existentialism, 7
Expectations:
   in dating, 278–281
   and health, 84–87
   for marriage, 319–337
Experience:
   complexity of, 71
   concept of, 69
   and the developmental task, 164–169
   expectations and, 75–77
   future in, 75
   and growth, 72
   influence of the past, 74–75
   and learning, 72
   peak, 123–125
   prenatal, 346–350
Experience cycle, 70

Failure:
   risk of, 164
   and success, 142
Faithfulness in dating, 287
Feelings in marriage, 331–332
Fellatio, 269
Frankl, Victor, 8
Freedom in dating, 292
Fromm, Erich, 27–29, 206
Frustration in developmental tasks, 162
Function:
   physiologic, 42, 62
   and relationships, 48

Function:
   and symbols, 62–65
   unity of, 87–88
   and values, 150–153

General adaptation syndrome, 101–102, 105–106
Generosity in dating, 285
Gibran, Kahlil, 35
Give-up-itis, 112
Giving-up complex, 111
Glasser, William, 53
Going steady, 290
Gonorrhea, 314
Good life, the, 5–6
Growth:
   and experience, 72
   resistance to, 215–216
   and response, 92–93
Guilt and adaptation, 130–131

Health:
   and affirmation, 88
   degrees of, 82
   and disease, 101–114
   dynamism of, 3–4
   and existentialism, 7
   and expectations, 84–87
   and function, 82
   a goal and a process, 83
   and humanness, 23–25
   misconceptions of, 80
   problems of understanding, 3–15
   promotion of, 10–12
   protection of, 10
   and purpose, 44
   a qualitative response, 14
   and relatedness, 48
   and symbols, 66
   and technology, 376

Health:
 traditional concepts of, 79
 and unity, 87–88
 and values, 102
Heterosexual relationships, quality of, 289
Hinkle, Dr. Lawrence, 356
Homeostasis, 98
Homosexual, fear of being, 262–263
Hospital, 351–354
Human, on being, 17–35
Humanness, basic qualities of, 37–55
Hutschnecker, Arnold, 63
Hypnosis, 154

Identity:
 and conflict, 191–207
 and developmental tasks, 169
 establishing an, 191–207
 formation of, 133–135
 and relationship, 46
 the search for, 192–194
 and sex, 256
 and symbols, 65
Institutionalization, 375
Intrauterine contraceptive device, 306

Jackel, Merl M., 112

Kindness in dating, 288
Kline, Nathan, 65

Labor in childbirth, 353
Lamaze, 355
Learning:
 and experience, 72–73
 and growth, 72–73

LeShan, Lawrence, 7, 107
Lewis, Faye, 64
Life, affirmation of, 88–89
Life style:
 and drugs, 235–236
 variables in, 6
Loneliness, 194–197
Love, 26–29
LSD, 124–125

Malcolm X, 76, 120
Marriage:
 attitudes and expectations, 319–324
 backgrounds, 332–336
 and children, 342–344
 and communication, 330–332
 the perfect, 336
 and readiness, 327–330
 roles in, 323–327
 successful, 338
 and values, 326
 work of, 330–332
Maslow, Abraham, 30–35, 123, 186
Maturity and self-control, 216–218
Meaning:
 and drugs, 237–238
 in life, 9
 will to, 8
Meir, William, 111–112
Menstruation, 263
Mononucleosis, 113
Morality, the new, 315

National Institute of Mental Health, 202
New York Addiction Services Agency, 243
Nursing, 357–359

Opiates, 239

Parent-child relationships, 138
Peak experience, 123–125
Perception of reality, 95
Personalities, idealized, 139
Phoenix House, 243–246
Pill, the, 305
Potential:
   and becoming, 50
   for living, 12
Preconditioning and suggestion, 154
Pregnancy:
   hospital experience, 351–354
   sex during, 350–351
   unmarried, 307–312
Premarital counseling, 335
Premarital sex, attitudes about, 264–267
Prenatal experience, 346–350
Progoff, Ira, 24
Promiscuity, 295–301
Promotion of health, 10–12
Psychedelic drugs, 124–125, 238–239
Psychogenic regional pain, 109
Psychology Today, 250
Purpose:
   biological, 41–44
   and health, 44
   and meaning, 43
   and satisfaction, 43–44
   and value, 147

Questioning, 5–6

Relatedness:
   and health, 48
   and identity, 46–48
   to others, 46

Relatedness:
   to physical environment, 45–46
Relationships:
   and function, 48
   heterosexual, 289
   parent-child, 138
   and symbols, 60
Reorganization, conflict resolution, 186–187
Repression, 112–113
Resistance, stage of, 101
Response:
   and adaptation, 39
   appropriateness of, 91
   and autonomy, 96
   and creativity, 97
   and cultural mores, 93
   evaluation of, 91–99
   and the future, 94
   and growth, 92
   and homeostasis, 98
   and learning, 39
   origin of, 92
   patterns of, 40
   and perception, 95
   quality of, 14
   and satisfaction, 99
   uniqueness of, 14
Role identification, 261–262
Rolebound, 261–262
Roles, identification of, 136
Rooming in, 356

Salinger, J. D., 26
Satisfaction, 99
Schulhofer, Edith, 113
Sedatives, 240
Self:
   belief in, 19–20
   discovery of, 24
   image of, 22
   the lost, 229

Self:
- relationship to goals, 22
- relationship to others, 21
- revolt against, 212–214
- sense of, 133–135

Self-acceptance, 211
Self-actualization, 30–35
Self-control, mature, 216–218
Self-criticism, 129–130
Self-determination, 19
Self-testing, 163
Selye, Hans, 98, 101, 105, 106
Sex:
- and the college campus, 295–297
- and conflict, 257–260
- and identity, 256
- and normalcy, 268–272
- during pregnancy, 350–351
- premarital, 264–267, 316
- repression versus freedom, 255
- and symbolism, 299

Sex act, the, 270–272
Sexual activity, premarital, 316
Sexuality, 135–138
Simeons, A. T. W., 102
Social committment, 372–375
Social factors in addiction, 235–236
Social surrender, 367–370
Spermacides, chemical, 304
Stressor, 101–102
Success and academic pressure, 222–225
Suggestion:
- and culture, 156–157
- the power of, 153–157
- and preconditioning, 154

Symbolism:
- beginnings of, 58
- and communication, 59
- and function, 62–65
- and growth, 58
- and health, 66–67
- and identity, 65
- and relationships, 60

Synanon, 249
Syphilis, 314

Technology and health, 376

Value conditioning, 147–157
Value structure, 147–148
Values:
- a concern for human, 378–380
- and function, 150–153
- and health, 102–103
- hierarchical structure of, 149
- and marriage, 326
- and purpose, 147

Vasectomy, 302
Venereal disease, 313

Walters, Allan, 108–109
Watchful self, 21–23
Wholeness, 24–26
Will to change, 130
Will to meaning, 7
Williams, Jesse Feiring, 79
Women's Liberation movement, 137
World Health Organization, 79